T0133387

WOMEN AND HEALTH:

Cultural and Social Perspectives

■ BODIES OF TECHNOLOGY

Women's Involvement with Reproductive Medicine

Edited by

Ann Rudinow Saetnan

Nelly Oudshoorn

and Marta Kirejczyk

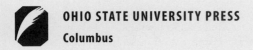 **OHIO STATE UNIVERSITY PRESS**
Columbus

Copyright © 2000 by The Ohio State University.
All rights reserved.

Library of Congress Cataloging-in-Publication Data

Bodies of technology : women's involvement with reproductive medicine / edited by Ann Rudinow Saetnan, Nelly Oudshoorn, and Marta Kirejczyk.
    p. cm.—(Women and health)
    Includes bibliographical references and index.
    ISBN 0-8142-0846-0 (hardcover : alk. paper)—ISBN 0-8142-5050-5 (paper : alk. paper)
    1. Human reproductive technology—Social aspects. 2. Human reproductive technology—Cross-cultural studies. 3. Women—Health and hygiene—Social aspects. 4. Women—Health and hygiene—Cross-cultural studies. I. Saetnan, Ann Rudinow. II. Oudshoorn, Nelly, 1950– III. Kirejczyk, Marta Stefania Maria, 1947– IV. Women & health (Columbus, Ohio)

RG133.5 .B625 2000
618.1′7806—dc21

00-032368

Text and jacket design by Diane Gleba Hall.
Type set in Adobe Garamond by Graphic Composition, Inc., Athens, Georgia.
Printed by Sheridan Books.

The paper used in this publication meets the minimum requirements of the American National Standard for Information Sciences—Permanence of Paper for Printed Library Materials. ANSI Z39.48-1992.

9 8 7 6 5 4 3 2 1

Contents

Series Editors' Foreword

Modern developments in reproductive science and technology present us with an amazing and frightening array of choices and possibilities. When anxious to conceive and experiencing difficulties, we can and do use procedures such as in vitro fertilization to enable pregnancy. Concerned about the health of a fetus, we undergo ultrasound and other diagnostic procedures in order to gain information. As individuals, we consider the new technologies emancipatory, but collectively we can see that they can be controlling and even oppressive.

Viewing reproductive technologies from many vistas, the social analysts in *Bodies of Technology* direct our attention to critical issues surrounding their development, implementation, and use. The authors cogently address the undeniable political and cultural significance of new procedures and technologies and show how they shape our understanding of gender, of technology, and of society. Their analyses document the complex interactions among medical technology, scientific culture, and medical culture. Equally important, the essays in this collection clearly demonstrate the view of multidisciplinary, multicultural critiques and investigate how understandings of technology and gender can be used to create a democratic society.

Acknowledgments

This volume was initially conceived as the first step in a joint research project. The idea for the project was to bring together concepts and research results from several research and policy networks in which we were involved—science and technology studies, cross-cultural studies, women's and gender studies, feminist and women's health networks—and bring them to bear on medical technology assessment and regulation. Although the project proposal never achieved funding, the idea of a book to sum up our starting point and point out a direction for future work took on a life of its own. Our thanks go first of all to the various networks through which we came to know of the empirical work and concepts that form the basis for this volume. Among these networks, special thanks go to the Society for Social Studies of Science (4S) and the European Association for the Study of Science and Technology (EASST). The 4S and EASST meetings were focal points where we most frequently met. And when the project application failed, it was the 4S/EASST joint meeting in Bielefeld in 1996 that provided a site for us to hold our first and only "project workshop" in the form of a series of paper sessions. We thank the organizers of the conference for providing us with this venue. In particular, we thank Sarah Franklin, who served as commentator for the IVF session. Having decided to attempt to publish the papers, we next went in search of a publisher. We are deeply grateful to Rima Apple, coeditor of the Women and Health Series at Ohio State University Press, for the enthusiasm and helpful advice with which she greeted our proposal. Likewise, the anonymous referee who reviewed the manuscript has been a source of inspiration. Her superlatives boosted our spirits and left us with a sense of urgency to complete the book, while at the same time her critical remarks pointed out weak points that needed to be reworked. Although the papers that form the basis to this volume were first written and presented nearly three years ago, the themes and arguments they forward remain timely. It is our hope that this collection will serve as a source of dialogue and debate in ongoing analyses of reproductive technologies in both global and local perspectives.

1

Women's Involvement with Reproductive Medicine: Introducing Shared Concepts

Ann Rudinow Saetnan

HOPES, FEARS, AND QUESTIONS

To many, new reproductive technologies (e.g., the Pill, in vitro fertilization, and sonograms) are among the great liberators of our time. Women have been spared the health risks and social burdens of unwanted pregnancy. Women and men have (sometimes) been spared the grief of involuntary infertility. Childbirth has become safer and less painful. Prospective parents now often have the option of terminating a pregnancy that would result in a handicapped child or of better preparing themselves to care for such a child.

And yet to others—or even at times to the same people who appreciate what new reproductive technologies offer them—these technologies are among the great oppressors of our time. Women have incurred grave health damage—have even lost their lives—through the use of contraceptives. Women have been pressured to endure painful and risky treatments in order to achieve pregnancy when they might otherwise have accepted infertility. Pregnant women, and to a lesser extent expectant fathers, have found themselves increasingly subjected to surveillance and control. For instance, women who have consumed alcohol or drugs during pregnancy have been prosecuted and imprisoned for child (fetus) abuse, as the embryo and fetus have gained technological visibility and have been ascribed rights and interests as individuals.[1]

Many of these technologies are no longer so new: The Pill has been in widespread use since the mid-1960s. Sonography was adapted for medical use shortly after World War II and has been used routinely in prenatal care in some countries since the late 1960s. In 1978 the first baby was born as a result of in vitro fertilization. Nevertheless, these technologies continue to be hotly debated. That is to say, they are not yet entirely taken for granted.

Critical positions toward these and other technological innovations in reproduction have been taken primarily by feminists, skeptical as to the technologies' impacts on women (e.g., Corea 1991a; Duden 1993; Rothman 1986, 1994). Primarily, but not exclusively. Protests have also been lodged by the World Health Organization (WHO) and other international agencies (e.g., WHO 1991, 1996), by national political bodies (e.g., the Health Council [The Netherlands] 1992, the Royal Commission on New Reproductive Technologies [Canada] 1993, the Norwegian Ministry of Health and Social Affairs 1992–93, the Denmark Council of Ethics 1995), by religious organizations (e.g., Catholic Church 1987), and by the mass media and the general public (see, for instance, the essays by Nelly Oudshoorn and Lise Kvande in this volume). These critical voices have been raised not only out of concern for the liberation or oppression of women but also for the technologies' impacts on men and masculinities, on cultural understandings of parenthood and kinship, etc.

How can a single technological artifact—a pill, a machine, a medical technique—have such manifold and contradictory impacts? Doesn't each technology have its own "true nature," its own particular and inevitable social consequences, which can be read out of the artifact itself? Or are there an infinite variety of possible consequences, all contingent on the variety of contexts in which the technology is used and understood? And if the latter, how can we then evaluate technologies? How can we make informed decisions regarding their development and usage?

The essays in this volume address such questions. They are concerned with how technologies come to have cultural and political meanings, with the implications of these particular technologies for the shaping of gender, and with how existing gendered cultures interact with the technologies as the meanings of technology and gender are (re)produced.

The contributors to this volume come from a number of academic disciplines. We are anthropologists, historians, sociologists, and natural scientists. We are active in the multidisciplinary field of women's studies and/or in the equally multidisciplinary field of science and technology studies. Thus we bring to the volume a variety of vocabularies and theoretical concerns. We also bring a variety of cultural experiences, political views, and values. However, we meet in this volume through a shared concern for certain social and technological policy issues. These issues can in turn be discussed with the help of a shared set of concepts. In this introduction, we will present the key concepts and issues that connect the essays in this volume.

OUR STARTING POINT: THE ONGOING SHAPING
OF GENDER AND TECHNOLOGY

Our collaboration began with a shared dilemma. We were concerned with the effects of (reproductive) technological change on gender identities, situations, and relations—and vice versa, with the influence of gender meanings and structures on the shaping of reproductive technologies. It would seem easiest to explore these effects if technologies could be dealt with as fixed artifacts with predetermined effects and genders as fixed categories with predetermined interests. One could then know precisely what the consequences of a technology would be in terms of the interests of one gendered group or another. And, conversely, one could know the effects on a given technology of involving one gendered group or another in the shaping of technological artifacts, policies, and practices. However, it was our shared conviction that this is not so.

Rejecting such determinist views, we see genders and technologies as mutually and continually reshaping one another.[2] Our first step in this introduction is to convey this perception to our readers. The next step will be to look at the questions this raises when technologies cross cultural borders. Finally, we discuss conceptual tools that we believe will help us to explore the politics of technologies once determinisms have been abandoned and questions of globalization and localization have been raised.

First, what do we mean by determinist views? One such view, known as technology determinism (Smith and Marx 1994), is that technologies arise as if from nowhere, for instance, through isolated acts of inventive genius. They arise simply because they work.[3] And then, given that they work, they will be used. According to this view, there are practical, material, and natural limits to the ways in which technologies can work. Technologies therefore place demands on the societies that use them, causing social change and social conflicts. We can sum up this view as based on two assumptions: (1) Technologies are, in their origins, autonomous from Society; (2) Society, on the other hand, is not autonomous from Technology. Technologies have clear and inevitable consequences—sometimes positive, sometimes negative—for Society.

This view is still commonly encountered in public discourse. Thus we might hear someone claim that the Pill produced a sexual revolution. However, technology determinism has fallen into discredit academically.

One problem with technology determinism lies in its first assumption. Technologies do not arise in a social vacuum. They are the products of social processes and social choices. The interpretation of Nature's capacities, the selection of which capacities to exploit technologically, the design of technological artifacts to do so—all are outcomes of social processes and social choices. Technological artifacts are made precisely for social (and thereby also political) reasons, in order to achieve certain social effects. Thus we may see technologies as being "socially shaped." This raises questions of which individuals and groups are making these social choices and which individuals and groups are affected by them. In other words, given the current social structure, who has the power to shape technology and thereby reshape (or, more likely, maintain the current shape of) society? And who must sit by, powerless, as their lives are changed?

Such questions are acutely relevant when examining social changes in reproductive technologies. Quite obviously, medical professionals and the biotechnological industry have more power to shape these technologies than do the men, women, and offspring who are (in different senses) their users. Equally obviously, users are bodily confronted with these technologies in the most personal and intimate spheres of their lives.

However, there are problems with the social shaping view. One problem arises because this view shares the second assumption of technology determinism—namely, that technologies, once designed and ready for production, have clear and inevitable consequences for the societies in which they are implemented.[4] From a technology determinist standpoint, this is simply a fact, not a result of political intentions. From the social shaping perspective, this means that a technology's social consequences, being foreseeable, can be intentionally designed. The social shaping position furthermore tends to be linked with structuralist views of society, for instance, Marxist theories or certain types of feminist theories. Structuralist theories view society as resiliently prestructured in terms of interests and power. This refers to the assumption that the parties involved in shaping technologies and the interests these parties represent are also foreseeable, say, in terms of established class or gender relations. One frequent claim is that technologies tend to be designed by men, with men's images of needs and solutions in mind, for use by women for whom those images and the resulting technologies may seem oppressive.[5]

But empirical studies based in constructivist approaches[6] have shown that the predictability of technologies' effects cannot be taken for granted. Technologies inevitably have unexpected and unintended effects (Winner 1986). Technologies, their usage, and their effects may be reshaped by their users (Akrich 1992; Lie and Sørensen 1996). In other words, technologies are *interpretatively flexible* (Bijker 1995), and they remain so, to a greater or lesser degree, throughout their "life cycles."[7] Thus we need to explore not only who are the primary shapers of technologies and who are affected by them but also how those affected can influence technological choices and shapes. We will return to this issue when we discuss the concept of "users."

Nor are social structures and interests entirely predictable. Social categories that seem fixed and pertinent in one context may be cross-cut, sidelined, or replaced by newly emerging categories in another context—not least in contexts involving technological change. For instance, Latour (1987) describes how a change in photographic technologies involved creating a whole new constituency of hobby photographers, or how acceptance of the microbe as an agent of disease involved redefining society in terms of infected vs. vaccinated rather than poor vs. rich. Society too, then, is interpretatively flexible.

In recent years, science and technology studies have been gravitating toward a common ground where structuralist and constructivist analyses meet (Sørensen 1997). It is now widely accepted that social groups—their boundaries, alliances, interests, and actions—are not entirely predictable. At the same time, it is also widely accepted that neither are they entirely unpredictable. Thus studies focusing on the effects of existing interest constellations can be seen to communicate with studies focusing on how social structures and interests change during processes of technological innovation. The contributions to this volume are situated in various spots within this common ground. For instance, in the model Naomi Pfeffer proposes for analyzing the political regulation of reproductive technologies, the structure of political discourse seems relatively stable. Adele Clarke applies a social shaping perspective to her study of the development of contraceptives: Since social groups interested in simple, woman-controlled contraceptives were marginalized early on, we now have few such contraceptives available. Since groups interested in science, "sophisticated" technology, and control came to dominate developments, we instead have a number of contraceptives that can be "imposed" on their users, leaving little scope for user influence. At a more constructivist spot in the shared territory we find the chapter by Lynn Morgan, in which she emphasizes the culturally constructed character of both "technoscientific" and "ethnoscientific" knowledge about reproduction.

As mentioned above, we are particularly interested in the influence of gendered social patterns on reproductive technologies and vice versa. Are gender categories examples of the interpretative flexibility of society?

Gender, too, has been subject to determinist, structuralist, and constructivist interpretations. In the case of gender, determinist views tend to see the social attributes of women and men as a dichotomy firmly rooted in biology. Furthermore, they tend to see biology as a given set of facts, not as a malleable set of social understandings. Taking a grammatical metaphor, we might say that in this view, gender takes the role of a noun (or rather, two nouns: man, woman). Gender becomes a matter of fate. We are born into one noun category or the other, and the fate of our birth determines certain key personality traits, behavioral tendencies, etc.[8] Such views of gender are also referred to as "essentialist" in that they build from an understanding that somewhere under the layers of historical and cultural differences in gendered experiences, behaviors, and values there is some universal "essence" of masculinity and femininity, somehow linked to biological sex—be it anatomically, hormonally, or genetically. This "essence" is then seen as autonomous from social processes.

In contrast, structuralist views would argue that we are not simply born woman or man, but must learn to take on the traits and behaviors expected of our gender. We must be socialized, through social interactions or through the constraints of institutionalized structures. In other words, we are socially shaped into our respective forms as woman or man. Gender then becomes adjectival and adverbial—a set of descriptive aspects that we learn to ascribe to ourselves and to act in accordance with. Gender is no longer a pair of nouns (man, woman) but a paired set of descriptive terms grouped under the headings "feminine" and "masculine."[9]

Like gender-as-noun, gender-as-adjective emphasizes stability, but it does so as a result of social process rather than as a biological (and thereby moral) imperative. Although our biology does not automatically create in us the expected traits and behaviors of a sex category, the content of the category is, at least in the short term, knowable in advance. We must learn, but what we must learn—for example, the hegemonic norms of gender (Connel 1987; Kimmel 1987; Lie 1995)—although changeable, are for the most part knowable at a given moment in time and cultural space. The focus of adjectival approaches to understanding has been on the short-term experience of how we "read" gender in current local culture and how we experience gendered identity formation as constrained, rather than on explaining how gender roles and images change, sometimes radically, over time.

If, however, we view gender as interpretatively flexible, then gender becomes a verb. The shape of gender at any given place or time emerges from collective and individual acts of interpretation. Gender is then performed,[10] as in the performance of a script.[11] Performances are instructed by the current script (i.e., by social norms and institutions). Thus we would still expect to find considerable influence from social structures, such as gendered power differentials. However, each performance represents a new reading, sometimes even a rewriting, of the script. Change in the script may be slow or rapid, but the script is certainly always changing, and any degree of permanence in the script is the outcome of constant maintenance, the outcome of both conscious and unconscious work. Even the seemingly universal dichotomy of gender is subject to and an outcome of interpretation, so we might equally conceivably interpret gender as some larger or smaller number of categories. Gender is no longer limited to a pair of nouns (man, woman) or a paired set of adjectives (masculine, feminine). Instead, there are potentially any number of performable femininities, masculinities, and possibly other genders for which we as yet have no established terms.

Biology has a place in constructivist and structuralist accounts of gender as well, not only in essentialist ones. In constructivist and structuralist accounts, biology—or at the very least, knowledge about biology—is socially constructed, just as are gendered symbols, structures, and identities. In fact, gendered symbols, structures, and identities play active roles in the social construction of biological knowledge. For instance, what we know about human fertility may depend on what materials are available for research, which may in turn depend on what categories of people are aggregated as patients in clinics where such materials might be obtained. Thus the existence of obstetrical and gynecological clinics and the nonexistence of andrological clinics have played a key role in the development of knowledge about human fertility (see Oudshoorn 1994; Laborie, this volume).

Again, the essays in this volume are arrayed within a common ground between structuralist and constructivist views of gender, our respective positions perhaps due as much to the cultural situation being described or the focus of analysis as to theoretical preferences. For instance, my own contribution examines competing Norwegian narratives about gender, knowledge, and interests regarding ultrasound diagnostics and therefore represents a constructivist account. In India, however, dominant structures of gender and class are more daunting. Thus it is not surprising that, in her chapter, Jyotsna Agnihotri Gupta presents a more structuralist account of IVF.

Although understandings of technology and gender run parallel, it does not necessarily follow that they are readily combinable. For instance, technology determinist and gender essentialist views share a similar view of Nature as playing a culturally autonomous and determinant role. However, there is also an inescapable tension between the two: If technologies are capable of determining social patterns, including gendered social patterns, then Nature's role as a determinant of the essence of femininity and masculinity would come into question. And if gendered values and behaviors shape how men and women relate to technologies, then Nature's role as a determinant of how technologies work would come into question.

There are similar tensions among structuralist and constructivist accounts of gender and technology. For instance, there are potential tensions between constructivist theories of technology and almost any theory of gender. The two dominant constructivist theories of technology (SCOT and ANT) hold as a methodological precept that the constitution of social groups relevant to a given technological innovation cannot be foreseen. It cannot be known in advance what social categories, or what attributes of those categories, will be invoked in or affected by the process of building a new sociotechnology. New categories may be created in sociotechnology building processes. Existing categories may be modified in their attributes. This would apply to gender categories as well: new versions of gender might arise. Even whole new genders might conceivably arise. Or, on the other hand, gender might be of no consequence in a given sociotechnical case.

However, for many feminists, regardless of whether they favor structuralist or constructivist approaches, gender (and as an aspect of gender, power) is so pervasive a social system as to be always implicated in any process of social change. Where we "see" gender in action depends, of course, on what we count as gender. If gender is only about differences between men and women, then single-sex contexts might not be about gender at all. Nor would technologies toward which men and women developed similar attitudes and practices tell us anything about gender. However, if gender is about the manifold meanings of femininity and masculinity, if gender is also about similarities between women and men, if gender is also about differences among women and among men, then all social phenomena—including all technologies—are relevant to our understanding of gender. Even for gender to appear as a nonissue in a given situation would, paradoxically, be part of the social process that defines the meaning of gender, as it would indicate what is deemed to be outside the boundaries of current gender meanings.

In spite of the tensions between technology-focused and gender-focused theories, a large body of research is emerging that seeks a common ground between structuralist and constructivist accounts of both gender and technology together. One definition of gender that works in this common ground is that of Sandra Harding (1986).[12] Harding parses gender up into interactions among three factors: symbol, structure, and identity. The gendered symbol system is the culturally (and thus locally and temporally) specific set of associations between sex and other human and nonhuman phenomena—for example, thinking of machines as masculine, or associating parenthood more with femininity than with masculinity. The gendered social structure organizes daily lives in sex-linked ways, most notably a sex-linked division of labor and the assignment of greater power to positions predominantly occupied by men. Individuals develop their own self-perceived identities and public images in reference to these structures and symbol systems, but note that "in reference" can also include "in opposition."

Sometimes these three systems reinforce one another, as for instance when computers are perceived as masculine, computer design is a predominantly male career, and women tend not to see themselves as computer scientists (Rasmussen and Håpnes 1991). But each of the three factors is dynamic, unstable, containing inconsistencies and paradoxes at any given time. Furthermore, although they interact, these three factors do not mirror one another perfectly and thus do not perfectly reinforce one another. For instance, computers may also be seen as feminine in that they resemble typewriters, or because they are small, clean machines rather than heavy, greasy ones, or in that they are often used by women in feminized jobs. These images and structural roles of computers are discordant with certain images of masculinity (Lie 1996). And finally, each factor may be more or less radically reshaped through the actions of individuals and groups. For instance, in recent years, the Norwegian University of Science and Technology has had some success in changing the gendered images of information science held by high school students and thus modifying the gendered recruitment of students to that field at the university. As these examples show, gender is constantly being reshaped, is constantly in need of maintenance and reproduction. For this reason, Harding's definition works well with constructivist theories of gender.

But the definition also includes the element of structure, and Harding points out that a male-favoring hierarchy—with that which is counted as masculine generally being more highly valued than that which is counted as feminine—has been a resilient part of gender structure, however much gender structures otherwise might vary. The inclusion of structure, and especially of relatively stable elements in that structure, invites a conversation between constructivist and structuralist views.

Harding's definition of gender also invites conversations with structuralist and/or constructivist accounts of technologies. Technologies too are ascribed symbolic meanings—not least gendered meanings (Lie 1998; Kline and Pinch 1996; Lohan 1998). Technologies are sites around which social relations, including gendered social relations, are performed. For instance, the Pill has been developed in such a way that responsibilities for contraception are delegated to women (Oudshoorn 1994; chapters by Clarke, Marks, Oudshoorn, and van Kammen in this volume). Technologies are objects that can be mobilized in identity projects, including gendered identity projects—for example, the mobile phone as an icon for a high-tech, mobile, masculine identity (Oudshoorn 1999). And vice versa: gendered symbols, gendered social structures, and gendered identities are resources that can be mobilized in connection with the shaping of technologies—such as when pornography, war, and football are mobilized to make video games and the Internet attractive for anticipated "early adopters," namely, midteen to middle-aged men, or when household machines are given a less high-tech image (e.g., simple icons rather than buttons with technical codes) so as to appeal to women buyers who are seen or who see themselves as having limited technical competence (Oudshoorn 1999). Thus gender and technology can be seen as mutually and simultaneously shaping one another.

Note that both femininity and masculinity are subject to the same three-part definition and that the definition allows a multitude of variations and contradictions between and within symbol, structure, and identity systems. In other words, this definition encourages us not only to study femininity, or even femininity in relation to masculinity, but to study the processes through which various femininities and masculinities arise in relation to one another and in relation to other phenomena that are enlisted into the process of creating, maintaining, and re-creating genders. In combining this definition of gender with structuralist and constructivist understandings of technology, we are also encouraged to examine the ways gender(s) is/are mobilized in the process of creating, maintaining, and re-creating technologies and, by the same token, the ways in which technologies are mobilized in creating, maintaining, and re-creating genders. Neither gender nor technology appears as an independent variable—as a cause that can explain the remaining dependent variable. Both are mutually dependent. Both are shaped and given social meaning simultaneously through the same social actions. We may say they co-construct each other.

The essays in this volume are all situated at various spots within the common ground described above, where structuralist and constructivist analyses of gender and technology meet. Some of the essays focus on how technological innovations affect gender, as when Oudshoorn and Laborie show how new technologies open up new relationships between masculinity and reproduction—namely, relationships of pain and risk. Some essays focus on how gender is mobilized in the shaping of technologies' "careers," as when Gupta shows how structures of gender and class in India combine to create a market for a multitude of fertility assistance services. Some focus on the immediate constraints that limit the interpretative flexibility of gender and/or technology, thus tending toward a structuralist account. The chapters by Neresini and Bimbi, Laborie, and Gupta are examples of this. Others focus on interpretative processes and changes, thus tending toward a constructivist account—for example, the chapter in which Kirejczyk discusses how changing Dutch sexual and reproductive norms have affected and been affected by debates on the regulation of fertility assistance services. Where within this common ground any given essay might be placed is as much a matter of the specific issues addressed in the essay as of the longer-term theoretical commitments of the authors.

With this common ground as our shared starting point—with a shared interest in the intertwinings of technology with gender, a shared concern for women's health and integrity in particular, and a shared abandonment of determinisms—we have sought to explore the implications of innovations in reproductive technologies as they cross cultural borders.

OUR AIM: LOCALIZING GLOBALIZATION

If gender is dynamically constituted as symbol, structure, and identity—as discussed above—this might tell us nothing more than that gender is an aspect of culture. Other phenomena, artifacts, traditions—in short, anything that we as members of a culture are capable of noticing and naming—could equally be described in those same three terms. Technologies, certainly, carry ascribed symbolic meanings—not least gendered meanings. For instance, Oudshoorn (this volume) describes the linking up of competing images of masculinity with images of male contraceptive injections—injections as symbols of pain are linked with images of men as egoistic and irresponsible; injections as symbols of science and progress are linked with images of men as willing to share responsibility for family planning and women's health. Technologies are also integral to the formation and reformation of social structures, as when IVF practices are shaped so as to reinforce and/or relax hegemonic norms of family structures and sexual and kinship relations (compare chapters by Kirejczyk and Neresini and Bimbi in this volume). And technologies are invoked as objects of identity projects, as when Greek women request a sonogram as part of the process of becoming a modern mother (see chapter by Mitchell and Georges, this volume). These symbols, structures and identity projects are gendered, but they are also "raced," "classed," "aged," "nationed," and "ethnicized." In other words, the observable phenomenon that technology and gender mutually shape one another is one crucial instance of a far broader cultural dynamic.

Not only is the mutual construction of technology and gender an instance of this larger dynamic. It is also inextricably situated *within* the larger dynamic. Technology and gender are shaped not only in reference to one another but also in reference to all other aspects of social symbolism, structure, and identity.[13] Thus if we set out to explore the relationship between changes in reproductive technologies and changes in perceptions and structures of genders, we will find not one such relationship but many different relationships contingent on class structures, religious understandings, etc.

Of particular relevance here is the notion that technologies are carriers for cultural-technical intersections—that cultural assumptions are built into technologies during development and production so that "technology transfer" (the movement of a technology from its place of origin to some new setting) also entails cultural transfer. Thus the spread of automobiles, mobile telephones, personal computers—or of contraceptive pills, techniques for assisted fertilization, fetal diagnostic technologies—would lead to the standardization (globalization) of culture. For example, if sonographic visualization of the fetus feeds into the separation and individualization of the fetus in Canadian culture, then it will do the same in Bolivian or Greek culture. However, careful empirical work (such as the essays in this volume by Mitchell and Georges, by Browner and Preloran, and by Morgan) demonstrates that this is not always the case.

As a hypothesis, globalization would be among the expectations of technology determinist approaches as well as of some social shaping approaches. Once shaped, the technology would remain stable and would discipline the practices surrounding its usage, thereby reshaping culture. However, technology- and gender-constructivist perspectives lead us to at least examine the extent to which the technological artifacts and practices are themselves *re*shaped in their encounters with new cultural environments. This is in large part a question of the scope for agency: Are local actors relegated to a passive, recipient, reactive position vis-à-vis global flows of technology, capital, and so forth? Or are local actors themselves agents in processes of social change? In other words, is the spread of technological artifacts a globalizing force, or are technologies also localized as they are moved from setting to setting?

A number of authors have therefore called for the cultural and historical contextualization of gender-technology case studies and for diachronic and cross-cultural comparative studies (e.g., Rapp 1994; Ginsburg and Rapp 1995). This volume is one of a number of recent works that answer those calls.[14] Responding to the calls, we aim in this volume to explore how meanings and material structures of reproductive technology and their linkage with gender are (re-)created in the various cultural and organizational contexts where attempts are made to implement the technology. Here we have gathered essays on the interactions of genders with materially similar technologies in culturally diverse settings. Some of the essays (those by Morgan, Mitchell and Georges, Brown and Preloran) are explicitly cross-culturally comparative. In addition, the juxtaposition of a number of both multiculturally and monoculturally contextualized accounts in a single volume invites the reader to generate further comparisons. For instance, both in Italy (Neresini and Bimbi, this volume) and in India (Gupta, this volume), IVF services are not subjected to government regulation. But the reasons for this and the systems of services resulting from this are quite different, as the essays show. Another form of invitation to generate further comparisons can be found in those essays, such as the ones by Pfeffer and by Blizzard, that propose and demonstrate models and/or metaphors for making such comparisons.

The essays in this volume generally use the nation-state as a roughly bounded cultural site. This is, of course, by no means unproblematic.[15] Even though we may be able to recognize certain national cultural traits at any given moment, national culture is constantly evolving, constantly being reenvisioned and structurally modified, not least in interaction with technological change. Thus, just as the gendering of technologies is not simply a matter of "add gender and stir" (Cockburn 1985), neither can we simply add culture and stir. We cannot add, say, a drop of Catholicism, a dash of fashion sense, and a *soupçon* of linguistic reverence and thereby make a Japanese sonogram machine French. What it means for a machine, or a pill, or a surgical technique to be, for example, "French" as opposed to "Japanese" is the outcome of a process of cultural appropriation. That same process also redefines the meanings of the cultures concerned and of the technology involved. Can a contraceptive be made Catholic? Proponents of the Pill thought so. They thought that a pill based on the natural hormone regulation of fertility might meet with Vatican approval (Oudshoorn 1994, 121). It did not. In choosing among several alternative understandings of "natural," the Vatican at once redefined the meanings of natural, of Catholicism, and of the Pill.

Furthermore, by the same tokens as discussed above for gender(s), nations are far from culturally homogeneous or monolithic. They are structurally, symbolically, and in terms of identity divided in any number of ways, giving rise to so-called subcultures, some of which cut across national cultural boundaries creating linkages and similarities. Thus gendered technological practices and meanings are developed not only at a national level but in parallel and intersecting subcultures within and between nations. For instance, Anglo Americans do not attach the same meanings to fetal diagnostics as do acculturated Mexican Americans, whose meanings again differ from those of recently immigrated Mexican Americans (Browner and Preloran, this volume).

And finally, technological practices and meanings are developed not only along the stripes of the sort of pluralistically parallel cultural "fabric" evoked above. Superimposed on those stripes is a network pattern with nodes, or foci, where interests meet and decisions are made which then form an infrastructure for our daily lives. For instance, science is conducted along a network of communication links among laboratories and other research institutions, and communications along these links are constrained by formal and informal rules regarding who may participate, in what ways, how must they formulate their statements to be taken seriously, and so forth. Political regulation of technologies forms another such network with other nodes (e.g., parliamentary committees, cabinets) and other rules of discourse. These two networks have points of contact with one another (political bodies often fund research, and research findings may be used in political debates), but they are not identical.

If the cultural meanings of technologies are the sum result of the ways we typically speak of them and relate to them, then the infrastructures within which we live out our daily lives (i.e., constrained within which we play out our relationships to technologies and gather our experiences of them) are key to the development of those meanings. Networks of discourse such as science or politics, and nodes such as laboratories or committees, are important sites in the development of cultural meanings and structures of gender and technology. But note that these nodes are not autonomous from culture. They are themselves entwined in national, subnational, and transnational cultures. They are themselves bearers of cultural symbols and structures, places where cultures are enacted.

In this volume we focus, rather broadly, on four such networks:

1. a research network, including laboratories where reproductive technologies are developed and field sites where they are tested (part one);

2. a governmental network, referring to the regulation of reproductive technologies and the forums where such regulations are officially discussed and decided (part two);

3. a clinical network, where clinicians and patients meet and their respective understandings of the technologies confront one another (part three); and

4. mass media, where debates from each of these networks (and potentially others as well) may be made available to a larger public (the chapters by Oudshoorn and Kvande).

Two other networks or nodes are discussed more briefly in some of the chapters. These are the commercial market for sale and purchase of medical products and services, and the conjugal partnership.

As mentioned above, each network and each node is subject to certain rules of discourse (Foucault 1969, 1971; Schaaning 1997). These rules vary, of course, between cultures and over time. But until they are challenged and changed, rules of discourse denote who (what categories of actors, and sometimes which specific actors) may participate in a discourse, what issues will be counted as important in that discourse, and what sort of statements will be taken seriously.[16] For example, in current Euro-American culture, physicians' statements about the body are to be taken seriously. Physicians' statements linking, say, tobacco smoke and health are considered relevant in a number of contexts: scientific literature, clinical encounters, lawsuits, formation of new laws, etc. That is to say, physicians are authority figures regarding health and healthy behaviors. However, their authority is limited to making certain statements. A physician who claims that smoking is *good* for your health would suffer an acute loss of credibility. In other words, ongoing discourse is always grounded in the discourses that have preceded it and that have left a "residue" of rules—formal and informal, locally and temporally knowable.

Some rules, in some discourses, have become international (global). Science, for instance, strives for global networks of communications with globally accepted rules of discourse. Nevertheless, local (e.g., national) styles of science can be observed (Traweek 1988; Hård and Knie 1999). And some discourses are less standardized across cultures (political structures are an obvious example of this).

In this volume, we are particularly interested in the roles allotted to technology "users" in the various networks and nodes of discourse. But why users? Other categories of actors may well be more prominent speakers in most of the networks and nodes mentioned above. In the next section we will explain why we have chosen to focus on users and what this focus entails.

FOCUSING ON USERS: AGENTS OF CULTURAL APPROPRIATION

Two of the basic issues that have brought us together in this volume also cause us to turn our gaze toward users. One is the question of cultural appropriation of technology. If cultures and technologies mutually adapt to one another, then the outcome of that adaptation process must be most apparent in the technology-related meanings and practices taken up by technologies' users at the grassroots level—that is, by the general public.

This is not to deny the roles played by various elites in shaping an agenda in which meanings are discussed or in scripting technology-usage patterns with which the general public is confronted. But it is, nevertheless, in the general public's acceptance of meanings and practices—be that acceptance grudging or enthusiastic—that the success (or failure) of elite actors' scripts can be read. Remember, too, that we are dealing with technologies that have crossed cultural borders and taken on somewhat different meanings and usages in the respective cultural settings. This should remind us to lend attention to the general public, since we will in most of these settings find ourselves some distance removed from the laboratories, industries, and so forth, where the artifacts and techniques were originally developed. If meanings and usages diverge thence forward, something important must be occurring at the user end of the scale.

We chose to focus on users, however, before discussing what a focus on cultural appropriation might entail. The now growing focus on users in science and technology studies was introduced to the field by feminist researchers (e.g., Cowan 1987) who have been major sources of inspiration for us.[17] In keeping with this line of research, our focus on users is at least as much grounded in our shared concern for the health and integrity of those (primarily women) to whose bodies and life situations reproductive technologies are applied. As Jessika van Kammen so plainly states in her essay: "Those who use a technology should have some say in its design."

But who are the users? The answer to this question is not obvious. For instance, consider the sonograph apparatus: Is the physician who refers a patient for sonography and receives the lab results the user? Or is it the state, which has sanctioned routine sonograms and pays their cost? What of the physician in charge of the sonography laboratory? Or the operator who conducts the examination? Or is the user the pregnant woman carrying the fetus being examined? Or her partner, who comes along to view the images? Or perhaps the fetus itself? In varying senses, they all use the technology.

We have chosen not necessarily to have our gaze on the user follow the shifting paths of who operates the equipment, pays for its use, or makes usage decisions. Our concern is primarily for those users on whose bodies the technologies are applied, whatever their decisional power may or may not be in each case. To mark these apart from users in other senses, we may refer to them as end users or, if we wish to highlight their relative exclusion from expert discourses, as "lay end users." The various health professionals and the state could then be called "intermediary users," that is, users on behalf of end users.

Even with this qualification, it may not be entirely clear who is, in the final instance, the end user. In the case of sonograms, would the end user be the pregnant woman? Or the woman and her fetus? Or the fetus alone? What about her partner? Is he another end user, or perhaps an "ancillary" user?[18] These questions are far from frivolous. In the case of in vitro fertilization, defining the couple as end users has legitimated treating male infertility by means of potentially dangerous interventions in women's bodies (as described in some detail in the chapters by Kirejczyk and by Laborie, this volume; see also Kirejczyk 1993; Kirejczyk and Van der Ploeg 1993). Or in the case of technologies used during pregnancy, defining the fetus as user allows us to posit an opposition between the interests of mothers and fetuses (Casper 1994, 1998). We may well wish to avoid ascribing such meanings to pregnancy. However, ignoring the fetus as user could blind us to severe health problems that may appear in future generations, for example, those caused by thalidomide or by diethylstilbestrol (DES). In the chapters in this volume, we will concentrate primarily on the immediate bodily users, that is, generally women, but at times we will broaden our gaze to encompass other lay end users.

What is it then that we wish to explore about lay end user involvement in the processes of reproductive technology innovation and cultural appropriation? Taking users as our focus while we examine different nodes of discourse, we ask ourselves to what extent and in what ways users are involved in the respective nodes. What user roles do the rules of discourse encourage in research, technology policy formation, clinical encounters, and the media?

In the research network, we have encountered users in three roles: as imaginary figures (we might call them "virtual users"), ascribed certain interests and anticipated behaviors in the scripts of the scientists and engineers developing the technology; as living, embodied users in clinical trials, not necessarily behaving as anticipated by those scripts; and as organized interest groups lobbying for research funds and for specific directions in research. These users—both imagined and living—are the focus of part one of this book.

In the technology policy network, we have encountered aggregated users: here, too, user interest groups may be active lobbyists. Users also appear here as voter constituencies, as an aggregated market made up of the sum of personal economic circumstances and consumer decisions, and (imagined in political scripts) as a mass-to-be-controlled and/or a mass-to-be-protected through regulatory interventions. This aggregated perspective on users is especially pertinent in part two.

In clinics, which are the primary focus of part three, we encounter users as individuals in direct interaction with medical service providers. Here users seek to achieve their own goals—including goals relating to the conjugal partnership—within the constraints of the services being offered them and in interaction with health professionals whose goals in the encounter may well be rather different (see also Cussins 1996). In some ways, these users play the same role as test users in clinical trials; however, their experiences are not being systematically summed up and applied to technology development or policy formation.

And finally, in the media (Oudshoorn, this volume; Kvande, this volume) we find users in whatever guise journalists have deemed newsworthy. User voices may reach a wide audience via the media, but only through the filter of journalistic judgment.

To gain some estimate of the efficacy of these user roles in influencing the shaping of technological meanings and practices, and to identify means of making user voices more powerful, we analyze our observations in terms of two other shared concepts: representation and negotiation. Who represents users in the different discourses? How are users portrayed? How may users themselves control their representatives? What decisions are being made that constrain users' choices? What scope is left for users to maneuver in seeking to achieve their own goals? How are gendered power relationships affecting and being affected by these processes? How are the shapes and shaping of technologies involved? In the final section of this introduction, we discuss how the concepts of representation and negotiation can help us explore these issues.

USER AGENCY: NO NEGOTIATION WITHOUT REPRESENTATION?

Why should we expect theoretical concepts to be useful to us? Putting a name to some assortment of events hardly seems to matter that much. It merely constitutes those events as a generic class by ascribing to them certain generic properties. But in making a generic class out of an assortment of events, those events and the properties in them that interest us become more visible to us. Our next step then would be to examine in historically specific detail how those events function in the world, how they vary, how their variations might be manipulated, and so forth.[19]

The events that concern us here are classed together in terms of relationships between grassroots interests and power. That is why making them visible as generic classes of events and exploring their various expressions and constellations becomes a useful scientific and political strategy. It can help us understand the role of users in (re-)shaping technology and society. It can help us empower users to do so more effectively. So what do we intend to explore about representation and negotiation?

Looking up *representation* and related words in an unabridged dictionary, I found fourteen meanings of *represent,* sixteen of *representation,* and twelve of *representative.* Among these, two are our main interest in this volume. On the one hand, representation carries a legal, political sense, as in "representative democracy." The Translation Theory term *spokesperson* evokes this same sense, as does the term *delegate,* although in a slightly different permutation (Latour 1987). In exploring the event of one person or thing representing (that is, speaking for) others, we would want to examine how the representative came to claim the mandate to speak on those others' behalf.[20]

To illustrate the importance of representation in this sense, consider the following example from my field notes from a Norwegian consensus conference on sonography in pregnancy.[21]

The conference organizers had been instructed by the Ministry of Health and Social Affairs to make the issue of selective abortions (i.e., abortion on the basis of a diagnosis of developmental aberrations in the fetus) a central theme in the conference. This was, in part, accomplished by inviting elected officers of patient interest groups to speak regarding the life circumstances of individuals living with now-diagnosable conditions for which abortions are now offered. Each of the three speakers—the mother of a child with Down's syndrome and officer of a support group for Down's parents, an officer of a broad-based interest organization for the handicapped, and a woman with osteogenesis imperfecta (congenital osteoporosis) and officer of a patients' support group—presented stories of pain and grief, but reported nevertheless valuing their lives. When the conference chair opened for questions from the audience, one pediatrician present challenged these stories. He characterized them as "sunshine stories" told by individuals with exceptional resources. He claimed that, based on his many contacts with patients, bitterness was more common and that many such patients wished they had never lived. The audience—an auditorium filled with some three hundred gynecologists, pediatricians, general practitioners, midwives, and other health professionals—applauded him enthusiastically. In doing so, they disclaimed the previous speakers: even as elected officials of the patients' own interest organizations, these women were (in the eyes of the health professionals present) less legitimate spokespersons for the handicapped—indeed, for themselves and/or their children—than were their physicians.

What are the ongoing relationships between speakers and those they speak for in the example above? In what ways can those spoken for control the spokesperson's mandate? The women who spoke for their organizations' members at the conference were elected officers of those organizations. The members could vote them out of office or participate in discussions at meetings instructing their officers what to say. The women also spoke on the basis of personal experience. Health professionals speak on behalf of patients on the basis of a different mandate, different sources of authority. They might claim to have more thorough and accurate knowledge of patients' bodies than patients themselves can glean from personal experience. They might also, as in the example above, claim to have information from more patients than are members of a support organization.

As the example shows, spokespersonship may be contested. Not only health professionals, patients, and officers of patients' organizations but also engineers, researchers, politicians, religious authorities, journalists, and others may claim to represent patients' best interests regarding a given technology.

Of course, who speaks would matter little if all would-be spokespersons said the same things. However, as the example above also shows, spokespersons may disagree about what constitutes the "truth," or the most relevant information, about those spoken for. This points to the other meaning of representation that interests us—namely, the artistic sense of the word, representation as in representational art. Here we intentionally conflate several of *Webster's* sixteen definitions of the word: "(10) presentation to the mind, as of an idea or image, (11) the act of portrayal, picturing, or other rendering in visible form, often representations, a description or statement, as of things true or alleged."

We conflate here traditionally artistic with realist/scientific senses of the word in order to emphasize that any presentation to the mind—be it presented as art or as science, as fiction or as documentary—is a selective and creative one. There are always other images that might have been presented, for instance, by other spokespersons.

So another aspect of spokespersonship to explore is precisely how spokespersons *portray* those they claim to speak for. In the example above, both the physician and the patient group officers portrayed these patients as suffering. However, the physician claimed that their suffering was so great that many wished they had not been born, whereas the patient group officers claimed to appreciate life in spite of their pain and other problems. How, then, do different portrayals arise? Do they vary from context to context as well as from spokesperson to spokesperson? And how do those portrayals correspond to self-portrayals (if any) by those spoken for? Could it be, for instance, that the same patients who speak of suffering to their physician will speak of enjoying life when at a patient group meeting? Could it be that when in pain they seek out a physician, but they attend meetings when feeling better? Could it also be that different portrayals arise on the basis of different (self-)interests on the part of competing spokespersons?

Bringing the two aspects of representation together, linking spokespersonship with portrayal: are those who are spoken for aware of how they are being portrayed, where, and by whom? Do patients know that their narratives of pain told to the physician at the clinic are being retold to a committee discussing abortion? If patients knew where and how their narratives were being retold, might they be provoked to speak more directly on their own behalf? (There at last, if not before, it should be clear why we imagine this to be a politically potent concept.)

Moving on to the concept of *negotiation,* we are again interested in two senses of the word—to deal or bargain with another or others, as in the preparation of a treaty; and to move through, around, or over in a satisfactory manner, e.g., to negotiate a dance step—or "negotiation-at-the-table" vs. "negotiation-as-navigation."[22]

In negotiations-at-the-table, we tend to encounter spokespersons. Our interest then (as democratically inclined feminists) would be to maximize the power of those spoken for, for instance, by increasing their control over their spokespersons or by opening up more direct access for them to the negotiation situation.

But user-focused, constructivist studies of technology have shown that negotiations-as-navigation also can have a significant impact on sociotechnical outcomes. Here we are talking about users who are not seated at the table where designs are drawn and "treaties" are signed. They meet the results of design and treaty negotiations as a limited set of consumer options or as infrastructures in their daily lives. And yet, in threading their personal paths through those infrastructures, lay end users also negotiate sociotechnical outcomes.

Concepts such as anti-program (Latour 1992), de-inscription (Akrich 1992), user scripts (Gjøen and Hård 1996), domestication or mutual taming (Silverstone and Hirsch 1992; Sørensen, Aune, and Hatling 1996), and choreography (Cussins 1996) all refer to this type of negotiation. Summing up the empirical results described with these terms, we find that lay end users are participants—often only indirectly or through "take-it-or-leave-it" choices and "voting with their feet"—but still effective participants in the sociotechnical shaping process.

Nevertheless, this is no cause for complacency. Lay end user involvement is often marginalized. Lay end user viewpoints and competencies are therefore often undereffective in the shaping process. Lay end users are often underinformed on what expert discourses represent them as choosing when they vote with their feet, underinformed on how their negotiations-as-navigation are represented by spokespersons during negotiations-at-the-table. Therefore, lay end user actions may at times lead to consequences diametrically opposed to their own understandings of the sociotechnology concerned.

An example of this could be the ways in which women appropriate and adapt to available reproductive technologies. For instance, in many places pregnant women are accepting, often seeking, fetal diagnostics. On the basis of this "foot-vote" of confidence, clinicians have claimed a mandate as spokespersons, not only for the interests and intentions of the women themselves but also for their partners and fetuses. One key advocate of ultrasound, for instance, discounts feminists, ethicists, and other critics as being out of touch with women's needs when they complain of ethical dilemmas that women face when asked to choose whether to continue or abort an abnormal pregnancy. The self-appointed spokesperson himself claims: "I'm not worried about the times we are entering, because I feel strongly that the women we are dealing with, they stand for these views. It's outsiders who are not in the situation themselves who talk about the 'terrible choices' we force women to confront. And I understand that we do. But, on the other hand, we have experienced so many women going through these choices. . . . They react differently. It's the whole spectrum of human reactions. But I think they all thought it was positive that they got their diagnosis and didn't have to go through with the pregnancy" (excerpt from an interview with a Norwegian ultrasound expert).

However, this attitude is not how I understood the statements of one woman who received such a diagnosis and chose an abortion. In her interview, she spoke of attending each ultrasound examination with the hope of finding some basis to continue the pregnancy, some indication that the fetus, though handicapped, might be viable. And she gave no indication that, in undergoing these examinations, she saw herself as authorizing the hospital staff to speak for her regarding ultrasound policy.

■

Summing up—taking together the indications that technologies and genders interact to reshape one another, the implications of this in terms of focusing on users and on cultural appropriation, and the proposal that concepts of representation and negotiation might help us understand those appropriation processes—all of this means that both empirical and political agendas are possible for constructivist, feminist science and technology studies. We could seek to map out affected groups: how, by whom, and to what extent are they represented in the shaping process? We could develop strategies for opening up discourses to admit underrepresented groups more directly to negotiations-at-the-table. We could address the empirically difficult but theoretically and politically vital task of identifying silenced voices, voices defined as irrelevant or otherwise excluded from ongoing discourses.[23] We could popularize our findings on lay user negotiations (both at-table and as-navigation). This might build self-awareness of competence and relevance among underrepresented groups. It might also lead them to apply pressure to spokespersons and gatekeepers that control more powerful discourse agendas. It might also help if we popularize "expert" discourses to make them available to affected lay groups.

This volume embarks on the first step in that process—the mapping of groups affected by or implicated in new reproductive technologies and of their representation(s) at nodes where negotiations occur. We hereby invite our readers to explore the volume. We hope some of you will be inspired to join us in further endeavors: to continue the mapping of interactions between users and technologies, to develop concepts to describe and understand those interactions, and to apply the results of such research to political projects of liberation and empowerment.

NOTES

This introduction was written on the basis of an outline developed in collaboration with Nelly Oudshoorn and Marta Kirejczyk, who have also served as the main critics and commentators as the introduction was drafted and revised.

1. For example, on 30 October 1997, the *New York Times* reported, "South Carolina's highest court this week upheld the criminal prosecution of pregnant women who used drugs, finding that a viable fetus is a 'person' covered by the state's child-abuse laws" (A17). See also Tsing (1990) and Balsamo (1996) for discussions of such cases.

2. The notion of the mutual shaping of gender and technology was first presented by Cockburn and Ormrod (1993), who in turn credit a larger collaborative network for the idea. This network was then in press with a collection of papers (Cockburn and Fürst-Dilić 1994) where the concept of mutual shaping was elaborated. The concept has since been applied and developed by Berg (1996), Berg and Lie (1995), Lohan (1998), and Saetnan (1996), among others.

3. This tale of a mystical event, of a technology appearing as out of nowhere or appearing as the product of an isolated act of genius, implies perhaps the invisible hand of Nature: Technologies work because Nature allows them to work. Geniuses invent through a peculiarly creative combination of an intuitive grasp of Nature's capabilities and limits together with an abundance of tinkering skills. Technologies need not be grounded in the institutions and practices of the natural sciences, but they are seen as grounded in Nature.

4. For instance, Langdon Winner (1986) writes that "because choices tend to become strongly fixed in material equipment, economic investment, and social habit, the original flexibility vanishes for all practical purposes once the initial commitments are made."

5. In one sarcastic example, Berit Schei (1989) presents a fictional medical technology invention she calls the "ballograph," an X-ray instrument that examines men's testes for tumors. Like the mammograph, this machine flattens the organ being examined between two spring-mounted glass plates. Sometimes the spring mechanism jams or applies more pressure than intended, but the discomfort is deemed acceptable given the number of lives potentially saved by early detection of cancers. These are claims Schei has translated to the "ballograph" directly from experts' lectures for a consensus conference on mammography screening. Schei thereby dramatizes the point that, had the male engineers who designed the mammograph themselves imagined having their breasts (or an equally sensitive organ) examined in this fashion, they might have paid more attention to patients' comfort and safety.

6. *Constructivism* refers here to theories which claim that social categories, scientific knowledge, and technological artifacts and practices all emerge from social processes. Currently, two such theories are major points of reference within science and technology studies—namely, Social Construction of Technology (or SCOT; see Bijker 1995) and Actor Network Theory (or ANT, also known as Translation Theory; see Latour 1987). For a discussion of similarities and differences between these and other constructivist theories, see Law and Bijker (1992).

7. A number of examples of this can be found in the collection by Lie and Sørensen (1996). For instance, one may at any given time observe numerous (re)definitions and usages of household technologies such as telephones, microwave ovens, computers, and televisions (Vestby 1996).

8. This metaphor was inspired by Rakow (1986), who uses the term *verb* to indicate gender as process rather than fixed category.

9. These terms are, furthermore, ranked hierarchically relative to one another so that the masculine is almost universally more highly valued, more powerful than the feminine.

10. Judith Butler (1993) emphasizes that this view of gender as performance implies substantial stability, in that it is repetitive, citational performance, the sum of perceived similarities among individual performances, which most strongly shapes gender, rather than individual performances each taken separately. Thus differences between "adjectival" and "verbial" approaches to gender are more on the scale of variations in focus (on processes of change or on sources of constraint), rather than differences in basic understandings of gender as a subject of study.

11. The word *script* is used here as a simple metaphor from everyday language: the text of a play, which disciplines the performances of the actors but nevertheless leaves them considerable leeway for creativity. This metaphor has been further elaborated as a concept within science and technology studies (e.g., Akrich 1992; Akrich and Latour 1992), where it points to the authorlike role of technology designers, who "write" (inscribe) into the shape of a technical artifact certain expectations about how and by whom it will be used. Here, too, users may "read" (or even contravene) the script whose performance entails some degree of interpretation by actors in creative ways. Thus some refer to users as "de-inscribing" the script from the artifact (Akrich 1992), or they refer to actions instructed by the script as a "program" which can be confronted with "anti-programs" (Latour 1992), or they refer to users as competing authors who write "user-scripts" (Gjøen and Hård 1996). All of these elaborations of the metaphor, however, refer back to the simple metaphor used here—that of the text of a play.

12. Harding's definition of gender has been used as a link between gender and technology in various ways by Berg (1996), Cockburn and Ormrod (1993), Lie (1991, 1998), Lohan (1998), Saetnan (1996), and others.

13. This point has been made by a number of authors. See, for example, Ruzek, Clarke, and Olesen (1997) and other essays in the same volume.

14. For other work in this vein, see collections by Ginsburg and Rapp (1995), Ruzek, Olesen, and Clarke (1997), and Lock and Kaufert (1998).

15. In fact, the whole notion of cultural "sites" is problematic. However, on this occasion we will let those problems lie. For a discussion of problems with the concept of sites, see Layne (1998).

16. Statements have the form of associations (*a* has somehow to do with *b*) that constitute the world for us (Foucault 1969, 1971; Schaaning 1997). Strathern (1992) also discusses how cultures as a whole can be described in terms of what they do or do not "bring together" in this way. Statements in this context are taken broadly to encompass not only spoken or written statements but also actions (which, as we have all heard, speak louder than words); not only language and action, but also artifacts. Artifacts and artifact usage are also associations of meaningful elements and thus serve as repositories of meaning. The deployment of an artifact (new or old) into a new (for that artifact) situation represents a new juxtaposition of meanings, ergo, a new associative statement. The use of an artifact in a customary fashion represents the reenactment and thereby the reinforcement of such an association. Discarding an artifact from usage represents the disassociation of the meanings of that artifact from the meanings otherwise associated with the usage context. For instance, sonar was first developed for locating submarines underwater. Taking it into use to examine fetuses in utero gave the instrument new social meanings in addition to a modified design and a new name (sonogram). The practices of examining fetuses by sonogram vary from country to country and clinic to clinic, implying somewhat different social meanings in each location. At many such locations these practices have become routine, each new examination reinforcing local social meanings. To change those routines (e.g., to discontinue the practice of examining all pregnancies with ultrasound) would imply the dissociation of certain meanings (e.g., safe, precise, inexpensive) from the artifact and replacing them with others (e.g., risky, inexact, costly).

17. The appeal for a focus on users has also been made by researchers (many of them also feminists) entering science and technology studies from a background in studies of work (see, e.g., Berg and Lie 1995).

18. Note that the various categories of users discussed in this section—end users, intermediary users, ancillary users, embodied users, imagined users, regulated users—are not mutually exclusive. The categories are separated not so much by characteristics of individuals observed as by the interests of the observer. In one context, a given individual may appear as an end user—for example, as a woman attending an IVF clinic. In another context, she may be aggregated into a larger group of users as observed through the imaginations of politicians seeking to regulate user safety or morality. In a third context, we might focus on her interactions with other users as mutual mediators of user experiences and thus as a type of intermediary user.

19. This is also the point of Michael Lynch's article "Representation Is Overrated" (1994), although the title is alarmingly disparaging.

20. Note that the "others" being spoken for may include not only persons but also things (technologies, natural phenomena). The same can also apply to the category of spokesperson: conceivably, there might also be "spokesthings," such as a sonogram representing the fetus.

The inclusion of nonhuman entities would entail a rather different set of answers to the questions that we propose to ask regarding the relationships between spokespersons and those spoken for, but the concept of spokespersonship, or representation, still opens up those relationships for exploration.

21. Consensus conferences are a forum for technology policy formation. For a description of consensus conferences, see Jacoby (1985) and Perry and Kalberer (1980). For an international comparison of different styles of consensus conferences, see the *European Newsletter on Quality Assurance* (1985).

22. Ginsburg and Tsing (1990) make this same distinction in similar terms.

23. One excellent example of empirical work on silenced voices is an article by Susan Leigh Star (1991). She uses the example that onion allergies (and other rare allergies) are rendered invisible in restaurant contexts. Two other examples, both addressing reproductive technologies, are an article by Gina Corea (1991b) on the registration and nonregistration of "side" effects of Depo-Provera, and an article by Adele Clarke and Theresa Montini (1993) concerning which perspectives on the "abortion pill" RU486 have been heard in different contexts.

REFERENCES

Akrich, Madeleine:
  1992 The De-Scription of Technical Objects. In Wiebe E. Bijker and John Law (eds.), *Shaping Technology/Building Society: Studies in Sociotechnical Change*, 205–24. Cambridge: MIT Press.
Akrich, Madeleine, and Bruno Latour:
  1992 A Summary of a Convenient Vocabulary for the Semiotics of Human and Nonhuman Assemblies. In Wiebe E. Bijker and John Law (eds.), *Shaping Technology/Building Society: Studies in Sociotechnical Change*, 259–64. Cambridge: MIT Press.
Balsamo, Anne:
  1996 Public Pregnancies and Cultural Narratives of Surveillance. Chapter 4 in Balsamo, *Technologies of the Gendered Body: Reading Cyborg Women*. Durham, N.C.: Duke University Press.
Berg, Anne-Jorunn:
  1996 *Digital Feminism*. Trondheim: Center for Technology and Society.
Berg, Anne-Jorunn, and Merete Lie:
  1995 Feminism and Constructivism: Do Artifacts Have Gender? *Science, Technology, and Human Values* 20(3): 332–51.
Bijker, Wiebe E.:
  1995 *Of Bicycles, Bakelites, and Bulbs: Toward a Theory of Sociotechnical Change*. Cambridge: MIT Press.
Butler, Judith:
  1993 *Bodies That Matter*. New York: Routledge.
Casper, Monica J.:
  1994 At the Margins of Humanity: Fetal Positions in Science and Medicine. *Science, Technology, and Human Values* 19(3): 307–23.
  1998 *The Making of the Unborn Patient: A Social Anatomy of Fetal Surgery*. New Brunswick, N.J.: Rutgers University Press.

Catholic Church, Congregatio pro Doctrina Fidei:
  1987   *Instruction on Respect for Human Life in Its Origin and on the Dignity of Procreation.* Vatican City: The Congregation.
Clarke, Adele, and Theresa Montini:
  1993   The Many Faces of RU486: Tales of Situated Knowledges and Technological Contestations. *Science, Technology, and Human Values* 18(1): 42–78.
Cockburn, Cynthia:
  1985   *Machinery of Dominance: Women, Men, and Technical Know-How.* London: Pluto Press.
Cockburn, Cynthia, and Ruza Fürst-Dilić:
  1994   *Bringing Technology Home: Gender and Technology in a Changing Europe.* Milton Keynes: Open University Press.
Cockburn, Cynthia, and Susan Ormrod:
  1993   *Gender and Technology in the Making.* London: Sage.
Connel, R. W.:
  1987   *Gender and Power.* Cambridge: Polity Press.
Corea, Gina:
  1991a How the New Reproductive Technologies Will Affect All Women. In Patricia Hynes (ed.), *Reconstructing Babylon: Essays on Women and Technology,* 41–60. Bloomington: Indiana University Press.
  1991b Depo-Provera and the Politics of Knowledge. In Patricia Hynes (ed.), *Reconstructing Babylon: Essays on Women and Technology,* 161–84. Bloomington: Indiana University Press.
Cowan, Ruth Schwartz:
  1987   The Consumption Junction: A Proposal for Research Strategies in the Sociology of Technology. In Wiebe E. Bijker, Thomas P. Hughes, and Trevor Pinch (eds.), *The Social Construction of Technological Systems: New Directions in the Sociology and History of Technology,* 261–80. Cambridge: MIT Press.
Cussins, Charis:
  1996   Ontological Choreography: Agency through Objectification in Infertility Clinics. *Social Studies of Science* 26(3): 575–610.
Denmark Council of Ethics:
  1995   *Assisted Reproduction: A Report.* Copenhagen: Council of Ethics.
Duden, Barbara:
  1993   *Disembodying Women: Perspectives on Pregnancy and the Unborn.* Cambridge: Harvard University Press.
European Newsletter on Quality Assurance 2(2) (1985).
Foucault, Michel:
  1969   *L'Archéologie du savoir.* Paris: Gallimard.
  1971   *L'Ordre du discours.* Paris: Gallimard.
Ginsburg, Faye D., and Rayna Rapp (eds.):
  1995   *Conceiving the New World Order: The Global Politics of Reproduction.* Berkeley: University of California Press.
Ginsburg, Faye, and Anna Lowenhaupt Tsing (eds.):
  1990   *Uncertain Terms: Negotiating Gender in American Culture.* Boston: Beacon Press.
Gjøen, Heidi, and Mikael Hård:
  1996   *Challenging the Engineering Script: The Mutual Appropriation of the Electric Vehicle*

and Its Drivers. Paper presented at the joint annual meeting of 4S and EASST, Bielefeld, October 1996.

Hård, Mikael, and Andreas Knie:

1999 The Grammar of Technology: German and French Diesel Engineering, 1920–1940. *Technology and Culture* 40(1): 26–46.

Harding, Sandra:

1986 *The Science Question in Feminism.* Ithaca, N.Y.: Cornell University Press.

Health Council:

1992 Annual Health Advice 1991. The Hague: Health Council.

Jacoby, I.:

1985 The Consensus Development Program of the National Institutes of Health: Current Practices and Historical Perspectives. *International Journal of Technology Assessment in Health Care* 1: 420–32.

Kimmel, Michael:

1987 Rethinking "Masculinity": New Directions in Research. In Michael S. Kimmel (ed.), *Changing Men: New Directions in Research on Men and Masculinity.* Newbury Park: Sage.

Kirejczyk, Marta:

1993 Shifting the Burden onto Women: The Gender Character of In Vitro Fertilization. *Science as Culture* 3(17): 507–21.

Kirejczyk, Marta, and Irma Van der Ploeg:

1993 Pregnant Couples: Medical Technology and Social Constructions around Fertility and Reproduction. *Journal of International Feminist Analysis* 5(2): 113–25.

Kline, Ronald, and Trevor Pinch:

1996 Users as Agents of Technological Change: The Social Construction of the Automobile in the Rural United States. *Technology and Culture* 37(4): 763–95.

Latour, Bruno:

1987 *Science in Action: How to Follow Scientists and Engineers through Society.* Milton Keynes: Open University Press.

1992 A Note on Socio-Technical Graphs. *Social Studies of Science* 22(1): 33–57.

Law, John, and Wiebe E. Bijker:

1992 Postscript: Technology, Stability, and Social Theory. In Wiebe E. Bijker and John Law (eds.), *Shaping Technology/Building Society: Studies in Sociotechnical Change,* 290–308. Cambridge: MIT Press.

Layne, Linda:

1998 Introduction to Special Issue: Anthropological Approaches in Science and Technology Studies. *Science, Technology, and Human Values* 23(1): 4–23.

Lie, Merete:

1991 Technology and Gender: Identity and Symbolism. In Anna-Maija Lehto and Inger Eriksson (eds.), *Proceedings of the Conference on Women, Work, and Computerization, Helsinki, June 30–July 2,* 425–46. Helsinki: Ministry of Health and Social Affairs.

1995 Technology and Masculinity: The Case of the Computer. *European Journal of Women's Studies* 2(3): 379–94.

1996 Gender in the Image of Technology. In Merete Lie and Knut H. Sørensen (eds.), *Making Technology Our Own? Domesticating Technology into Everyday Life,* 201–23. Oslo: Scandinavian University Press.

1998   *Computer Dialogues: Technology, Gender, and Change.* Trondheim: Center for Women's Studies.

Lie, Merete, and Knut H. Sørensen (eds.):

1996   *Making Technology Our Own? Domesticating Technology into Everyday Life.* Oslo: Scandinavian University Press.

Lock, Margaret, and Patricia A. Kaufert (eds.):

1998   *Pragmatic Women and Body Politics.* Cambridge: Cambridge University Press.

Lohan, E. Maria:

1998   The Transvestite Telephone: A Male Technology Dressed Up in Feminine Clothes? Ph.D. diss., University of Dublin, Trinity College.

Lynch, Michael:

1994   Representation Is Overrated: Some Critical Remarks about the Use of the Concept of Representation in Science Studies. *Configurations* 2(1): 137–49.

Norwegian Ministry of Health and Social Affairs:

1992–93 *On Humans and Biotechnology.* Parliamentary report no. 25. Oslo: Ministry of Health and Social Affairs.

Oudshoorn, Nelly:

1994   *Beyond the Natural Body: An Archaeology of Sex Hormones.* London: Routledge.

1999   On Gender and Things: Reflections on an Exhibition on Gendered Artefacts. *Science and the Public.* Amsterdam: New Metropolis.

Perry, S., and J. T. Kalberer:

1980   The NIH Consensus-Development Program and the Assessment of Health-Care Technologies: The First Two Years. *New England Journal of Medicine* 303(3): 169–72.

Rakow, Lana F.:

1986   Rethinking Gender and Communication. *Journal of Communication* 36: 11–26.

Rapp, Rayna:

1994   Women's Responses to Prenatal Diagnosis: A Sociocultural Perspective on Diversity. In Karen H. Rothenberg and Elizabeth J. Thomson (eds.), *Women and Prenatal Testing: Facing the Challenges of Genetic Technology.* Columbus: Ohio State University Press.

Rasmussen, Bente, and Tove Håpnes:

1991   Excluding Women from the Technologies of the Future? A Case Study of the Culture of Computer Science. *Futures,* December: 1107–19.

Rothman, Barbara Katz:

1986   *The Tentative Pregnancy: Prenatal Diagnosis and the Future of Motherhood.* New York: Viking.

1994   The Tentative Pregnancy: Then and Now. In Karen H. Rothenberg and Elizabeth J. Thomson (eds.), *Women and Prenatal Testing: Facing the Challenges of Genetic Technology,* 260–70. Columbus: Ohio State University Press.

Royal Commission on New Reproductive Technologies

1993   *Final Report: Proceed with Care.* Ottawa: Royal Commission on New Reproductive Technologies.

Ruzek, Sheryl Burt, Adele E. Clarke, and Virginia L. Olesen:

1997   What Are the Dynamics of Difference? In Sheryl Burt Ruzek, Virginia L. Olesen, and Adele E. Clarke (eds.), *Women's Health: Complexities and Differences,* 51–95. Columbus: Ohio State University Press.

Ruzek, Sheryl Burt, Virginia L. Olesen, and Adele E. Clarke (eds.):
  1997 *Women's Health: Complexities and Differences*. Columbus: Ohio State University Press.
Saetnan, Ann Rudinow:
  1996 Speaking of Gender . . . : Intertwinings of a Medical Technology Policy Debate and Everyday Life. In Merete Lie and Knut H. Sørensen (eds.), *Making Technology Our Own? Domesticating Technology into Everyday Life*, 31–63. Oslo: Scandinavian University Press.
Schaaning, Espen:
  1997 *Vitenskap som skapt viten: Foucault og historisk praksis*. Oslo: Spartakus.
Schei, Berit:
  1989 Ballografiscreening [It Should Save Lives]. *Tidsskrift for den Norske lægeforening* 109: 1088.
Silverstone, R., and E. Hirsch:
  1992 *Consuming Technologies: Media and Information in Domestic Spaces*. London: Routledge.
Smith, Merritt Roe, and Leo Marx (eds.):
  1994 *Does Technology Drive History? The Dilemma of Technological Determinism*. Cambridge: MIT Press.
Sørensen, Knut H.:
  1997 *Social Shaping on the Move? On the Policy Relevance of the Social Shaping of Technology Perspective*. STS working paper 9/97. Trondheim: Center for Technology and Society.
Sørensen, Knut H., Margrethe Aune, and Morten Hatling:
  1996 *Against Linearity: On the Cultural Appropriation of Science and Technology*. STS working paper 9/96. Trondheim: Center for Technology and Society.
Star, Susan Leigh:
  1991 Power, Technology and the Phenomenology of Conventions: On Being Allergic to Onions. In John Law (ed.), *A Sociology of Monsters: Essays on Power, Technology and Domination*, 26–56. London and New York: Routledge.
Strathern, Marilyn:
  1992 *Reproducing the Future: Anthropology, Kinship, and the New Reproductive Technologies*. Manchester: Manchester University Press.
Traweek, Sharon:
  1988 *Beamtimes and Lifetimes: The World of High Energy Physicists*. Cambridge: Harvard University Press.
Tsing, Anna Lowenhaupt:
  1990 Monster Stories: Women Charged with Perinatal Endangerment. In Faye Ginsburg and Anna Lowenhaupt Tsing (eds.), *Uncertain Terms: Negotiating Gender in American Culture*, 282–99. Boston: Beacon Press.
Vestby, Guri Mette:
  1996 Technologies of Autonomy? Parenthood in Contemporary "Modern Times." In Merete Lie and Knut H. Sørensen (eds.), *Making Technology Our Own? Domesticating Technology into Everyday Life*, 65–90. Oslo: Scandinavian University Press.
Webster's Encyclopedic Unabridged Dictionary of the English Language:
  1994 New York: Gramercy Books.

Winner, Langdon:
  1986   *The Whale and the Reactor: A Search for Limits in an Age of High Technology.* Chicago: University of Chicago Press.
World Health Organization/Human Reproduction Program:
  1991   *Creating Common Ground: Women's Perspectives on the Selection and Introduction of Fertility Regulating Technologies.* Report of a meeting between women's health advocates and scientists, Geneva, 20–22 February. Geneva: World Health Organization.
  1996   *Women's and Men's Perspectives on Fertility Regulating Methods and Services.* Report of a meeting in Geneva, 29 November–1 December 1995. Geneva: World Health Organization.

■ PART ONE

CONCEPTIONS AND COUNTERPERCEPTIONS:
User Involvement in the Development of
Contraceptive Technologies

Nelly Oudshoorn

USERS IN CONTRACEPTIVE DEVELOPMENT

Ever since the first modern contraceptives for women were introduced, questions of control and choice have been of central concern, particularly for women's health advocates who have critically monitored and protested against the potential abuse of contraceptives (Hartmann 1987; van Kammen 1998; Oudshoorn 1996). Criticism and controversies surrounding contraceptives have also included issues of safety. In this respect, contraceptives are a very peculiar type of drugs. Unlike other pharmaceuticals, which are used by people who suffer from specific illnesses, contraceptives are used by healthy people. Since contraceptives are not developed for treating or preventing diseases, the tolerance of health risks is much lower than for other drugs (Oudshoorn 1999). In the 1970s, safety issues became of central concern because feminist health advocates and physicians reported serious side effects of both oral contraceptives and intrauterine devices (Seaman and Seaman 1978; Boston Women's Health Book Collective 1971). These critics suggested that the reproductive sciences and industry had shown inadequate concern for the health of women (Gelijns and Pannenborg 1993). Due to advocacy of the women's health movement, women's reproductive health has become the major focus in policy documents of national and international family planning and public health organizations, as is exemplified by the Program of Action adopted at the 1994 United Nations International Conference on Population and Development in Cairo in 1994 (United Nations 1994).

Given this background of controversies, it is not surprising that the role of users in contraceptive development has become an important theme in feminist science and technology studies. This theme also connects the four chapters of this section, which address the various ways in which users are involved in contraceptive technological development. The authors all share the view that the design phase of a technology is an important site to understand technology-users relations. Or to use Jessika van Kammen's felicitous phrase from her chapter, "Users do not matter only once a technology is in use."

Adele Clarke discusses users of contraceptives in terms of "implicated actors." By introducing this notion, she emphasizes that, although women as the primary users of reproductive technologies are usually not very involved in the process of technological development, they are "clearly targeted and thereby configured by technoscience." She describes how women's health organizations have been important as spokespersons for women consumers in the world of contraceptive technological innovations both at the beginning and the end of the twentieth century.

Jessika van Kammen and Nelly Oudshoorn set out to map how users are represented in the design of two contraceptives that are currently being developed: immunological contraceptives and male hormonal contraceptives. Their chapters nicely illustrate the recent shift in attention in feminist studies of technologies from the role of users in a social sense (i.e., identifiable persons as such involved in the diffusion of technologies) toward users in the semiotic sense (i.e., users as imagined by actors involved in the design of technologies). This approach broadens our scope to take into account a wide variety of spokespersons of users in the struggle to shape the design of contraceptives. This shift toward including the "virtual user" is an important theoretical and political move because it enables us to understand how issues such as safety and the cultural feasibility of contraceptive innovations may be related to implicit or explicit choices in the design process that prioritize specific representations of users and use over others.

Lara Marks focuses on the role of users in a social sense. In her study of the testing of the first oral contraceptive for women in the 1950s, she views the trial participants as active subjects, rather than passive, "unwitting guinea pigs." She describes how women have made important contributions to the development of the pill that are usually not acknowledged in previous historical research on the first oral contraceptive.

AN OVERVIEW OF THE SECTION

Chapter 2 provides an intriguing account of the development of modern contraceptives. Adopting a social worlds approach, Adele Clarke portrays reproductive scientists who worked on contraceptives as "mavericks": scientists who often operated on the margins of the scientific community to be able to pursue their own work. Most scientists refused to work on contraceptives because, Clarke says, they believed it was "not legitimate research, basic research, proper research, good science, or even to be viewed as science at all." She distinguishes five generations of "maverick" reproductive scientists. It was only in the 1970s that contraceptive research became accepted as a legitimate scientific practice. However, this does not imply that the legitimacy of research in contraceptive technologies is no longer questioned. The development of these technologies continues to be the subject of severe contests, particularly by users and spokespersons for potential users. Since the 1960s, three generations of women's health advocates have discussed the many issues raised by the use of contraceptives: safety, potential for abuse, side effects, and the almost exclusive focus on the development of contraceptives for women. Questions of how contraceptive technologies can be developed to match the needs and perspectives of (women) users therefore remain of central concern for feminist scholars of science and technology.

In chapter 3, Jessika van Kammen suggests that if we wish to make women's voices more powerful we need to understand how the involvement of users is sustained and constituted in the design of contraceptives. In line with Madeleine Akrich, she conceptualizes the role of users in the design of technology in terms of "projected users": users as imagined by the designers who ascribe specific interests, preferences, and behaviors to the future users and "inscribe" these views into the material content of the technology-in-the-making. As the "projected user" is not a single entity but often consists of a variety of different representations of end-users, van Kammen is particularly interested in understanding how certain representations of users become more influential than others. Based on a thorough analysis of the early research on immunological contraceptives, she describes how experts such as biomedical scientists, clinicians, representatives of states, and to a lesser extent social scientists became the major spokespersons for potential users. Representations of users as constructed by family planning organizations and women's health groups were not taken into account in the design of these new contraceptives. Van Kammen ascribes this choice to scientists' need to reduce the complexities of the problems to be addressed. Family planning organizations and women's health groups provided a "more contextualized and therefore more complex set of user representations" that were considered to be constraints on the process of innovation. Van Kammen shows that there is still a long way to go before representations of users, as voiced by women's health advocates, are no longer marginalized in the design process.

Adopting the view that the construction of the cultural authority of science and technology can no longer be regarded as the exclusive domain of scientists,

I propose to extend the analysis of user representations to yet another group of nonexperts: the media. Focusing on the development of new hormonal contraceptives for men, I claim that journalists as well as feminists have been, and still are, important actors in constructing and contesting specific·representations of masculinities and male users. Ever since the demand for new male contraceptives was first articulated, experts and lay people have wondered whether men would be willing to use a contraceptive pill or injection if one were available. I suggest that these debates are an important site for studying the co-construction of a technology and its users. I describe how feminists, scientists, and journalists have constructed a conflicting set of user representations. I conclude that an analysis of user representations is relevant to understanding how scientists construct the technical feasibility of technologies and that images of users can function as powerful tools in enhancing or denouncing the cultural feasibility of a technology. Journalists and feminist opponents of male contraceptives used specific representations of masculinities to argue that new male contraceptives would never be accepted, either by potential users or by women. Scientists and feminist advocates of male contraceptives have constructed representations of male users to articulate the need for the new technology. Most important, this chapter challenges the view that dissenting voices that refute hegemonic representations of male identities are restricted to feminist discourse. I reveal how scientists can act as "cultural entrepreneurs" by being active participants in the construction of new meanings of masculinities, thus providing an intriguing view of the role of scientists in our culture today.

In chapter 5, Lara Marks discusses the agency of "test users" in contraceptive development. In her history of the testing of the first oral contraceptive for women, Marks adopts a critical position toward previous feminist and historical studies of the development of the pill in which the trial participants are depicted as passive victims. Reflecting on the psychologically and physically demanding conditions of the first trials of the pill, Marks concludes that the pill could not have been developed without "the dedication and commitment of women who risked swallowing it." Marks thus provides an important contribution to an understanding of users as coproducers of technologies by including the women on whose bodies technologies are tested. Moreover, she describes the crucial role women have played as initiators and sponsors, as technicians, and as doctors who supervised the trials of the pill. By doing so, she challenges the myth that the pill was "fathered" solely by male scientists. This last chapter thus provides an important contribution to the history of women in medicine by making visible the many roles that women have played in the making of the pill. Equally important, her focus on women's contributions to the development of the pill also bears relevance for understanding the role of expertise and knowledge in technological innovation. Marks convincingly shows that historical accounts that only focus on the expertise and knowledge of key scientific experts seriously misrepresent and undervaluate all the work of equally important but often silenced actors.

Taken together, the chapters in this section exemplify the importance of looking at the discourses of scientific experts, technicians, and doctors as well as the discourses of feminists and journalists as important sites for understanding the mutual shaping of gender, users, and technologies.

REFERENCES

Boston Women's Health Book Collective:
  1971   *Our Bodies, Ourselves.* New York: Simon and Schuster.
Gelijns, A., and C. Pannenborg:
  1993   The Development of Contraceptive Technology: Case Studies of Incentives and Disincentives of Innovation. *International Journal of Technology Assessment in Health Care* 9(2): 210–32.
Hartmann, B.:
  1987   *Reproductive Rights and Wrongs: The Global Politics of Population Control and Contraceptive Choice.* New York: Harper and Row.
Oudshoorn, N.:
  1996   The Decline of the One-Size-Fits-All Paradigm; or, How Reproductive Scientists Try to Cope with Postmodernity. In Nina Lykke and Rosi Braidotti (eds.), *Between Monsters, Goddesses, and Cyborgs: Feminist Confrontations with Science, Medicine, and Cyberspace,* 153–69. London: Zed Books.
  1999   *Drugs for Healthy People: The Culture of Testing and Approving Hormonal Contraceptives for Women and Men.* London: Wellcome Institute.
Seaman, B., and G. Seaman:
  1978   *Women and the Crisis in Sex Hormones: An Investigation of the Dangerous Uses of Hormones: From Birth Control to Menopause and the Safe Alternatives.* Brighton: Harvester.
United Nations:
  1994   *International Conference on Population and Development: Program of Action.* Cairo.
van Kammen, J.:
  1998   Integrating Users into the Design of Anti-Fertility Vaccines. Unpublished manuscript. University of Amsterdam.

2

Maverick Reproductive Scientists and the Production of Contraceptives, 1915–2000+

Adele E. Clarke

[A] woman possessing an adequate knowledge of her reproductive functions is the best judge of the time and conditions under which her child should be brought into this world. We further maintain that it is her right, regardless of other considerations, to determine whether she shall bear children or not, and how many children she shall bear if she chooses to become a mother.
  —*Margaret Sanger*

But there is agreement that in science is power.
  —*Frank Lillie*

Where there is power, there is resistance.
  —*Michel Foucault*

Modern contraceptives are products of the combined efforts of the reproductive sciences, birth control/population control/eugenics movements, and major private philanthropic organizations. In sharp contrast to the comparatively limited overall investment in research on reproduction, its technoscientific products such as contraceptives have likely affected more individuals per penny on the planet than almost any other technologies. Despite intervention in billions of human lives in even the most remote corners of the globe (e.g., Tsing 1993), the reproductive sciences themselves have been relatively ignored.[1] For most of the twentieth century, during the formation, coalescence, golden age, and retrenchment periods of the reproductive sciences, most such scientists refused to pursue research explicitly on contraceptives of any kind. They did so because they believed it was not legitimate research, basic research, proper research, good science, or even to be viewed as science at all. But during each of these periods, some maverick reproductive scientists did so for various reasons, using diverse approaches and producing a wide assortment of technoscientific results. This chapter examines their efforts.

To contextualize this analysis, it is crucial to remember how very radical birth control was in the early twentieth-century United States. Women were not full citizens with voting rights until five years after Margaret Sanger's first arrest in 1915 for distributing contraceptives. Distribution to unmarried people was not fully legal in all states until 1972, the year before the U.S. Supreme Court legalized abortion. For most of the twentieth century, the birth control issue has been at least as charged and controversial as the abortion issue is today. The modern reproductive sciences began about 1900. European scientists were the major contributors until World War I; then, for the next half century, American reproductive scientists reigned (Clarke 1998). Because of the social and scientific impropriety of the reproductive sciences, the reproductive sciences and contraceptive research have been pursued almost exclusively through the fiscal sponsorship of private philanthropy, with limited government sponsorship after 1965.[2] While contraceptives have been distributed globally since the 1930s, engendering elaborate distribution networks, the scientific infrastructures of research as well as production have also been globalized since the late 1970s, largely through philanthropic investments moving along the sinews of maternal and child health infrastructures dating back as far as the 1930s.[3] Yet even after one hundred years of reproductive science, such work remains marginalized and illegitimate.

Foucault is among a very few major social theorists to address reproduction as a central phenomenon of human life, much less contraception (e.g., Ginsberg and Rapp 1995). Certainly in the reproductive domain we see struggles concerning what Foucault (1980, 103–55) termed the "socialization of procreative behavior" and the construction of "the Malthusian couple" as the target and anchorpoint "for the ventures of knowledge" production. Yet I argue strongly, contra Foucault, that the reproductive sciences are marked on the one hand by incredible potency in the world and on the other hand by shame due to their enduring illegitimacy, marginality, and controversial status as science. Here I am both contradicting and complicating Foucault's analysis of the relations between the reproductive sciences and what we now call sexology. Foucault's assertion that the reproductive sciences proceeded apace while sexology was hampered in its development by social and cultural constraints is, in short, only half right. Both lines of work were and remain considerably hampered due to their scientific and social/cultural illegitimacy,[4] and contraceptive research has taken the brunt of the consequences. Even today, according to an Institute of Medicine committee, contraception is a "topic that remains sensitive, controversial, and even somewhat unfashionable" (Harrison and Rosenfield 1996, vii).

Reproductive scientists were unable to create the separation between science and society often desired by scientists. Reproduction is too much at the core of human social life for any tinkering in its processes to be ignored (e.g., Haraway 1995; A. F. Robertson 1991). The status of reproductive sciences vis-à-vis other sciences has always been low, and they have been routinely marginalized in ways that have been deeply consequential for the nature of their work. Against this now routine disparagement within the sciences, reproductive scientists and contraceptive researchers have struggled time and again. I am arguing here that this is a contributing factor to the consistent bias across the twentieth century against the simple, low-technology contraceptives that feminist birth control advocates initially sought, toward endocrinological and other "more scientific" means and, along the way, to profound resistance against taking users seriously, much less engaging them/us in technology design processes. Here Foucault (1980, 11–12) again makes immense sense: "What knowledge [savoir] was formed as a result . . . my main concern will be to locate the forms of power, the channels it takes, and the discourses it permeates in order to reach the most tenuous and individual modes of behavior."[5] Like other scientists, reproductive scientists have fought hard for their autonomy; unlike most other scientists, they have had to fight for status within the sciences as well as in other domains.

CONCEPTUAL FRAMEWORK

My conceptual framework centers on the concepts of social worlds/arenas and mavericks and implicated actors. I view the reproductive sciences and the other major social groupings with which they related in the broader American reproductive arena this century (philanthropic and birth/population control/eugenic groups) as social worlds—communities of practice, discourse, and meaning-making.[6] Social worlds form fundamental "building blocks" of collective action and organize social life. All the social worlds that focus on a given issue typically come together in an arena of concern and action. For example, the many heterogeneous social worlds concerned with contraception "live" in a broader reproductive arena, prepared to act/intervene in some way.[7]

Participation in social worlds usually remains fluid. Some participants cluster around the core of the world and mobilize those around them (Hughes 1971, 54). Becker (1963) refers to them as "entrepreneurs." Usually on the margins are what Becker (1982) has called "mavericks," those who participate on their own terms, taking the sometimes considerable risks of following their own convictions against the grain of local or disciplinary conventions. Becker (1982, 233) says that mavericks

> propose innovations the . . . world refuses to accept as within the limits of what it ordinarily produces. Other participants in the world—audiences, support personnel, sources of support, or distributors—refuse to cooperate in the production of those innovations. Instead of giving up and returning to more acceptable [approaches], . . . mavericks continue to pursue the innovation without support. . . . Not surprisingly, mavericks get a hostile reception when they present their innovations to other . . . world members. Because it violates some of the . . . world's conventions in a blatant way, the work suggests to others that they will have trouble cooperating with its maker.

Mavericks too can be individuals or small groups, marginalized by others within their shared social world.

We can also ask whether there are implicated actors in a social world or arena, individuals and/or groups or nonhuman entities who, while they do not actively participate (for whatever reasons, including exclusion), are the targets of or will likely be considerably affected by actions taken within the social worlds or arenas (Clarke and Montini 1993). For example, women as the primary users/consumers of the technoscientific products of the reproductive sciences are usually implicated actors in that arena—historically not present at technology design stages but clearly targeted and thereby configured by technoscience. In this essay, women consumers are also represented by feminist and women's organizations at the beginning and end of the twentieth century.

The word *generations* usually refers to cohorts born within some era of wider social significance, such as baby boomers or Gen X in the United States. Here I translate *generation* to refer less to chronological age in the broader society than to one's era of entry into a particular social world such as the reproductive sciences. In social worlds, within particular eras, distinctively "situated knowledges" (Haraway 1991) are produced within specific historical parameters in terms of the science itself. Thus I view the reproductive sciences as a social world composed of a series of generations that produced distinctively situated knowledges appropriately examined within the broader arena in which they were historically formed and where they "matter" most (Butler 1993). Social and cultural constructions of science also matter here. To most scientists, basic research has higher status and is more important than applied science or technology development. Further, in the prestige hierarchy of the sciences, physics was at the pinnacle until recently displaced in late capitalism by biotechnologies—flexible hybrids of molecular biology, genetics, and related technologies of transformation. The reproductive sciences have been and remain quite low on the totem pole.

This chapter is also illustrative of several emphases in the social construction of technology.[8] Especially important here are (1) examining the earliest design stages in the making of the technology and its subsequent use by consumers, (2) analyzing the interests and commitments that are built into the actual design of the technology by analyzing all the engaged social worlds, including their interpretations of the technology itself (interpretative flexibility), (3) interpreting the technology as including the eventual institutional distribution, regulatory, and other related systems or networks involved in delivery and consumption, and (4) attending to processes of closure when interpretive flexibility supposedly vanishes. Both Woolgar's (1991) key point that we can examine how technologies configure their users (and I would add also configure discursive constructions of users) and Latour's (1991) notion that technology is society made durable have long histories in feminist technoscience studies. Here Cowan (1987) first drew our attention to the consumption junction, and a number of analysts have attended to how users are imagined across a range of technologies.[9] Thus, technology here is used in the Foucauldian sense as "not only machines and devices, but also as social, economic and institutional forces" (Balsamo 1996, 159), forces which include the construction of social positions such as users.[10] Feminists have long noted the exclusion of women users from design stages of most technologies, most certainly contraception,[11] even recently, at the very same time that inclusion of users/clients in application-oriented research in computing and information systems is experiencing "ubiquitous support" because it is "widely believed to benefit system development" (Weedman 1998, 315). Callon's (1991) darker point that these are often techno-economic networks and often close to irreversible also pertains. Contraceptives are, after all, what Foucault (1977) termed "disciplinary technologies."

HISTORICAL BACKGROUND

Because of controversy and illegitimacy, the relations of reproductive scientists with other social worlds have been of fundamental importance to their existence and survival. The social worlds that have mattered most to their development in the twentieth century have been those of birth control and population control advocates and philanthropists. Birth control/population control groups have included feminists, physicians, eugenicists, demographers, and others. Serious philanthropic sponsorship of the reproductive sciences and contraceptive research began c. 1920 and continues extensively to this day.[12] Contraception was and remains very much part of the modernist project of the reproductive sciences—achieving control over reproductive processes.[13]

In 1915, in a "frenzy of renown" well covered by the media, birth control advocates began speaking out, organizing, setting up clinics, distributing illegal birth control information and devices, and getting arrested.[14] They also actively sought improved means of simple, woman-controlled contraception—their specific *contraceptive advocacy* (Berkman 1980). Then, from 1920 to 1945, reproductive scientists used several strategies vis-à-vis their often insistent market audiences of birth control and population control advocates to assert their legitimacy, scientific autonomy, and authority. First, they carefully distinguished reproductive research from contraceptive research and refused to participate in studies of simple contraceptives (such as spermicides, douches, and diaphragms), making any reproductive scientists who did so marginal within the profession.[15] Second, they argued with birth control advocates for basic research as the ultimate source of modern contraception and made token offerings from their "basic" research work to the birth control cause (such as accurate information on the timing of ovulation). Third, they redirected contraceptive research toward modern scientific methods that would utilize basic reproductive science—their continuing contraceptive advocacy. In short, reproductive scientists successfully insisted on the culture of science, which has operated as what Bijker (1987) calls a "technological frame" around contraceptive research and development ever since. By 1945, the very nature of what would constitute modern contraception had been negotiated, and reproductive scientists had captured definitional authority. After endless petitioning by feminist birth control advocates to produce and test improved simple contraceptives, some reproductive scientists finally capitulated *if instead* the new contraceptives were properly scientific, such as new endocrinological means like the Pill and injectables, new plastic IUDs, and so on. During the Great Depression, eugenicists and other social conservatives began to find contraception attractive, especially as birth control advocates exploited the issue of skyrocketing welfare costs. They talked much less of women controlling their bodies and much more of the need to "democratize" contraceptive practice— to spread it "down" from the upper and middle classes, who had the best access to such technologies in the United States and Europe, to the lower classes globally.[16] The contraceptive advocacy of population control worlds and philanthropists who funded such research after 1920 centered on new, more effective means of contraception controlled not by users but by clinicians. I call such means "imposables."

Configuring women as the primary users of contraceptive technologies— implicated actors—was, in fact, a core goal of certain birth control and population control groups. It is important here to remember that Margaret Sanger and other feminists initially sought explicitly woman-controlled means of contraception specifically to enhance women's sexual autonomy (Chesler 1992). Population control advocates targeted women because it is women who bear children and therefore women who, in their logics, should be controlled (e.g., Gordon 1990; Dixon-Mueller 1993b). By 1945, Sanger and others in what had become Planned Parenthood had shifted their contraceptive advocacy to include modern scientific means, including imposables.

By 1950, in an intimate dance of realignment, these once distinctive and often oppositional social worlds of reproductive sciences, contraceptive philanthropy, birth control, and population control advocates were reconstituted and transformed through a quid pro quo that focused on the development of "properly scientific" forms of contraception.[17] This quid pro quo reigned essentially unchallenged until the late 1960s, when feminists from emergent women's health movements began major sustained and increasingly international campaigns for safe and effective woman-centered contraception. That quid pro quo still predominates today, although it is now also challenged by a new generation of "mavericks" *within* the reproductive sciences as well as heterogeneous feminist and other groups. Since the 1960s, feminists have offered various bottom-up rather than top-down interpretations of "democratization" of birth control to mean the inclusion of women as users in contraceptive research, design, development, testing, framing of informed consent, and distribution, attempting to turn this vision into concrete practices, locally and globally.[18]

FIRST-GENERATION MAVERICKS: PRODUCING THE FEMALE CYCLE, 1915–1930

When the American reproductive sciences were forming after 1910, there were hardly any reproductive scientists at all. It was then a maverick act—a radical social, political, cultural, and moral act—to pursue any reproductive topics in scientific venues, much less contraception, because they were so deeply controversial (Clarke 1990a, 1998, chap. 8). Moreover, most American reproductive scientists were deeply committed to basic research on mammals to reveal universal laws and functions, pursuing "normality studies" (Fletcher et al. 1981) through morphological, anatomical, physiological, endocrinological, and other biochemical approaches. By the early 1930s, some of the research done by first-generation scientists produced the first seemingly accurate understanding of the female reproductive cycle, fundamental to development of most subsequent means of contraception from rhythm and other "natural" modes to the Pill, injectables, and so-called vaccines.[19] The newly constructed female cycle was, in fact, contrary to earlier conceptualizations of the time of fertility, which had often asserted that as the time of menstruation. Earlier rhythm methods of contraception had thus favored unprotected intercourse in the week just after menstruation (when pregnancy was most likely) whereas abstinence was advocated during menstruation (Langley 1973).

The maverick reproductive scientists most responsible for producing this new knowledge of the female cycle were founders and giants of the emergent discipline (Gruhn and Kazer 1989). George Washington Corner (1889–1981), a physician and fledgling reproductive scientist, began pursuing the cycle in about 1915, culminating in a series of experiments on the monkey *Macaca rhesus* at Johns Hopkins Medical School to determine the parameters of the menstrual cycle (Corner 1981, 164). This work led to Corner's understanding of the action of progesterone, an essential hormonal actor in the menstrual cycle, and subsequently an actor in birth control pills (Corner and Allen 1929a, 1929b). George Bartelmez (1885–1967), based in the anatomy department at the University of Chicago, broke new ground in the scientific study of menstruation (Bartelmez 1933, 1935, 1937). He too was linked with the Carnegie Department of Embryology at Johns Hopkins (e.g., Bartelmez, Corner, and Hartman 1951). Carl Hartman (1879–1967) first published on the female cycle in the opossum, moving on to primates at Johns Hopkins in the late 1920s (Hartman 1932, 1939). In a long series of publications, Hartman (1933, 1936, 1937, 1962) explicitly transformed this knowledge into a method of contraception. Called the "rhythm method," it requires menstrual charting of some kind plus abstinence or the use of a barrier method during the vulnerable interlude of fertility. An array of users have long been interested, from Roman Catholics to those who cannot or will not take medications or use devices for whatever reasons. Hartman's 1933 article was entitled "Catholic Advice on the Safe Period," published in the *Birth Control Review,* journal of the American Birth Control League. The key to using this method successfully is accurate knowledge of the time of fertility. In the 1930s, this was deemed achievable only by timing the fertility cycle. The mucus method of assessing rhythm, a very simple, woman-controlled method discussed below, was not pursued at this time despite extensive knowledge of the mucus-based vaginal smear developed by George Papanicolaou (the Pap smear) and elaborated by many others starting in 1917 (see Clarke 1998, 82–85; Casper and Clarke 1998). Paths that were not pursued for possible contraceptives are also significant.

SECOND-GENERATION MAVERICKS: PRODUCING SPERMICIDES AND STERILIZATION, 1930–1950

In the United States, birth control was essentially illegal from 1873 until 1936—and until much later in some states. The federal Comstock Act of 1873 made it illegal to put through the mails any contraceptive advice, device, or information. Aimed largely at controlling vice and prostitution, the Comstock Act explicitly defined "the prevention of conception" as obscene, and the law prohibited the mailing of obscene matter. The mails had been (and may well have continued to be) the primary means of distribution of birth control (including abortifacients) for some decades. But the subject of contraception was therefore omitted from new editions of books in which it had formerly appeared so they could be legally mailed. A variety of state and local statutes also prohibited distribution of contraceptive devices and information.

American philanthropists committed to birth control therefore sponsored research that was pursued elsewhere. Although many British scientists were also unenthusiastic about applied research on simple contraceptives (Soloway 1995), two major projects centered on spermicides were conducted in the British Isles. They led to successfully tested spermicides effective especially in conjunction with diaphragm use, but the two British investigators were punished for their research. One was forced into an applied department from a basic one, and the other left the academy entirely.

Cecil Voge did one study under the direction of F. A. E. Crew of the Animal Breeding Research Department of the University of Edinburgh. Voge's work focused on tests of extant spermicides to determine if there was a safe, highly effective one that would also work as a prophylactic against venereal diseases (a search that continues to this day). Voge's project was sponsored by the National Committee for Maternal Health (NCMH), an American physicians' birth control advocacy group, funded by the Rockefeller-supported Bureau of Social Hygiene (BSH). Interestingly, just before the spermicide research, Crew's department at Edinburgh was transformed between 1927 and 1930 into the Institute of Animal Genetics by a matching grant from the Rockefeller International Education Board, providing an endowed chair, buildings, and equipment (Hogben 1974, 139). Crew's approval of Voge's contraceptive research project was grudging and may well have been induced by his prior grant.

The NCMH's contraceptive advocacy here was for an "easily available chemical in a form that should keep in good condition over a long period of time and in all climates, and be so easy to use that the most ignorant woman in the Orient, the tropics, the rural outposts or the city slums might be protected."[20] The Voge study, published in 1933, did not produce such a miracle, but sponsors considered it a great research success in establishing standards of safety and effectiveness.[21] Dr. Crew, however, had a very different reaction, stating that Voge had been "a traitor to science."[22] Despite his Ph.D. in immunology, Voge (1933, 11) had somehow crossed the invisible and shifting border into "applied" research. Crew then recommended that the NCMH cease to support Voge's work because his future as a research chemist was being jeopardized.

Voge ultimately "fulfilled the worst fears of his colleagues" when he went into business as a consulting industrial chemist (Reed 1984, 243). There was also some controversy about Voge's use of Baker's early research (Soloway 1995).

Baker's was the other spermicide study in Britain, sponsored by the Birth Control Investigation Committee, part of the British activist clinic movement, along with the British Eugenics Society and the American BSH and NCMH. Initially, reproductive scientist F. H. A. Marshall, then president of the Cambridge birth control clinic, tried to place the project in a lab at Cambridge University, where he was on the agricultural faculty, but he was unsuccessful (Soloway 1995). Instead, in the late 1920s, John R. Baker, an ardent eugenicist based in the zoology department at Oxford, began examining the spermicidal value of pure chemicals as well as testing extant means and vehicles used to convey them vaginally (Baker 1930a, 1930b, 1931a, 1931b, 1935). According to one source, Baker assembled at Oxford a team of scientists in zoology, chemistry, physiology, and bacteriology and related both clinical and laboratory findings.[23]

In 1930, Baker specified that the ideal contraceptive should be small, inexpensive, and require no special appliance for insertion into the vagina; that it should be unaffected by the ordinary range of climates, should leave no trace on skin or fabrics, contain no volatile or odorous substance, and not irritate the vagina, cervix, and penis; that it should be without pharmaceutical effect if absorbed into the bloodstream, contain a substance reducing surface tension to ensure that the smallest crevices of the folds of the vagina are reached, kill sperm at 5/8 or lower concentration in the alkaline and acid test, and diffuse rapidly out of the vehicle into the semen (W. H. Robertson 1989, 84–85). These remain the key requirements for this common and simple contraceptive today.

By the late 1930s, this work had produced a popular and very effective spermicide called Volpar for *vol*untary *par*enthood (Borell 1987). Baker, however, was forced to leave the zoology department at Oxford when the director discovered the purpose of his experiments. He was allowed to relocate in the pathology department. His contraceptive research was thus "rather prejudicial to his career" (Porter and Hall 1995, 176). It was "permanently symbolized in his recollection of assembling his apparatus and reagents on a handcart and trundling this from department to department," although he did remain in academic chemistry (Reed 1984, 243).

To "complete the work done by Voge and Baker" and focus on spermicides available in the United States, Dr. Clarence Gamble of the NCMH then funded a research fellowship in chemistry at New York University in 1934 to work on the "Standards Program" for testing contraceptive product effectiveness, including the establishment of state and federal product regulations. Led by Leo Shedlovsky, the research focused on measuring the physical and chemical properties of the more than forty contraceptives then on the market (mostly spermicides). This was the first laboratory study of contraceptives in the United States. Reprints of Shedlovsky's work were sent to 1,500 teaching physicians throughout the United States as part of the NCMH effort to get the AMA Council on Pharmacy and Chemistry to issue reports on contraceptives as they already did on other drugs; the effort succeeded, and a major report was published in 1943 (Reed 1984, 243–46).

The surgeries of sterilization for males and females were technically developed in the late nineteenth century (thanks to anaesthesia and asepsis), largely for medical purposes rather than as means of contraception.[24] However, when such surgeries were utilized with prisoners and those institutionalized as "feeble-minded" or "insane," their contraceptive side effects were commonly valued for this eugenic effect.[25] After World War II, surgical sterilization was (re)produced as a permanent contraceptive. The major medical birth control advocate of his generation, gynecologist Robert Latou Dickinson, promoted it in *Human Sterilization: Techniques of Permanent Conception Control* (Dickinson and Gamble 1950).

Before 1960, it was available on a very limited basis (Langley 1973). Subsequently, for white women, the 120-rule was used informally by American physicians to determine eligibility: a woman's age times the number of live children she had must exceed 120 (Clarke 1984). No such rule obtained for women of color, and coercive sterilization practices were and likely remain widespread. Today, "sterilization is the most used contraceptive in virtually all the world's regions, including the United States" (Harrison and Rosenfield 1996, 7). About 39 percent of contraceptors in the United States use sterilization as their method (Piccicino and Mosher 1998, 5); globally, it is about 22 percent (Biegelmann-Massari and Bateman 1998).

The career trajectories of reproductive scientists who undertook research on simple contraceptives vividly demonstrated that there was an applied/basic boundary that could not be crossed without negative consequences. Physicians were seemingly not subjected to the same standards.

THIRD-GENERATION MAVERICKS: PRODUCING THE FIRST "MODERN SCIENTIFIC CONTRACEPTIVES," 1950–1977

Third-generation maverick reproductive scientists produced the Pill, IUDs, and a different kind of maverick product—a proposal for transdisciplinary approaches to reproduction.

The Pill: Pincus, Chang, Marker, and Djerassi

In the United States, no explicitly contraceptive research was undertaken other than the spermicide studies until after 1950, although many reproductive scientists did note how the outcomes of their work pointed to ways in which the female cycle could be interrupted.[26] They were not at all interested in barrier methods, dismissed as "messy makeshifts" (Reed 1984, 243), but instead dreamed of "truly scientific" means of contraception, mostly endocrinological. Medical efforts to take over the feminist birth control movement had succeeded by 1950 (McCann 1994), and as birth control became more legitimate and "scientific," both suited to medical *science* and increasingly under its professional control, hostility within the medical profession ebbed. Significantly, it was not until the 1950s that American reproductive scientists pursued explicit research on "scientific" means of contraception, and even then these third-generation mavericks did so outside the hallowed walls of academe.

When Gregory Pincus began explicit work on the Pill, he was already "a refugee from academic biology" (Reed 1984, 316), denied tenure at Harvard during the era when "proper" biology departments were getting out of the reproductive science business—and actively expressing anti-Semitism.[27] After leaving Harvard and setting up the Worcester Foundation, Pincus and his colleague M. C. Chang received $14,500 from the Planned Parenthood Federation of America (PPFA, the nonfeminist successor organization to the American Birth Control League) in 1948 and 1949 for work on the mammalian egg. In 1951, he conferred with Sanger regarding hormonal contraception, successfully reapplied to the PPFA, and received $3,100 in 1951 and $3,400 in 1952. Pincus then sent in a most promising report of this research, which was ignored by the man then directing Planned Parenthood, William Vogt, who wanted organizational expansion to be focused on his administrative functions rather than on animal testing of new contraceptives. When she saw the report, Sanger, in one of the preemptive moves for which she was famous (McCann 1994), simply bypassed Vogt. She got Katherine McCormick, heir to the International Harvester fortune and longtime suffragist and birth control advocate, to accompany her on the now-famous visit to Pincus and Chang at the Worcester Foundation in 1953. Sanger had discussed with McCormick how she could contribute to research into "a fool-proof contraceptive" (Watkins 1998, 26). At the end of their conversation with Pincus, McCormick promised him $10,000/year on the spot; this expanded to $150,000 per year and more during her life (totaling about $2 million), and she left the Foundation $1 million in her will (Reed 1984, 340; Chesler 1992, 432). Sanger and McCormick were both in their seventies at the time.

Developments in steroid chemistry were key to the Pill. Russell Marker's and Carl Djerassi's chemical efforts were based at different times in Syntex, an industrial pharmaceutical company. Marker had analyzed plant steroids for the first time, and he realized that hormones could be synthetically produced using a Mexican yam. Unable to locate support, he then left academia (Pennsylvania State University) in frustration and went to Mexico to pursue the yam, joining with others in Syntex to produce estrogen. Djerassi joined Syntex after Marker left, and with colleagues he produced an orally active estrogen, which he then sent to Pincus and others for testing. Both Searle (with whom Pincus was already working) and Syntex eventually produced birth control pills.[28]

Not all reproductive scientists were thrilled with the Pill, and the clinical trials were problematic.[29] Carl Hartman, then chairman of the medical committee of Planned Parenthood, expressed reservations about the Pill's systemic properties and predicted that it would take fifteen to twenty years before its safety could be assessed. This was about the same period estimated by women's health activists (Seaman 1969; Boston Women's Health Book Collective 1971; Seaman and Seaman 1977).[30] But Sanger and McCormick were "so confident . . . of the Pill's revolutionary consequences that they seemed positively immune to any objections to it whatsoever, and interpreted reasonable concerns about the liabilities of experimenting with so potent a drug as just one more round in the arsenal of opposition that birth control advocates had confronted for years" (Chesler 1992, 434, 445). Sanger was, after all, a licensed nurse and ardent believer in scientific medicine, and McCormick held the first Ph.D. in biology from MIT granted to a woman. Then as now feminists have held multiple positions about the Pill as a contraceptive.

Maverick scientists Pincus, Chang, and Marker all left academia to pursue their work on their own terms in industrial or semi-industrial venues. They may have laughed all the way to the bank, but academic reproductive scientists were still refusing to do explicitly contraceptive research. These three had, in fact, gone beyond the scholarly pale of their era—and become more or less commercial.[31] By 1970, 9 million American women were using the Pill. Currently about 10.5 million do so in the United States, and 60 million women do so globally.[32] Pill users are configured as active participants in contraception, as a Pill must be taken daily.

The IUD: Tietze, Lippes, and Margulis

Intrauterine devices (IUDs) are objects made of various substances (silk coils, rubber, metal, and after c. 1958 plastic) that are placed in the uterus through the cervix. It is surmised that they prevent conception by creating a hostile uterine environment, one too irritated or inflamed for implantation to occur (Mishell 1998). Physicians have traditionally inserted them (Langley 1973, 336–37). IUDs are obviously directed at women as implicated users.

By the late nineteenth century, IUDs were in use for contraceptive purposes and were patented devices. Dr. Robert L. Dickinson, leader of the National Committee on Maternal Health, began promoting such devices in the United States in 1916 (Southam 1965, 3). IUDs were also discussed at the Fifth International Conference on Birth Control in 1922 (Pierpoint 1922, 275–77). The first modern developer was Ernest Gräfenberg, a German gynecologist, who began experimenting with various types in 1909 and began publishing on IUDs in 1928 (Langley 1973, 336).[33] Gräfenberg reported great success with the method in 1930 at the Seventh International Birth Control Congress, and considerable experimentation followed with what were then called "Gräfenberg rings" (Reed 1984, 275).

But IUDs also generated considerable debate *within* the medical community. In the 1930s and after, many physicians vehemently opposed their use largely on grounds of risk of infection.[34] It was even difficult to publish on this method in the United States where physician hostility to it was strongest.[35] "No physician who himself had used IUCDs published a report in any medical journal of the Western countries between 1934 and 1959" (Tietze 1965b, 1148). As with surgical sterilization, the increasing availability of antibiotics after World War II helped to overcome these fears as well as to overcome infection (Bullough 1994, 186).

In 1952, the Population Council was established and funded by John D. Rockefeller III as a free-standing research institute when, during the McCarthy era attack on the Rockefeller Foundation, he could not convince the Foundation's board to support population control research. The Population Council later provided grants covering about 95 percent of development costs of a new IUD (Notestein 1982, 678). Drawing on work done in Israel and Japan (Tietze 1965b) between 1958 and 1960, Dr. Lazar Margulies of the obstetrics department of Mt. Sinai Hospital in New York and Dr. Jack Lippes of the University of Buffalo pioneered a plastic product as a new modern means of "scientific" contraception. Christopher Tietze of the Population Council candidly stated: "It was a very exciting period . . . we were working with something that had been *absolutely rejected by the [American medical] profession. . . .* There was such a feeling of urgency among professional people, not among the masses, but something had to be done. And this was *something that you could do to the people* rather than *something people could do for themselves.* So it made it very attractive to the doers" (Reed 1984, 307, emphasis added). This approach, seeking means of contraception "you could do to the people," which I have termed "imposables," has guided much if not most subsequent research within the population control framework.

Dugdale (2000) beautifully points out how the reinvented plastic IUD reconfigured IUD users from Grafenberg's earlier focus on white upper-class women, especially in Germany, to women of color in what was known as the Third World. These reconfigured users of the IUD are women who do not want to or supposedly cannot actively contracept successfully.[36] Meldrum (1996, 294–95) notes: "The women who participated in the trials . . . are anonymous to us . . . but their story speaks to us nevertheless. They refused to be randomized, insisted on making choices, insisted on changing those choices when it suited them, stubbornly refused to adhere to statistical models or to give up all control of their contraceptive practice." Women's resistance efforts were clear from the outset. Meldrum chronicles how innovative statistical techniques needed to be constructed that could erase such resistance, not only to the IUD but to any method.

As predicted by physicians in the 1930s, downstream problems did manifest for all IUDs, especially infection and "traveling." Seemingly all IUDs are capable of causing infections that can lead to infertility. One device, the Dalkon Shield, was a major disaster associated with an estimated seventeen deaths and extensive morbidity, including permanent infertility.[37] Only a couple of IUDs are currently marketed in the United States due to steep product liability largely due to the Dalkon Shield case (Mastroianni et al. 1990). About 12 percent of the world's contraceptors now use IUDs (Biegelmann-Massari and Bateman 1998). In the United States, it was less than 1 percent in 1995 (Piccinino and Mosher 1998, 5).

A Maverick Transdisciplinary Proposal: Shelesnyak

I have argued with others (e.g., Bijker 1994; Bijker et al. 1987; Bijker and Law 1992) that technologies can and should conceptually be viewed as including all related elements of the "delivery systems" that bring them to users and users themselves, elements from which they are practically—in practice—inextricable. Amid all the efforts to develop new scientific contraceptives, only one proposal by a reproductive scientist addressed this. M. C. Shelesnyak suggested taking a transdisciplinary "biodynamics" approach to reproduction including contraception. In a paper entitled "Biodynamics and the Population Explosion," Shelesnyak (1966, 21–22, 23–24) argued that it was

> important at the outset to dispel any oversimplification that the matter can
> be reduced to a race between the swelling number of the world's inhabitants
> and adequate expansion of food supplies and space. . . . [T]o appreciate the
> extent of related factors, reproduction must be viewed beyond the limits of
> the biology of reproduction: it must be viewed from a broad ecological
> stance, since the assessment of reproductive capacity entails more than the
> physiological parameters. It must include demographic, social, cultural, eco-
> nomic and anthropological aspects.

Further, Shelesnyak's proposal for the "fullest achievement of fertility regulation" from birth control to infertility treatment was based on his assumption of heterogeneity: "It can be accepted as fact that there will not be a single universally accepted method" of fertility control (32–33). He called for local (national) leadership, the development of inter- and multidisciplinary approaches, and distinctive transdisciplinary centers for the study of reproduction. His writings certainly reflected the fact that he was a biologist, but he saw vividly that reproduction is also a social, cultural, and economic phenomenon.[38]

In sum, most of the third generation of American reproductive scientists who focused on contraceptive development worked outside the academy, and the transdisciplinary proposal came from the margins. But in the development of the Pill and new IUDs, we can also see the elaboration of method-based and institutional competition among contraceptive researchers, pitting the Pill against the IUD, the Worcester Institute against the Population Council (Onorato 1991), in a pattern of "product championship" that continues today.[39] The concept of "advocate researchers" clearly applies (Gallagher 1992).

PRODUCTION INTERLUDE: A CHANGING CONTRACEPTIVE R&D SCENE

It was not until well into the 1960s that "population" funding from foundations and the federal government filtered into academia on a scale massive enough to involve basic reproductive scientists in research related, both directly and indirectly, to contraception (Greep et al. 1976, 1977). Such research was almost exclusively undertaken in medical settings and pharmaceutical companies. Finally, half a century after Margaret Sanger was first jailed for distributing birth control information, it was legitimate to do academic scientific research in the field.

In the 1970s, major changes took place in the organization of contraceptive research and development involving new forms and locations. The "great men" era of contraceptive development had ended (insofar as it ever really existed) and, as elsewhere in science, broader teams of researchers were routinely involved. Further, these teams were then and continue to be based not only in academia, pharmaceutical companies, and biomedical research institutes but also in population control organizations and in international public organizations such as the World Health Organization of the United Nations (Oudshoorn 1997a, 1997b).

This shift came in partial response to the reduction of pharmaceutical company interest in such R&D because of their extensive regulation and liability for health problems with the Pill and IUD (Oudshoorn 1997b, 45). But it is also due to the reduction in profits from contraception, since the major "purchasers"/"users" are often governmental or international organizational units buying large amounts at discount for free or cheap distribution (Charo 1991). In the United States only one pharmaceutical company, Ortho, continues major contraceptive R&D, while European companies now do more, including Organon, Schering AG, and Roussel-Uclaf (Oudshoorn 1994, 1997a, 1997b; Mastroianni et al. 1990). A movement for federal sponsorship of private pharmaceutical contraceptive research and development has been growing.[40]

Last, this shift included very early articulations on the part of producers of the need for more than one "perfect" contraceptive. From the 1950s to the 1970s, the policy had been what Oudshoorn (1996a) wonderfully calls "one-size-fits-all," capturing the dream of a universal contraceptive for the universal woman. However, in 1976, Roy Greep and his colleagues published in a major survey of the field: "The heterogeneity of personal, cultural, religious, and economic circumstances of human life, as well as the varying need of individuals at different stages in the life cycle, impose diverse demands upon the technology" (4). This marks the beginning of the end of modernity in contraceptive R&D; in postmodernity lies increasing acknowledgment of difference (Clarke 1995).

FOURTH GENERATION: PRODUCING MORE MODERN SCIENTIFIC CONTRACEPTIVES, 1977–1990

Contraceptive research had finally been made truly scientific. At the core of earlier objections lay the culture of scientific medicine revealed in physicians' dislike of available simple methods of contraception. A medical journal editor had declared in 1943, "Caustic self-analysis leads to only one honest conclusion: candid physicians are ashamed of these messy makeshifts . . . these disreputable paraphernalia. . . . The messy little gadgets . . . [were simply] an embarrassment to the scientific mind" (Reed 1978, 132). Endocrinology was not.

Endocrinology as Paradigm

I have argued elsewhere (Clarke 1998) that it was the newly "discovered" and named reproductive "hormones" which seduced American academic scientists into the study of reproductive phenomena in the late teens and early twenties. Reproductive scientists then linked reproductive endocrinology with general endocrinology, riding the coattails of the biochemical bandwagon in the life sciences through the 1920s, 1930s, and 1940s (coattails resembling those of genetics today). Neena B. Schwartz's presidential address to the Endocrine Society at its sixty-fifth annual meeting in 1983 captured the spirit of the century in the American reproductive sciences with her title "Endocrinology as Paradigm, Endocrinology as Authority." Moreover, when Schwartz asserted "endocrinology as paradigm," she meant it in the full Kuhnian sense of achieving status as the reigning paradigm that characterized the normal science of the era. It still does. Thus, the fourth generation of reproductive scientists and contraceptive researchers are not really mavericks. They operate within a well-established scientific paradigm in pursuit of technological elaborations rather than moving in wholly new directions.

More Endocrinological Contraceptives

It was easy to anticipate that the Pill was, therefore, only the first in a long series of hormonally based contraceptives. The next generation products, however, are not controlled by users but by providers—imposables. Depo-Provera, a long-acting injectable, was developed in the 1960s by researchers in the American pharmaceutical company Upjohn and tested predominantly in what was then called the Third World. Like earlier contraceptives, Depo-Provera was challenged using various safety criteria. Feminist women's health groups fought against U.S. Food and Drug Administration (USFDA) approval of Depo-Provera as a contraceptive for many years, as many other countries rely on the USFDA for their own drug regulation policy. It was first proposed to the FDA in the early 1980s but not approved until the early 1990s (Rakusen 1981; NWHN 1985; Moskowitz and Jennings 1996). An array of injectables are available today, many developed by the WHO, which now patents its products and licenses pharmaceutical companies to distribute them (Oudshoorn 1997a, 1997b). In the United States in 1995, only 3 percent of contraceptors used injectables (Piccinino and Mosher 1998, 5); globally it appears to be under 2 percent (Biegelmann-Massari and Bateman 1998).

Recently, even greater controversy has surrounded implants (notably Norplant) and so-called vaccines. Norplant consists of a set of six silastic rods containing the progestin hormone levonorgestrel, effective for about five years. It was developed, like plastic IUDs, by scientists at the Population Council and produced since 1983. About half a million women had used it by 1990 by having the rods implanted in their upper arms via outpatient surgery. In poorer countries, risks center around anemia and liver problems, plus coercion (also found in the West). Difficulties of removal are common (usually due to extensive scar tissue buildup at implant sites). Testing protocols were also controversial in terms of adequately informed consent.[41] In the United States in 1995, only 1.3 percent of contraceptors used implants (Piccinino and Mosher 1998, 5); globally it appears to be under 2 percent (Biegelmann-Massari and Bateman 1998).

Within months of Norplant's approval by the USFDA, proposals were made for punitive applications for women accused of crimes and for women to obtain welfare, highlighting its parallel potential for abuse with surgical sterilization (e.g., Pies 1997; Moskowitz and Jennings 1996; Kuo 1998). A 1996 article entitled "Implant for Birth Control 'Killed Off'" reported that in Britain, prescriptions for Norplant had "dwindled from up to 5,000 per month to fewer than 20, as allegations of side-effects and threats of legal action against the drug company have grown" (Hunt 1996). Provider refusal to remove Norplant during clinical trials in Egypt despite repeated requests was documented (Morsy 1995). Implicated actors responded individually as pragmatic women demonstrating selective resistance and compliance (Lock and Kaufert 1998; Kuiper et al. 1997) and collectively as activists.

Vaccination against pregnancy has long been both a fantasy and a focus of contraceptive research in the United States. Reproductive scientists viewed immunology as a logical and exciting research path and sought means of immunizing women against pregnancy starting in the 1930s. The means of effecting immunity at that time was subcutaneous injection of the female with a serum or "spermatoxin" derived from fresh sperm of the same or different species. Mention was made of the possibilities of contraceptive autoimmunity in the male, but as in the lay and medical birth control movements, focus was much more on female means of contraception at that time (Sanger and Stone 1931, 112–13). Two aspects of spermatoxin contraception became especially attractive during the Great Depression—its simplicity and its cost: "Think of how wonderful it would be if one could immunize a patient by simple hypodermic injection once every six months, just as we today immunize children against diphtheria. It will indeed be a new and wonderful era in the practice of preventive gynecology" (Daniels in Sanger and Stone 1931, 111). The appeal of injectable hormonal means is clear here as well.[42]

Since c. 1967, there has been a renaissance of interest in what is now called "immunoreproduction," with considerable focus on finding male as well as female means. Several new so-called vaccines focused on intervening in the action of sperm, eggs, and (especially) hormonal action are coming into use at this juncture.[43] However, national and transnational women's health groups have raised serious questions in terms of both the safety and efficacy of immunocontraception.[44] Their concerns begin with the discursive use of the term *vaccine,* which resituates use of such means of family planning away from their usual and accepted place in maternal and child health/family planning services and places them instead in a "preventive health" framework along with diphtheria shots and other public health measures. This is a radically different transnational technoscientific infrastructure, one with little or no experience of women's health, further endangering women users. Specific concerns center on inadvertent autoimmune diseases, the consequences of contraceptive-caused immunorepression or immune system compromise because of the AIDS epidemic and, for many women who are already malnourished, because of unwanted permanent sterile response, risks for unknown or subsequent pregnancy, and complete lack of protection against STDs and AIDS. Both implants and "vaccines" require more elaborate health systems than are available in much of the world. Van Kammen (1999, and this volume) illuminates additional important user issues.

Other lines of current immunological contraceptive research continue to seek what Max Mason of the Rockefeller Foundation called "antihormones" during the 1930s, "vaccines" to block hormones needed for very early pregnancy and a "vaccine" to block the hormone needed for the surface of the egg to function properly (Mastroianni 1990, 33; Alexander 1995). Some women's health groups have called for research on such "vaccines" to be stopped completely, especially because of the increased risks of AIDS and other STDs.[45] All of the above are long-acting hormonal means of contraception. All of these methods raise major ethical and moral policy challenges because of their potential and actual—already demonstrated—coercive use (e.g., Moskowitz and Jennings 1996; Morsy 1995).

Last is a molecular endocrinological development, RU486, known first as "the French abortion pill" but also as a "morning after" pill—a very early pill preventing implantation. The name RU486 comes from its original maker, Roussel-Uclaf Paris, a pharmaceutical subsidiary of the large German company Hoechst. Longtime Roussel-Uclaf consultant Etienne-Emile Baulieu, a French endocrinologist and head of his own state-supported (INSERM) laboratory, promoted the work that led to RU486. In the late 1960s, Baulieu was urged by Gregory Pincus and the Ford Foundation to "participate in the worldwide efforts to improve birth control methods." He then began to search for the sites of steroid receptors because "[w]here Pincus had worked in physiology, we could now do molecular endocrinology" (Baulieu 1991, 67). In 1962 Baulieu was invited to head research for Roussel-Uclaf, but he chose instead to consult for them. In c. 1980, Philibert and others at Uclaf working with Baulieu constructed RU486, a drug that would act as a nonsurgical abortifacient. Baulieu and others have worked diligently for research on and dissemination of this first new abortion technology since the late 1960s, when vacuum aspiration and suction methods were developed as abortion legalization gained momentum (Ruzek 1978). Today this drug is also being studied as a possible contraceptive (Baulieu 1997).

Many reproductive scientists have historically chosen to exit or been pushed out of the laboratory/closet into the public limelight of contention around reproductive phenomena. Gregory Pincus became known as a "product champion" for the ways in which he relentlessly promoted the Pill internationally (Reed 1984, 346). His protégé Baulieu, in choosing to pursue endocrine receptor research over twenty-five years ago, also intentionally constructed a career path that combined work in his laboratory with active reproductive product championship—most recently of RU486.[46] Baulieu's construction of RU486 and related drugs is that they should be viewed as "contragestives" instead of "abortifacients." Arguing that since many methods of fertility control are not strictly "contraceptive" in that conception may well occur (e.g., the Pill and IUD), Baulieu notes:

> Indeed, postfertilization interruption is an everyday process that most women have experienced at some time, even though they may not be aware of it. Therefore I propose a new word: "contragestion" (a contraction of contra-gestation), stressing the quite natural aspects of fertility and the control thereof. . . . [T]he drug itself may give women greater ability to exercise responsibility in matters of fertility control. We must offer people the best that science can provide so that there may be more flexibility and personal initiative in the control of familial and social problems. (1989, 1356)

For Baulieu (1991, 19), RU486 is "the second generation pill."

■

Much of the research and contraceptive product development done by this fourth generation of reproductive scientists was, for the first time, considered relatively legitimate. Some of it was even undertaken in the academy or in state-sponsored scientific labs such as INSERM. It was "scientific" enough to satisfy the (perhaps changing) standards for proper scientific research.

RESISTANCE INTERLUDE: CONSEQUENCES OF WOMEN'S HEALTH ACTIVISM, 1969–2000+

> There is not, on the one side, a discourse of power, and opposite it, another discourse that runs counter to it. Discourses are tactical elements or blocks operating in the field of force relations; there can exist different and even contradictory discourses within the same strategy.
> —*Michel Foucault*

Explicitly feminist voices were widely influential at the beginning of the twentieth century in placing birth control in the public forum and in forming the lay and medical birth control movements. Yet these voices were co-opted and silenced in the shift from birth control to family planning and population control by the end of the Depression (McCann 1994, chaps. 5 and 6). The negotiated quid pro quo discussed at the outset left feminist birth control advocates out of the contraceptive R&D loop once Sanger and her allies were displaced. The Pill was that generation of feminists' last contribution. The next generation of feminists appeared by the late 1960s, responding not only to the problematics of contraception per se but much more broadly to the treatment of women by biomedicine.[47]

In formulating their contraceptive advocacy strategies (Berkman 1980), many feminists tacitly or explicitly have drawn on the "three contraceptive axioms" stated by Dr. Mary Calderone (1964, 153) when she was still medical director of Planned Parenthood–World Population:[48]

1. *Any* method of birth control is more effective than no method.
2. The most effective method is the one the couple will use with the greatest consistency.
3. Acceptability is the most critical factor in the effectiveness of a contraceptive method.

Focus was and remains deeply on users' assessments, and users are assumed to be intelligent, capable, and rational—i.e., fully human. User studies began under Sanger (e.g., Kopp 1933; Meldrum 1996), seeking to understand what women wanted and thought about extant methods. In sharp contrast, within population control frames, compliance with providers' dictums rather than meeting women's needs and desires was and remains the research focus (e.g., Tietze 1962, 1965a, 1965b; Meldrum 1996). The first feminist user study of "modern scientific contraception" was Barbara Seaman's (1969/1980) inflammatory *Doctor's Case against the Pill,* based on public testimony of users. This volume, along with *Our Bodies, Ourselves,* contributed to the coalescence of the feminist women's health movements nationally and internationally and their ongoing skepticism regarding "modern scientific contraception."[49]

An ambitious national and transnational infrastructure of women's health groups has emerged, largely of nongovernmental organizations committed to improving the situations of women vis-à-vis contraception and reproductive health broadly conceived.[50] Part of their task is technology assessment and organizing resistance as appropriate. To date, about three generations of women and men have protested against everything from the means of testing the birth control pill on Third World women of color to the Pill itself, to IUDs, to Depo-Provera and other injectables, to Norplant and other implants, and most recently to contraceptive vaccines. Problems have included safety, irreversibility, fetal damage, undesirable to life-threatening side effects (from headaches to acne, obesity, infertility, and death), and lack of protection from STDs and HIV.[51] Equally significant with such organized movements of resistance is the fact that globally women have pragmatically voted with their feet (Lock and Kaufert 1998), resisting and rejecting means of contraception that do not meet their needs, even at great personal cost. One major study found that women respondents from seven countries "aspire to control their own fertility, child-bearing and contraceptive use, although social, institutional and legal barriers may prevent them from succeeding. Often this sense of entitlement is acted upon in conscious transgression of community and religious norms and—prompted by fear of violence or harsh reprisals—in secrecy from parents, husbands, partners and authorities" (Petchesky and Judd 1998, 300). Feminist interventions also contributed to the shift from the modernist, standard-ized "one-size-fits-all" approach to a more postmodern individualized, niche-oriented "cafeteria approach" offering an array of means of contraception ide-ally suited to the highly varied health care and living situations of prospective users—men as well as women—including changing reproductive needs and goals across the life course. However, the modernistic "one-size-fits-all" pattern remains dominant in many southern countries while the postmodern "cafe-teria" is largely available in northern nations.[52] Specifically, while recognizing that no one method can serve all and that method selection always involves risks and trade-offs, women's groups have been calling for several changes. First, they have sought improved woman-controlled barrier means of contraception since 1915 and ever more loudly since 1980. For example, the International Women's Health Conference for Cairo stated the following in their mission (Organizing Committee 1994, 6):

> Item 12. In the area of contraceptive technology, resources should be redi-rected from provider-controlled and potentially high-risk methods, like the vaccine, to barrier methods. A significant proportion of the participants also felt strongly that Norplant or other long-term hormonal contraceptives should be explicitly mentioned as high-risk methods from which resources should be redirected. Female controlled methods that provide both contracep-tion and protection from sexually transmitted diseases, including HIV, as well as male methods, should receive highest priority in contraceptive research and development. Women's organizations are entitled to indepen-dently monitor contraceptive trials and ensure women's free, informed consent to enter the trial. Trial results must be available for women's organiza-tions at the different stages of such trials, including the very early stages.

Second, it also seems to many feminists as though it is no accident that there are no hormonal or implantable methods for men (Lissner 1992; Ouds-hoorn 1997a, 1997b, 1999). Given that thirty-five years have passed since the start of the "Contraceptive Revolution," many believe the nearly exclusive focus on women reflects sustained intentionality that women should bear the brunt of contraception as well as that of pregnancy, birth, and childcare. Certainly the many agencies sponsoring contraceptive research during these decades have not strongly promoted development of male methods (Oudshoorn 1997a, 1997b, 1999, 2000, in prep.; Ringheim 1996; World Health Organization 1996).

Third are the larger issues of user and user group involvement in contraceptive research and development—the "democratization" of R&D per se—and participation in national and transnational reproductive health policy arenas. Finally, in the 1990s, some combination of individual women's resistance and the activism of feminist and other women's health organizations is becoming consequential. Over the past decade or so, a rethinking of approaches to contraception has begun among reproductive scientists, philanthropists, and the many organizations involved (e.g., Alexander 1995; Heise and Elias 1995; Harrison and Rosenfield 1996). This shift was also triggered by the AIDS epidemic and the epidemic proportions of sexually transmitted diseases and related maternal mortality and morbidity. Finally, many feminist groups are participating in some venues where family planning and population concerns are translated into health care policy and foreign policy.[53]

Specifically, in the words of a National Academy of Science volume:

[A] construct referred to as a "woman-centered agenda" has evolved, its source an expanding dialogue within a number of national and international women's groups, and between some of those groups and scientists working in reproductive and contraceptive research. The agenda reflects a more expansive view of contraception that attempts to integrate concerns for contraceptive efficacy into concerns for the overall reproductive health and general well-being of the primary users of contraceptives, that is, women. The notion of a woman-centered agenda for contraceptive research and development does not imply that there is some "universal woman" or some necessary, unitary view of women's preferences, it is simply that the field should refocus itself toward approaches in areas where the needs of women are still unmet by existing methods.[54]

This shift is also deeply predicated on scientists' and policymakers' dawning recognition of the actions of millions of pragmatic women (Lock and Kaufert 1998) who have ceased or refused to use undesirable methods. The same report stated, "There is also growing and powerful evidence that *users can drive the demographics:* It has been suggested that family planning programs that truly enable individuals to achieve their reproductive objectives actually have more impact on reducing fertility than do programs driven solely by demographic goals" (Harrison and Rosenfield 1996, 5–6, emphasis added).

Yet despite more than twenty-five years of such efforts, some feminist women's health activists in interaction with reproductive scientists do not feel they have been heard or understood. A recent paper was entitled "Are We Speaking the Same Language? Women's Health Advocates and Scientists Talk About Contraceptive Technology" (Germain 1993). In these spheres of activity, controversy is quite unlikely to abate.[55]

FIFTH-GENERATION MAVERICKS ON THE VAGINAL AND MALE FRONTIERS, 1990–2000+

Two new-in-practice frontiers of contraceptive research and action that contemporary maverick scientists have pursued are nonhormonal vaginal approaches and male approaches. Moves toward nonhormonal female contraception recently got a huge boost from the finding that in monkeys, use of progesterone as a contraceptive "dramatically increases their risks of getting AIDS, opening the possibility that women given a related synthetic hormone, progestin, for birth control, could face the same increased risk" (Garrett 1996, 3). This connection between contraceptive hormone-induced thinning of the vaginal wall and easier transmission of AIDS was made in 1994 by Dr. Nancy Alexander, now chief of the contraceptive development branch of the National Institute of Child Health and Human Development.[56] The fact that having other STDs seems to make women more vulnerable to AIDS has also triggered reevaluation of other means of "modern scientific contraception" such as IUDs, which make women more vulnerable to PID; the prolonged and/or irregular bleeding common with the use of Norplant and Depo-Provera may also make women more vulnerable to STDs and HIV (Stratton and Alexander 1993). Only barrier methods clearly do not make matters worse and directly address such problems; moreover, spermicides may actually reduce vulnerability to transmission of HIV and other STDs.[57]

Thus some members of the current generation of reproductive scientists have turned maverick and begun moving in on the vagina as the "new contraceptive frontier," almost a century after Sanger and colleagues first called for such work. Endocrinology as paradigm still reigns, however, and challenges to it (that are not molecular, of course) are still looked at askance or even squashed—even despite AIDS. Not surprisingly, many mavericks challenging the endocrinological paradigm are younger, marginal, women and/or they do not challenge it categorically but instead call for *additional* new approaches to contraception to supplement the "contraceptive cafeteria." In this section I can merely note the wide array of such new approaches.

"Natural" Birth Control: Technoscientific Rhythm

The rhythm method has endured as a disparaged contraceptive option across the twentieth century. Carl Hartman (1936, 1962, vii) twice devoted an entire monograph, intentionally written for a more popular rather than scientific audience, "to evaluating the various methods that are recommended for determining the approximate duration of the fertile period."[58] In the late 1960s and 1970s, refinements of a basal temperature method and a cervical mucus assessment method were developed. DeNora (1996, 369) has noted, "[T]he physicality of mucus is . . . culturally subversive, at least to the extent that it lends itself to alternative configurations of the human body." Users of the mucus method were portrayed by method developers (Billings et al. 1972, 1980) as active—even agentic—"normal" women fully capable of assessing their own symptoms. At the end of the twentieth century, a host of new technologies that assist in assessing the time of fertility are hitting the consumer market, most of them over-the-counter technologies. Desires for contraception are driving these devices much less than desires for conception, the flip side of applied rhythm. Hormonal assays, special thermometers, mucus assays, urinary dipsticks, electroconductivity, and ultrasound approaches are all developed or in research. DeNora (1996, 370) characterizes these as "the body in the dipstick or the clinic in the home" as such conventional "medical modes" reconventionalize the female body as passive and in need of technoscientific assistance. Such products do, of course, become part of the contraceptive cafeteria requisite to meet women's heterogeneous needs.

The Female Condom and New Cervical Caps

Most reproductive scientists positioned themselves at some distance from condoms across the twentieth century. Nor did these "messy little gadgets" seduce physicians very much as contraceptives, although they were (barely) acceptable for disease control. Today, there is a major shift in the United States to condom use (Piccinino and Mosher 1998). "Only the condom provides protection against both conception and STD transmission," including HIV (Harrison and Rosenfield 1996, 8). For most of the twentieth century, condoms have been solely a male prerogative. In 1992, this situation changed when a new female condom was approved by the USFDA. The Reality or Femidom Vaginal Pouch is designed to protect against *both* pregnancy and disease. It is sold without prescription in ten countries; like other barrier methods, when used consistently and properly, it is quite effective, but much less so when not so used (Trussell 1998).

Variations on the cervical cap have existed for centuries. A rubber cap was developed in the mid-nineteenth century and was varyingly available through-out the twentieth century. American feminists seeking alternative simple meth-ods sought USFDA approval for contraceptive use for three types of caps reintroduced into the United States in the late 1970s, produced in London by Lamberts (Dalston) Ltd. The process was arduous and successful for only one type of cap, the Prentif Rim. The account of the process highlights some of the struggles that feminist health providers have experienced with the FDA (Gallagher 1992). A related product somewhere between a cervical cap and a diaphragm is the Lea's Shield, a one-size-fits-all barrier method. It is shaped like a bowl, made of silicon, and has a one-way valve so that cervical fluids can flow out but sperm cannot enter, allowing it to be worn for longer periods. It was still under review by the USFDA in 1998 (Bell et al. 1998, 289).

New and Better Prophylactic Spermicides/Microbicides

Part of the strategy to reduce transmission of AIDS/STDs is to produce new and better prophylactic spermicides/microbicides—chemical barrier methods against *both* conception and disease. "To prevent infection by the AIDS-causing human immunodeficiency virus or other microbes, a chemical barrier would, at minimum, have to coat the entire vaginal wall and cervix, be nonirri-tating and be nontoxic to beneficial microbes in the vagina. These features alone might be enough to reduce infection significantly, but agents intended to kill harmful microorganisms actively could be added as well" (Alexander 1995, 139–40). Existing spermicides have never been evaluated in these terms. Recently their effectiveness against chlamydia has been demonstrated (Alexan-der 1995, 140), and other tests are under way. An International Working Group on Vaginal Microbicides (1996) was formed and made recommendations for development before it dissolved (Bell 1999).[59] Remembering both the contra-ceptive advocacy of early twentieth-century feminists and the research of both Voges and Baker on spermicides, it is not unreasonable to speculate that *had this path been followed* at the time, countless agonies could have been avoided and HIV/AIDS might have been an epidemiological blip rather than a global disaster of as yet unfathomable magnitude. It is precisely here that the dangers of the contraceptive culture of science become highly visible.

Microbicides without Spermicide

Some women are also very interested in a microbicide that will prevent disease transmission but without spermicidal effects. That is, they want healthy sperm to be able to survive bathing in the microbicide in order to be able to fertilize them. In (too) many sociocultural contexts, having children is requisite for women's lives to be reasonable, regardless of their partner's disease status. Such products would protect vulnerable women from disease while permitting them to fulfill cultural expectations of motherhood. These are politically fascinating products as they are not contraceptives but they are very woman-identified (Petchesky and Judd 1998).

Male Methods-in-Progress

Oudshoorn (1995, 1996a, 1997a, 1997b, 1999, 2000, in prep.) has argued that simply working on contraception for men has been a marginalized activity in the already marginalized reproductive sciences and contraceptive development worlds. A reproductive scientist I interviewed actually reported that advocates of male contraception were intentionally punished by the power brokers in those worlds through lack of support and derogation in the 1970s and 1980s. One result of this double marginalization has certainly been the very slow development of modern scientific means of contraception for men. Almost a half century since the women's Pill was tested, no male Pill is yet on the market. Led by work at the World Health Organization (note *not* in pharmaceutical companies), male pills, injectables, and implantables paralleling women's hormonal methods are now in trials around the globe.[60] Research on male means has not been driven by a "demand from women for equity but by the perseverance of a small biomedical research community supported primarily by public sector donors" (Ringheim 1996).

Ringheim (1996) argues that acceptance of an effective, reversible hormonal contraceptive for men hinges on how it is perceived not only by men but also by women. Oudshoorn (this volume) demonstrates that not only women but also feminists hold multiple positions vis-à-vis male contraceptives, arguing that the media are already and will be even more deeply implicated in configuring male users (and their female partners) through discursive constructions of various masculinities in association with various means of contraception or their absence.

A Biotechnology of Desire: The Molecular Transgender "Condom"

Mavericks who are part of the new generation have begun moving in new but long fantasized directions. They are seeking methods of contraception that bridge the desires of women for safe, local, and seemingly simple nonsystemic means, the desires of scientists for "scientific" means, and the desires of all for disease prevention. Such emerging technologies are intended to be *both* spermicidal and prophylactic against sexually transmitted diseases, including AIDS. They require something still very scientifically radical—an understanding of the vaginal environment. After almost a century of reproductive science, the vagina is a "new" frontier, especially in terms of molecular biology.

While many avenues are being explored in this new biotechnological domain, among the most fascinating is what Cone and Whaley (1994) call a "molecular condom." The fantasized product would prevent both pathogens and sperm from entering mucus cells to which particular molecules have bound, disseminating rapidly through the cervical/vaginal mucus membranes. The product could also be used to coat the penis (and hence whatever the penis is in contact with). In effect, then, such a product would be an invisible, molecular condom usable by *any* sexed/gendered person. The very movements of sex would distribute the molecular condom more effectively! Note that this is a nonsystemic, locally acting product that is preventative rather than interventive or curative—rare on all three counts. What is required to produce such methods is an understanding of mucus and sperm. Mucus has been "understudied" despite its having been an important part of the technical repertoire of reproductive science since 1917, as discussed above.

Broad spectrum mucosal protection would constitute primary prevention, which is most radical, since mucus is "the primary route of transmission of sperm and germs in the reproductive tract" (Cone and Whaley 1994, 114). Extant natural antibodies in mucus already play a major role in preventing mucosal transmission. Human monoclonal antibodies (mAbs) can now be engineered to work *with* extant mucosal antibodies as protective agents. Human monoclonals may soon be economically feasible for sustained use as protection. They might also prevent or attenuate maternal/fetus disease transmission.[61]

The new molecular condom offers the possibility of a new quid pro quo. As a bioengineered molecular product, it is clearly "scientific enough" for scientists. As a local/nonsystemic product that is protective against both pregnancy and STDs, it addresses the demands that women users and feminist activists have made for nearly a century. Birth control advocates will be delighted at another viable means of contraception that seems safer than many if not most other means and that is unlikely to alienate many actors in the wider reproductive arena. And population control advocates may be happy enough because of the sustained release aspect (do it *to* them) of the method (Sherwood et al. 1996). This aspect will also please some users.

CONCLUSIONS

> Power is not so much a matter of imposing constraints upon citizens as of "making up" citizens capable of bearing a kind of regulated freedom. Personal autonomy is not the antithesis of power, but a key term in its exercise.
> —*Miller and Rose*

The [C]ommittee [on Contraceptive Research and Development, Division of Health Sciences Policy, Institute of Medicine] also finds an agenda for

contraceptive research and development that is "woman-centered" to be reasonable, just and also market worthy.
—*Harrison and Rosenfield*

For most of the twentieth century, contraceptives have been produced only by
maverick reproductive scientists working "beyond the pale" of their discipline.
They have been variously committed to women's autonomy, health, and population control. Their status vis-à-vis other sciences has been important to them,
and their professional denigration has contributed to a consistent bias against
simple, low-technology contraceptives and toward endocrinological and other
"more scientific" means. Effectiveness rather than safety has been the primary
technical commitment within their scientific frame. The "cultures of science"
that have been produced by five generations of scientists are cumulative—previous discourses remain lively as resources into the future—as well as hegemonic and difficult to negotiate and displace, even by maverick scientists.
Mavericks themselves have been varyingly reputable scientists as foci of institutional location or position in the academy and the broader scientific/industrial
complex. Most, however, seem to feel they have paid dearly for their maver-
ickhood and for choosing reproduction and contraception in terms of their
scientific careers.

Women as feminist birth control advocates and individual users have
fought for change since at least 1915. Here we must ask how the concerns of
women vis-à-vis contraception have been occluded. The tensions among scientists, population controllers, physicians, eugenicists, feminists, women's health
advocates, pharmaceutical companies, and the plethora of regulatory and distribution as well as policy organizations can be felt throughout these sagas.
Recently, a new version of the quid pro quo among birth control advocates,
population control advocates, reproductive scientists, and research support
groups has begun to be articulated. The earlier quid pro quo, achieved by the
1950s around "modern scientific contraception," was that women would get
new means of contraception—but *only* scientific means that would contribute
to the scientific legitimacy, autonomy, and authority of the reproductive sciences. These scientific means (pills, IUDs, injectables, implantables) also satisfied philanthropists and population controllers as something "done to people,"
in Tietze's terms, rather than something that people—read women—did for
themselves. They clearly have not satisfied a significant proportion of implicated actors—women users. These pragmatic women (Lock and Kaufert 1998)
mounted resistances that took two major forms: (1) voting with their feet by
walking away from unwanted methods, and (2) organizing around women's
reproductive health nationally and internationally. Since Cairo, at least, women
as users are more clearly "at the table" in the flesh—inside the world of contra-

ceptive research as living rather than implicated actors.[62] How and when this participation will manifest itself in concrete contraceptive R&D more broadly remains to be seen (International Working Group 1996).

Overall, the reproductive science I found across the twentieth century was peculiarly (however normatively) disengaged from its objects as agentic subjects. It is peculiar because of the very transparency of the reproductive sciences to most people: While many if not most other sciences are opaque, the purposes and goals of the reproductive sciences are transparent if controversial. The prolonged insularity of the reproductive sciences from society, from almost a century of demands of birth controllers, feminists, women users, etc., is really quite startling. The contraception/family planning literature has been rife with reports of user rejection for decades—and quite relentlessly since *The Doctors' Case against the Pill* (Seaman 1969). It seems to have taken all these decades for scientists and policymakers to grasp that it is not only privileged white northern women and uppity feminists who are capable of mounting serious and sustained resistances to inadequate technologies. In the words of renowned feminist theorist Janis Joplin, "Freedom's just another word for nothing left to lose."

Yet inclusion in R&D and policy processes will not solve all problems. Instead, this will create new ones (Clarke and Olesen 1998). For example, Weedman (1998, 315) examined design and client/user roles in computing where there have been strong commitments to extensive cooperation; she found that costs to users are unexpected, often not assumable, and that there are asymmetries inherent in the user/designer relationship that can easily destabilize the collaboration. Mere presence at the table will not suffice.

For one hundred years, contraceptives have been evaluated within the family planning/population control arena by individuals and organizations with "prior" commitments to these technologies, "advocate researchers" (Gallagher 1992). An alternative process has recently been framed in science and technology studies (Rip 1986; Rip et al. 1995; Koch 1995; Walsh 1995) called "constructive technology assessment," arguing for the inclusion of societally desirable criteria in the innovation and design decision-making process, shaping technologies as they develop. While I remain dubious of the possibility of societal consensus, such democratizing practices could certainly target implicated users and transform them from virtual users to embodied agentic actors in design processes. Living, breathing, sexually active, contracepting women and men users could thus be new mavericks.

The reproductive sciences and contraceptive and related technologies are today at least as controversial as they have been over the past century (Clarke 1990, 1998). In concert with the expansion of new technologies to manipulate genetic outcomes, controversy is also likely to expand rather than abate.

Certainly many feminists are more hopeful than we have been over the past half century. However, if we use the field of science and technology studies as a barometer regarding speed of acceptance of feminist contributions, or if we look at most articles on various means of contraception in the scientific literature in 1998, our hopefulness attenuates rather rapidly.[63] I would argue that it will take several more generations, and likely one or two more centuries, before the attitudes of most reproductive scientists are aligned with some version of a "woman-centered agenda." Ironically, some new contraceptive technologies may meet more women's—and men's—needs more safely, effectively, and rapidly.

NOTES

1. Feminist science and technology studies have avidly examined the applications of the reproductive sciences, especially conceptive technologies, but few have studied the science in production per se (with exceptions such as Oudshoorn 1994; Borell 1987; Hall 1978; Dugdale 2000). There is a strong and expanding literature on the history of contraception focused more on social movements, public culture, and use. For pre-nineteenth-century modes, see Himes (1936), W. H. Robertson (1989), and Riddle (1992). An excellent new work on the nineteenth-century United States is Brodie (1994). On the twentieth century see esp. Reed (1984), Gordon (1990), Chesler (1992), Greenhalgh (1995, 1996), Halfon (1997), Hodgson (1990), and McCann (1994). There is a History of Contraception Museum in Toronto at Ortho-McNeil, Inc., 19 Greenbelt Drive, Don Mills, Ontario, M3C 1L9, Canada. Open by appointment: 416-449-9444.

2. American philanthropic groups involved with contraception have included Rockefeller-sponsored and funded organizations such as the Bureau of Social Hygiene, the National Committee on Maternal Health, the National Research Council's Committee for Research in Problems of Sex, and the Rockefeller, Macy, Markle, Ford, and Packard Foundations. Not until the 1960s did the U.S. government fund contraceptive research, and even internationally, government funding of such research has not been extensive. See Clarke (1998, chap. 7), Greep et al. (1976), Mastroianni et al. (1990), and Harrison and Rosenfield (1996). McCabe (1998) reports that the Packard Foundation, long a contributor, has marked population control as its major focus for the next five years, donating $375 million to the cause.

3. See Hertz (1984), Mastroianni et al. (1990), and Harrison and Rosenfield (1996).

4. See Clarke (1998, 18–21) for a more meticulous handling of this argument. Nye (1994) makes essentially the same argument I do, even quoting the same passage of Foucault. I only wish I had read him earlier. See also Oudshoorn (1996b).

5. On the rationalization of sexual behavior, rather pertinent today as well, see Weingart (1987).

6. See Strauss (1993), Blumer (1958), and Clarke (1990, 1991, 1998).

7. For studies of different arenas in the arts, sciences, and computing, see Becker (1982), Clarke (1990a, 1990b), Clarke and Montini (1993), Casper and Clarke (1998), Fujimura (1988), and Star and Griesemer (1989).

8. See Bijker, Pinch, and Hughes (1987), Bijker and Law (1992), and Clarke (1998).

9. See Cowan (1987), Akrich (1992, 1995), Cockburn (1985, 1993), Cockburn and Fürst-

Dilić (1994), Berg (1994), Forsythe (1992), Chabaud-Rychter (1994), and Wajcman (1991). On users of contraception, see Bruce (1987, 1990), Cottingham (1997), and Reproductive Health Matters (1993, 1995, 1996).

10. Thanks to Laura Mamo for reminding me of Balsamo here.

11. See, e.g., Bruce (1987), Cottingham (1997), Germain (1993), Holmes et al. (1980), and Reproductive Health Matters (1993, 1995, 1996).

12. See n. 3.

13. The postmodernist project involves enhancing scientific capacities to transform reproductive bodies. In contrast to modernist applications such as contraception and hormonal interventions to control menstruation and menopause, postmodernist applications such as the new reproductive technologies are accessible to very few people (Clarke 1995).

14. In 1914, there were only three articles on birth control in the *New York Times,* and in 1915 there were only fourteen. But in 1916–17 there were ninety, and news magazines had similar coverage. See Chesler (1992, 129–30).

15. Certainly some reproductive scientists were also active in birth control (detailed below). But the positions these activists themselves articulated vis-à-vis contraceptive research were more parallel to those of other reproductive scientists than birth control advocates.

16. On this use of the term *democratize,* see Himes (1936), Pierpoint (1922), and Sanger (1920).

17. The story of these changes is rife with contradictions and conflicts. It is important to note that none of the multiple worlds involved were monolithic, nor were they ever fully segregated, as their boundaries were highly permeable. See Clarke (1998, chap. 6).

18. The term *democratization* also carries full participatory connotations in science and technology studies. See Edge (1995, 10–11).

19. Only the IUD, which is believed to "work" by creating a hostile environment in the uterus, does not depend on understanding the female cycle. Early IUDs, called Grafenberg rings, predated the revised standard cycle. See Langley (1973), Mishell (1998), and Dugdale (2000).

20. From the foreword to Voge's book (1933, 12) by Dr. Robert Latou Dickinson of the NCMH. Dr. Robert T. Frank was the director of research for the NCMH at this time, and the manuscript was also reviewed by Carl Hartman of Johns Hopkins.

21. See File Memoranda: Crew Spermaticide Study, Rockefeller Archives Center (Tarrytown, New York), Bureau of Social Hygiene Papers SIII-2 B7 F174.

22. As reported by Ruth Topping of the Bureau of Social Hygiene staff: File Memorandum RT. Subject: Crew Study and Interview with Dr. Crew. 12 September 1932. Rockefeller Archives Center, Bureau of Social Hygiene Papers SIII-2 B7 F174.

23. Memo to Mr. Dunham from Ruth Topping, Subject: Contraceptive Research, 30 September 1931. Rockefeller Archives Center, Bureau of Social Hygiene Papers SIII-2 B7 F166. See also Soloway (1995). Porter and Hall (1995, 176) assert that Solly Zuckerman received some American funding with Baker. Subsequently, they also report, Baker relied on funding from the (British) Eugenics Society and from the pharmaceutical company British Drug Houses, Ltd.

24. A form of tubal ligation was performed in 1880 in Ohio. Women were also sterilized by oophorectomy or uterectomy/hysterectomy, both of which were done in the nineteenth century for other medical purposes. Vasectomy was developed in 1899 by Dr. Harry C. Sharp in Indiana and initially used on prisoners there (Paul 1973, 28–29; Meyers 1970, 29; Guttmacher 1973).

25. Eugenicists' contraceptive advocacy had focused since the early twentieth century on negative eugenics via involuntary surgical sterilization of the "unfit," with institutionalized criminal, insane, and "feeble-minded" people as special targets. By the mid-1930s, such laws met with considerable opposition, especially after the Nazis copied and used them. Harry Laughlin's "Model Eugenical Sterilization Law" (Laughlin 1976, 138–45) was almost directly translated as the Nazi law of 1933. On eugenic sterilization and other sterilization abuse in the United States, see Kevles (1985), Robitscher (1973), Shapiro (1985), Reilly (1991), and Clarke (1984).

26. On earlier publications pointing to possible hormonal interventions for contraceptive purposes, see Cooper (1928, 120) and several articles on the interruption of pregnancy via administration of estrogens (Smith 1926; Makepeace et al. 1937; Parkes et al. 1938). H. Taylor reported on hormonal contraceptive research at Edinburgh in 1930 (in Sanger and Stone 1931, 98–104). See also Dickinson (1931), Dickinson and Morris (1941a, 1941b), Sanger (1934), and Sanger and Stone (1931).

27. While at Harvard, Pincus had done research on mammalian sexual physiology supported by both the NRC/CRPS and the Macy Foundation (Reed 1984, 319–20). See Reed (1984, chaps. 25–27) for a fuller account of Pincus's career and his work with Chang on Pill development. See Pincus (1965) for his summary work on control of fertility. Pincus did his undergraduate work at the Cornell School of Agriculture focusing on biochemistry and animal breeding. For Pincus as a disciple of Jacques Loeb's biological engineering ideology, see Pauly (1987, 182–98). See also Djerassi (1992) and W. H. Robertson (1989).

28. Considerable controversy surrounded Syntex for some years; Marker went into seclusion. On the development of the Pill, see Pramik (1978), Djerassi (1981, 1992), Applezweig (1975), Marker (1986), National Science Foundation–TRACES (1968), National Science Foundation–Batelle (1973), Goldzieher (1993), Perone (1993), Ramirez de Arellano and Seipp (1983), Oudshoorn (1994), Courey (1995), Marks (this volume), and Watkins (1998).

29. See Bloom and Parsons (1994) and note 20. On the clinical trials, see Hartman (1959), Tietze (1962, 1965a, 1965b), Meldrum (1996), Marks (1998, and this volume), Watkins (1998), and Courey (1995).

30. In the major current feminist analysis of the Pill, Bell et al. (1998, 314–15) discuss the following categories of problems that are currently manifest with the Pill: cancer, nausea or vomiting, breast changes, changes in menstrual flow, breakthrough bleeding, headaches, depression, change in intensity of sexual desire and response, urinary tract infections, vaginitis and vaginal discharges, cervical dysplasia, skin problems, gum inflammation, asthma and epilepsy, interactions with other medications, liver and gallbladder diseases, virus infections, and other problems.

31. This analysis differs radically from those of Pill development done for the National Science Foundation by TRACES (1968) and Batelle (1973), which offered an individualist "technical scientific entrepreneur" account focused on Pincus. Such accounts ignore both 120 years of activity by birth control advocates, including their recruitment of scientists, the crucial structural positions of the major developers outside of the academy, and the private philanthropic funding base. For a more fully developed analysis that takes all of the significant actors into account, see Courey (1995, chap. 1). On Djerassi, see Djerassi (1992).

32. See Piccicino and Mosher (1998, 5) and Biegelmann-Massari and Bateman (1998). Watkins (1998) argues that the role of the physician in family planning was transformed by the Pill from incidental participant to essential player, while patients also had to become more active to obtain and calibrate the Pill or other modern scientific means of contraception, changing the overall balance of physician/patient power as well.

33. For a good example of Gräfenberg's work, see his 1931 article reprinted in Langley (1973, 340–56). Dugdale (2000) is the major study of the development of IUDs.

34. For examples and accounts of these debates, especially in the 1930s, see Langley (1973, 336–39, 357), Sanger and Stone (1931, 33–71), Sanger (1934, 86–93), and Tietze (1962, 1965b).

35. Dr. Mary Halton, Margaret Sanger's gynecologist, showed Dickinson more than one thousand case histories in 1924. Dickinson wanted a full investigation of the method, but not until 1947 was there serious effort to publish Halton's results. Then her "Contraception with an Intrauterine Silk Coil" was rejected by the *American Journal of Obstetrics and Gynecology*. The NCMH refused to sponsor the paper; Earl Engle and Howard Taylor Jr. said, "This was too hot to be [easily] cleared." The article was finally published in 1948 in *Human Fertility*, the journal of Sanger's Clinical Research Bureau, with editorial warnings. Ironically, in 1964, Taylor hailed the IUD as a "contribution to . . . the freedom of mankind" (Reed 1984, 275–76).

36. In the development sagas of the Pill and the IUD, there seems to have been competition between sponsoring organizations and between physician-developers of the IUD versus the biologist-developers of hormonal contraception. For example, Gregory Pincus was "profoundly uninterested" in participating in evaluation of conventional barrier methods, and Reed (1984, 375) also found that "the IUD remains the butt of jokes at the Worcester Foundation, while representatives of the Population Council make vague references to the 'commercial interests' that control distribution of the Pill." Onorato (1991) compared the organizational styles and successes of the Population Council and the Planned Parenthood Federation of America in terms of contraceptive research.

37. On the Dalkon Shield controversy, see Mintz (1985), Grant (1992), and Hicks (1994). On IUDs more broadly, see Dugdale's excellent history (2000).

38. At the time of the proposal, Shelesnyak was director of the Institute of Biodynamics, Weizmann Institute of Science, Rehovoth, Israel, which received major grants from the Ford Foundation in support of the development of the reproductive sciences (Hertz 1984). Between 1962 and 1983, the Weizmann Institute directed by M. C. Shelesnyak and later by H. R. Lindner received $3,442,500 from Ford. Their focus was on the role of histamines in nidation, radioimmunoassays of steroids and other hormones, and ovulation processes. See Shelesnyak (1963, 1964, 1974, 1986).

39. See, e.g., Baulieu (1997) and Mishell (1998).

40. See Greep et al. (1976), Djerassi (1981, 1989), Segal (1987), and Mastroianni et al. (1990).

41. See Hardon (1992), Moskowitz and Jennings (1996), Pies (1997), Hardon et al. (1997a, 1997b), Kuiper et al. (1997), and Kuo (1998).

42. Sanger quoted a Dr. McCartney as saying: "Devices are all very nice for those who can afford them. The poor people with whom we are really concerned in this [Depression] recovery program cannot afford them. . . . [I]t is quite necessary to be concerned with something that can be applied very much more cheaply. Spermatoxins . . . are one of the methods" (1934, 111). Women here were configured as semiactive users as they would need to come for injections at regular intervals. In the late 1930s, the NCMH again supported spermatoxin research through grants from Squibb and Sons, but the method was found ineffective (Eastman, Guttmacher, and Stewart 1939, 151).

43. See Mastroianni et al. (1990, 33). A summary is offered in Harrison and Rosenfield (1996, app. C).

44. On immunocontraception, see Richter (1993), Reproductive Health Matters (1993, 1995, 1996), and Schrater (1992).

45. See Hardon (1992), Schrater (1992), and Ravindran and Berer (1995).

46. Interview by Clarke with Dr. Baulieu, December 8, 1991, Washington, D.C. Baulieu won the prestigious Lasker Prize in 1989. Some have argued that he might win the Nobel for RU486. However, the Nobel has never been awarded for explicitly and exclusively reproductive research, even "discovery" of sex hormones (Clarke 1998), and it seems highly unlikely that it would be awarded for an abortifacient.

47. See Ruzek (1978), Zimmerman (1987), Ruzek, Olesen, and Clarke (1997), and Clarke and Olesen (1998).

48. Calderone was one of the feminists eased out of the planned parenthood/population control movement. She left to join SEICUS. See Reynolds (1994) and Meldrum (1996).

49. See Boston Women's Health Book Collective (1971, 1984, 1992, 1998), Bell (1984, 1994a, 1994b, 1994c, 1998, 2000), and Bell et al. (1980).

50. For a list of such organizations, see Boston Women's Health Book Collective (1998, 680–754). See also Correa (1994), Petchesky and Judd (1998), and Hardon et al. (1997)

51. See Vaughan (1970), Ruzek (1978), Holmes et al. (1980), Riessman (1983), Arditti et al. (1984), Gunn (1987), Hartmann (1987/1995, 1992), Holmes (1992), Watkins (1998), and Ruzek (1978), Zimmerman (1987), Ruzek, Olesen, and Clarke (1997), Weisman (1998), and Clarke and Olesen (1998) on women's health movements.

52. See, e.g., Oudshoorn (1995a, 1995b, 1996a, 1996b), Petchesky and Judd (1998), Sen et al. (1994), Dixon-Mueller (1993a, 1993b), and Sen and Snow (1994).

53. See, e.g., Boston Women's Health Book Collective (1992), Sen et al. (1994), Dixon-Mueller (1993a, 1993b), Holmes (1992), Hartmann (1987/1995), Sen and Snow (1994), Cottingham (1997), Reproductive Health Matters (1993, 1995, 1996), Petchesky and Judd (1998), Hardon, Mutua, Kabir, and Engelkes (1997), Hardon and Hayes (1997), Coliver (1995), Correa with Reichmann (1994), and Biegelmann-Massari and Bateman (1998). There is also a website for the Global Reproductive Health Forum: www.hsph.harvard.edu/Organizations/healthnet.

54. Quote from Harrison and Rosenfield (1996, 2). See also Berkman (1980), Holmes et al. (1980), and Reproductive Health Matters (1993).

55. See, e.g., Germain and Dixon-Mueller (1993), the journal *Reproductive Health Matters,* no. 3 (1995), Dixon-Mueller (1993), Sen et al. (1994), and Holmes (1992). The issue of AIDS and heterosexual intercourse has become central to feminist concerns, especially internationally. See, e.g., Boston Women's Health Book Collective (1998). On resistances, see also Bloom and Parsons (1994), Petchesky and Judd (1998), Barroso and Correa (1995), and Correa (1994).

56. On the thinning of vaginal walls due to ingested hormones, see Marx et al. (1996) and Alexander (1996).

57. See, e.g., Moench et al. (1993), Saltzman et al. (1994), Sherwood et al. (1996), and Whaley et al. (1993).

58. This work extensively criticized other rhythm-based systems as inadequate, including those of Knaus and Ogino, both of whom had offered models using shorter fertile periods. See Knaus (1934a and 1934b), and Ogino (1934).

59. See also Alexander et al. (1996), Moench et al. (1993), Whaley et al. (1993), and Zeitlin et al. (1997).

60. See, e.g., Clermont (1991), Alexander (1995), Lissner (1992), Oudshoorn (1995,

1996a, 1997a, 1997b, 1997c, 1999/2000), Setchell (1984), Mastroianni et al. (1990), Harrison and Rosenfield (1996), and Ringheim (1996). A summary is offered in Harrison and Rosenfield (1996, app. B).

61. See Sherwood et al. (1996), Castle et al. (1998), Randomsky et al. (1992), Saltzman et al. (1994), and Wyatt et al. (1998). A summary is offered in Harrison and Rosenfield (1996, app. D).

62. For example, Judy Norsigian of the Boston Women's Health Book Collective served on the Committee on Contraceptive Research and Development, Division of Health Sciences Policy, Institute of Medicine (Harrison and Rosenfield 1996).

63. For a recent popular debate, see Westoff (1994) and Chesler (1994). Westoff was asked, "What's the world's priority task?" He replied, "Finally, control population." Chesler responded, "No, the first priority is stop coercing women."

REFERENCES

Akrich, Madeleine:
   1992 The De-Scription of Technical Objects. In Wiebe E. Bijker and John Law (eds.), *Shaping Technology/Building Society: Studies in Sociotechnical Change*, 205–24. Cambridge: MIT Press.
   1995 User Representations: Practices, Methods, and Sociology. In Arie Rip, Thomas J. Misa, and Johan Schot (eds.), *Managing Technology in Society: The Approach of Constructive Technology Assessment*, 167–84. London and New York: Pinter/St. Martin's Press.

Alexander, Nancy J.:
   1995 Future Contraceptives. *Scientific American,* September, 136–41.
   1996 Sexual Spread of HIV Infection. *Human Reproduction* 11(7): 111–20.

Alexander, Nancy J., V. Alexander, S. Allen, L. Dorflinger, et al.:
   1996 Recommendations for the Development of Vaginal Microbicides. *AIDS* 10(8): 1–6.

Applezweig, Norman:
   1975 *Russel Marker to Gregory Pincus: The Mexican Steroid Industry and the Development of Modern Contraceptive Technology.* Based on a lecture given at the Symposium on the Historical Development of Anticonceptive Methods, First Chemical Congress of the North American Continent, Mexico.

Arditti, Rita, Renate Duelli Klein, and Shelley Minden (eds.):
   1984 *Test-Tube Women: What Future for Motherhood?* Boston: Pandora/Routledge and Kegan Paul.

Baker, J. R.:
   1930a The Spermicidal Power of Chemical Contraception. I. Introduction: Experiments on Guinea Pig Sperm. *Journal of Hygiene* 29: 323–29.
   1930b The Spermicidal Power of Chemical Contraception. II. Pure Substances. *Journal of Hygiene* 30: 273–94.
   1931a Chemical Contraceptives. Proceedings of the Second International Congress for Sex Research.
   1931b The Spermicidal Power of Chemical Contraception. III. Pessaries. *Journal of Hygiene* 31: 309–20.
   1935 *The Chemical Control of Conception.* London: Chapman and Hall.

Balsamo, Anne:
1996 *Technologies of the Gendered Body: Reading Cyborg Women.* Durham, N.C.: Duke University Press.
Barroso, Carmen, and Sonia Correa:
1995 Public Servants, Professionals, and Feminists: The Politics of Contraception in Brazil. In Faye D. Ginsberg and Rayna Rapp (eds.), *Conceiving the New World Order: The Global Stratification of Reproduction,* 292–322. Berkeley: University of California Press.
Bartelmez, George W.:
1933 (with C. Cuthbertson) Histologic Studies of Menstruating Mucus Membrane of the Human Uterus. *Carnegie Contributions to Embryology* 24(142): 141–86.
1935 The Circulation in the Intervillous Space of the Macaque Placenta. *Anatomical Record* 61(4): Suppl. A.
1937 Menstruation. *Physiological Reviews* 17(1): 28–72.
Bartelmez, George W., George W. Corner, and Carl G. Hartman:
1951 Cyclic Changes in the Endometrium of the Rhesus Monkey. *Carnegie Contributions to Embryology* 34: 99–144.
Baulieu, Etienne-Emile:
1989 RU-486 as an Antiprogesterone Steroid: From Receptor to Contragestion and Beyond. *Journal of the American Medical Association* 262(13): 1808–14 (supplement).
1991 (with Mort Rosenblum) *The "Abortion Pill": RU486, a Woman's Choice.* New York: Simon and Schuster.
1997 RU486 (Mifepristone): A Short Overview of Its Mechanisms of Action and Clinical Uses at the End of 1996. *Annals of the New York Academy of Sciences* 828: 47–58.
Becker, Howard S.:
1963 *Outsiders: Studies in the Sociology of Deviance.* New York: Free Press.
1982 *Art Worlds.* Berkeley: University of California Press.
Bell, Susan:
1984 Birth Control. In Boston Women's Health Book Collective (eds.), *The New Our Bodies, Ourselves,* 220–62. New York: Simon and Schuster.
1994 Birth Control for Women in Midlife: Update. In Paula Doress-Worters and Diana Siegel (eds.), *The New Ourselves Growing Older,* 101–7. New York: Simon and Schuster.
1994 Translating Science to the People: Updating *The New Our Bodies, Ourselves. Women's Studies International Forum* 17(1): 9–18.
1999 Empowering Technologies: Connecting Women and Science in Microbicide Research. Unpublished manuscript.
Bell, Susan, Paula Garbarino, Jeanne Hubbich, Adrienne Ingram, Lyn Koehnline, and Jill Wolhandler:
1980 Reclaiming Reproductive Control: A Feminist Approach to Fertility Consciousness. *Science for the People,* January–February, 6–9, 30–35.
Bell, Susan (with Suzannah Cooper-Doyle, Judy Norsigian, and F. Stewart):
1992 Birth Control. In Boston Women's Health Book Collective (eds.), *The New Our Bodies, Ourselves,* 259–307. New York: Simon and Schuster.
Bell, Susan, and Lauren Wise (with Suzannah Cooper-Doyle and Judy Norsigian):
1998 Birth Control. In Boston Women's Health Book Collective (eds.), *The New Our Bodies, Ourselves,* 288–340. New York: Simon and Schuster.
Berg, Anne Jorun:
1994 Technological Flexibility: Bringing Gender into Technology (or Was It the Other

Way Around?) In Cynthia Cockburn and Ruza Fürst-Dilić (eds.), *Bringing Technology Home: Gender and Technology in a Changing Europe,* 94–110. Buckingham, England: Open University Press.

Berkman, Joyce Avrech:
   1980   Historical Styles of Contraceptive Advocacy. In Helen B. Holmes et al. (eds.), *Birth Control and Controlling Birth: Women-Centered Perspectives,* 23–26. Clifton, N.J.: Humana Press.

Biegelmann-Massari, Michele, and Simone Bateman (Novaes):
   1998   Panorama of Fertility Control in the World. In J. Rose (ed.), *Human Population Problems.* London: Gordon and Breach.

Bijker, Wiebe E.:
   1994   Socio-Historical Technology Studies. In Sheila Jassanoff, Gerald Markle, James Petersen, and Trevor Pinch (eds.), *Handbook of Science and Technology Studies,* 229–55. Thousand Oaks, Calif.: Sage.

Bijker, Wiebe E., Thomas P. Hughes, and Trevor Pinch (eds.):
   1987   *The Social Construction of Technological Systems.* Cambridge: MIT Press.

Bijker, Wiebe E., and John Law (eds.):
   1992   *Shaping Technology/Building Society.* Cambridge: MIT Press.

Billings, E., J. Billings, J. B. Brown, and H. G. Burger:
   1972   Symptoms and Hormonal Changes Accompanying Ovulation. *Lancet* 1: 282–84.

Billings, Evelyn, and Ann Westmore:
   1980   *The Billings Method: Controlling Fertility without Drugs or Devices.* New York: Penguin.

Bloom, Amy S., and P. Ellen Parsons:
   1994   Twenty-fifth Anniversary of *The Doctor's Case against the Pill. National Women's Health Network News,* November–December, 1, 3.

Blumer, Herbert:
   1958   Race Prejudice as a Sense of Group Position. *Pacific Sociological Review* 1: 3–8.

Borell, Merriley:
   1987   Biologists and the Promotion of Birth Control Research, 1918–1938. *Journal of the History of Biology* 19(1): 51–87.

Boston Women's Health Book Collective:
   1971   *Our Bodies, Ourselves.* Boston: South End Press.
   1984/ *The New Our Bodies, Ourselves: A Book by and for Women.* 3d and 4th eds. New York:
   1992   Simon and Schuster.
   1998   *Our Bodies, Ourselves for the New Century: A Book by and for Women.* New York: Simon and Schuster.

Brodie, Janet Farrell:
   1994   *Contraception and Abortion in Nineteenth-Century America.* Ithaca, N.Y.: Cornell University Press.

Bruce, Judith:
   1987   Users' Perspectives on Contraceptive Technology and Delivery Systems: Highlighting Some Feminist Issues. *Technology in Society* 9: 359–83.
   1990   Fundamental Elements of the Quality of Care: A Simple Framework. *Studies in Family Planning* 21(2): 61–91.

Bullough, Vern L.:
   1994   *Science in the Bedroom: A History of Sex Research.* New York: Basic Books.

Butler, Judith:
   1993   *Bodies That Matter.* New York: Routledge.

Calderone, Mary Steichen:

1964   *Manual of Contraceptive Practice.* Baltimore: Williams and Wilkins.

Callon, Michel:

1991   Techno-economic Networks and Irreversibility. In John Law (ed.), *A Sociology of Monsters: Essays on Power, Technology and Domination,* 132–64. New York: Routledge.

Canguilhem, George:

1978   *On The Normal and the Pathological.* Translated by Carolyn R. Fawcett. Dordrecht: Reidel.

Casper, Monica, and Adele E. Clarke:

1998   Making the Pap Smear into the Right Tool for the Job: Cervical Cancer Screening in the United States, c. 1940–1995. *Social Studies of Science* 28(2/3): 255–90.

Castle, Philip E., Timothy E. Hoen, Kevin J. Whaley, and Richard A. Cone:

1998   Contraceptive Testing of Vaginal Agents in Rabbits. *Contraception* 58: 51–60.

Chabaud-Rychter, Danielle:

1994   Women Users in the Design Process of a Food Robot: Innovation in a French Domestic Appliance Company. In Cynthia Cockburn and Ruza Fürst-Dilić (eds.), *Bringing Technology Home: Gender and Technology in a Changing Europe,* 77–93. Buckingham, England: Open University Press.

Charo, R. Alta:

1991   A Political History of RU-486. In K. E. Hanna (ed.), *Biomedical Politics,* 43–93. Washington: National Academy Press.

Chesler, Ellen:

1992   *Woman of Valor: Margaret Sanger and the Birth Control Movement in America.* New York: Simon and Schuster.

1994   No, the First Priority Is Stop Coercing Women. *New York Times Magazine,* February 6, 31–32.

Clarke, Adele E.:

1984   Subtle Sterilization Abuse: A Reproductive Rights Perspective. In Rita Arditti, Renata Duelli Klein, and Shelley Minden (eds.), *Test-Tube Women: What Future for Motherhood?* 188–212. Boston: Pandora/Routledge and Kegan Paul (2d ed. 1989).

1990a Controversy and the Development of Reproductive Sciences. *Social Problems* 37(1): 18–37.

1990b A Social Worlds Research Adventure: The Case of Reproductive Science. In Susan E. Cozzens and Thomas F. Gieryn (eds.), *Theories of Science in Society,* 15–42. Bloomington: Indiana University Press.

1991   Social Worlds Theory as Organization Theory. In David Maines (ed.), *Social Organization and Social Process: Essays in Honor of Anselm Strauss,* 119–58. Hawthorne, N.Y.: Aldine de Gruyter.

1995   Modernity, Postmodernity, and Human Reproductive Processes c. 1890–1990, or "Mommy, Where do Cyborgs Come From Anyway?" In Chris Hables Gray et al. (eds.), *The Cyborg Handbook,* 139–55. New York: Routledge.

1998   *Disciplining Reproduction: Modernity, American Life Sciences, and "the Problems of Sex."* Berkeley: University of California Press.

Clarke, Adele E., and Theresa Montini:

1993   The Many Faces of RU486: Tales of Situated Knowledges and Technological Contestations. *Science, Technology, and Human Values* 18(1): 42–78.

Clarke, Adele E., and Virginia L. Olesen (eds.):
  1998   *Revisioning Women, Health, and Healing: Feminist, Cultural, and Technoscience Perspectives.* New York: Routledge.
Clermont, Y.:
  1991   Four Decades of Research on the Biology of the Male Reproductive System: A Few Landmarks. *Annals of the New York Academy of Sciences* 637: 17–25.
Cockburn, Cynthia:
  1985   *Machinery of Dominance: Women, Men, and Technical Know-How.* Boston: Northeastern University Press.
  1993   *Gender and Technology in the Making.* Thousand Oaks, Calif.: Sage.
Cockburn, Cynthia, and Ruza Fürst-Dilić (eds.):
  1994   *Bringing Technology Home: Gender and Technology in a Changing Europe.* Buckingham, England: Open University Press.
Coliver, Sandra (ed.) for Article 19:
  1995   *The Right to Know: Human Rights and Access to Reproductive Health Information.* Philadelphia: Article 19 and University of Pennsylvania Press.
Cone, Richard A., and Kevin J. Whaley:
  1994   Review Article: Monoclonal Antibodies for Reproductive Health: Part I. Preventing Sexual Transmission of Disease and Pregnancy with Topically Applied Antibodies. *American Journal of Reproductive Immunology* 32: 114–31.
Cooper, James F.:
  1928   *Technique of Contraception.* New York: [American Birth Control League].
Corner, George W.:
  1951   Our Knowledge of the Menstrual Cycle, 1910–1950. Fourth Annual Addison Lecture, delivered at Guy's Hospital, London, July 13, 1950. *Lancet,* April 28, 919–23.
Corner, George W., and Willard M. Allen:
  1929a Physiology of the Corpus Luteum 2. Production of a Special Uterine Reaction (Progestational Proliferation) by Extracts of the Corpus Luteum. *American Journal of Physiology* 88: 326–29.
  1929b Physiology of the Corpus Luteum 3. Normal Growth and Implantation of Embryos after Very Early Ablation of the Ovaries, under the Influence of Extracts of the Corpus Luteum. *American Journal of Physiology* 88: 340–46.
Correa, Sonia (with Rebecca Reichmann):
  1994   *Population and Reproductive Rights: Feminist Perspectives from the South.* London: Zed Books.
Cottingham, Jane:
  1997   Introduction. *Beyond Acceptability: Users' Perspectives on Contraception.* London: Reproductive Health Matters for the World Health Organization.
Courey, Renee:
  1995   Participants in the Development, Marketing and Safety Evaluation of the Oral Contraceptive, 1950–1965: Mythic Dimensions of a Scientific Solution. Ph.D. diss., University of California, Berkeley.
Cowan, Ruth Schwartz:
  1987   The Consumption Junction: A Proposal for Research Strategies in the Sociology of Technology. In Wiebe Bijker, Thomas Hughes, and Trevor Pinch (eds.), *The Social Construction of Technological Systems,* 261–80. Cambridge: MIT Press.

DeNora, Tia:
 1996 From Physiology to Feminism: Reconfiguring Body, Gender, and Expertise in Natural Fertility Control. *International Sociology* 11(3): 359–83.

Dickinson, Robert Latou:
 1931 *Control of Conception.* New York: National Committee on Maternal Health.

Dickinson, Robert Latou, and Clarence James Gamble:
 1950 *Human Sterilization: Techniques of Permanent Conception Control.* New York: National Committee on Maternal Health.

Dickinson, Robert Latou, and Woodbridge Edwards Morris:
 1941a *Techniques of Conception Control: A Practical Manual Issued by the Birth Control Federation of America, Inc.* Baltimore: Williams and Wilkins.
 1941b *Techniques of Contraception.* New York: Day-Nichols.

Dixon-Mueller, Ruth:
 1993a The Sexuality Connection in Reproductive Health. *Studies in Family Planning* 24(5): 269–82.
 1993b *Population Policy and Women's Rights: Transforming Reproductive Choice.* New York: Praeger.

Djerassi, Carl:
 1981 *The Politics of Contraception: Birth Control in the Year 2001.* San Francisco: W. H. Freeman.
 1989 The Bitter Pill. *Science* 245 (July 28): 356–61.
 1992 *The Pill, Pygmy Chimps, and Degas' Horse: The Autobiography of Carl Djerassi.* New York: Basic Books.

Dugdale, Ann:
 2000 *Devices and Desires: Contraceptive Technology and Women's Sexuality.* London: Zed Books.

Eastman, N. J., A. F. Guttmacher, and E. H. Stewart:
 1939 Experimental Observations on Sperm Immunity in the Rat. *Journal of Contraception* 4(7): 147–51.

Edge, David:
 1995 Reinventing the Wheel. In Sheila Jansanoff et al. (eds.), *Handbook of Science and Technology Studies,* 3–23. Thousand Oaks, Calif.: Sage.

Fletcher, Suzanne W., Robert H. Fletcher, and M. Andrew Greganti:
 1981 Clinical Research Trends in General Medical Journals, 1946–1976. In Edward B. Roberts, et al. (eds.), *Biomedical Innovation,* 284–300. Cambridge, Mass.: MIT Press.

Folbre, Nancy:
 1994 *Who Pays for the Kids? Gender and the Structures of Constraint.* New York: Routledge.

Forsythe, Diana E.:
 1992 Blaming the User in Medical Informatics. In David J. Hess and Linda L. Layne (eds.), *Knowledge and Society: The Anthropology of Science and Technology,* 9. Greenwich, Conn.: JAI Press.

Foucault, Michel:
 1977 *Discipline and Punish.* Harmondsworth: Penguin.
 1980 *The History of Sexuality.* New York: Vintage.

Fujimura, Joan H.:
 1988 The Molecular Biological Bandwagon in Cancer Research: Where Social Worlds Meet. *Social Problems* 35: 261–83.

Fukui, N.:
1923 On a Hitherto Unknown Action of Heat Ray on Testicles. *Japanese Medical World* 3: 27–28.

Gallagher, Dana:
1992 Cervical Caps and the Women's Health Movement: Feminists as "Advocate Researchers." In Helen Bequaert Holmes (ed.), *Issues in Reproductive Technology I: An Anthology,* 87–94. New York: Garland.

Garrett, Laurie:
1996 Monkey Study Shows Hormone Raises HIV Risk. *San Francisco Chronicle,* May 17: A3.

Germain, Adrienne:
1993 Are We Speaking the Same Language? Women's Health Advocates and Scientists Talk about Contraceptive Technology. In *Four Essays on Birth Control Needs and Risks.* New York: International Women's Health Coalition.

Germain, Adrienne, and Ruth Dixon-Mueller:
1993 Whose Life Is It, Anyway? Assessing the Relative Risks of Contraception and Pregnancy. In *Four Essays on Birth Control Needs and Risks.* New York: International Women's Health Coalition.

Ginsberg, Faye D., and Rayna Rapp (eds.):
1995 *Conceiving the New World Order: The Global Stratification of Reproduction.* Berkeley: University of California Press.

Goldzieher, Joseph W.:
1993 The History of Steroidal Contraceptive Development: The Estrogens. *Perspectives in Biology and Medicine* 36(3): 363–68.

Gordon, Linda:
1990 *Woman's Body, Woman's Right: A Social History of Birth Control in America.* 2d ed. New York: Viking.

Gräfenberg, E.:
1931 Intrauterine Methods: An Intrauterine Contraceptive Method. In Margaret Sanger and Hannah M. Stone (eds.), *The Practice of Contraception: An International Symposium and Survey,* 33–47. Baltimore: Williams and Wilkins.

Grant, Nicole J.:
1992 *The Selling of Contraception: The Dalkon Shield Case, Sexuality, and Women's Autonomy.* Columbus: Ohio State University Press.

Greenhalgh, Susan (ed.):
1995 *Situating Fertility: Anthropology and Demographic Inquiry.* Cambridge: Cambridge University Press.

Greenhalgh, Susan:
1996 The Social Construction of Population Science: An Intellectual, Institutional, and Political History of Twentieth-Century Demography. *Comparative Studies in Society and History* 38(1): 26–66.

Greep, Roy O., M. A. Koblinsky, and F. S. Jaffe:
1976 *Reproduction and Human Welfare: A Challenge to Research.* Boston: MIT (Ford Foundation).

Greep, Roy O., and Marjorie A. Koblinsky:
1977 *Frontiers in Reproduction and Fertility Control: A Review of the Reproductive Sciences and Contraceptive Development.* Boston: MIT (Ford Foundation).

Gruhn, John G., and Ralph R. Kazer:

1989   *Hormonal Regulation of the Menstrual Cycle: The Evolution of Concepts.* New York: Plenum.

Gunn, A. D. G.:

1987   *Oral Contraception in Perspective: Thirty Years of Clinical Experience with the Pill.* Park Ridge, N.J.: Parthenon.

Guttmacher, Alan F.:

1973   General Remarks on Medical Aspects of Male and Female Sterilization. In Jonas Robitscher (ed.), *Eugenic Sterilization.* Springfield, Ill.: Charles Thomas.

Halfon, Saul:

1997   Overpopulating the World: Notes toward a Discursive Reading. In Peter Taylor, Saul Halfon, and Paul N. Edwards (eds.), *Changing Life: Genomes, Ecologies, Bodies, Commodities,* 121–48. Minneapolis: University of Minnesota Press.

Hall, Diane Long:

1978   Sex, Fertility, and Taboo: The Committee for Research on Problems of Sex, 1920–1940. Paper presented at Workshop on Historical Perspectives on the Scientific Study of Fertility in the United States, American Academy of Arts and Sciences.

Haraway, Donna:

1991   Situated Knowledges: The Science Question in Feminism and the Privilege of Partial Perspective. In Haraway, *Simians, Cyborgs, and Women: The Reinvention of Nature,* 183–202. New York: Routledge.

1995   Universal Donors in a Vampire Culture: It's All in the Family: Biological Kinship Categories in the Twentieth-Century United States. In William Cronon (ed.), *Uncommon Ground: Toward Reinventing Nature,* 321–78. New York: W. W. Norton.

Hardon, Anita:

1992   Norplant: Conflicting Views on Its Safety and Acceptability. In Helen Bequaert Holmes (ed.), *Issues in Reproductive Technology I: An Anthology,* 11–30. New York: Garland.

Hardon, Anita, and Elizabeth Hayes (eds.):

1997   *Reproductive Rights in Practice: A Feminist Report on the Quality of Care.* London: Zed Books.

Hardon, Anita, Ann Mutua, Sandra Kabir, and Elly Engelkes:

1997   *Monitoring Family Planning and Reproductive Rights: A Manual for Empowerment.* London: Zed Books.

Harrison, P. F., and A. Rosenfield (eds.):

1996   *Contraceptive Research and Development.* Washington, D.C.: National Academy Press.

Hartman, Carl G.:

1932   Ovulation and the Transport and Viability of Ova and Sperm in the Female Genital Tract. In Edgar Allen (ed.), *Sex and Internal Secretions,* 647–732. Baltimore: Williams and Wilkins.

1933   Catholic Advice on the Safe Period. *Birth Control Review* 17 (May): 117–19.

1936   *Time of Ovulation in Women.* Baltimore: Williams and Wilkins.

1937   Facts and Fallacies of the Safe Period. *Journal of Contraception* 2: 51–61.

1939   Studies on Reproduction in the Monkey and Their Bearing in Gynecology and Anthropology. *Endocrinology* 25: 670–82.

1959   Annotated List of Published Reports on Clinical Trials with Contraceptives. *Fertility and Sterility* 10(2): 177–89.

1962   *Science and the Safe Period: A Compendium of Human Reproduction.* Baltimore: Williams and Wilkins.

Hartmann, Betsy:
1987/   *Reproductive Rights and Wrongs: The Global Politics of Population Control and Contra-*
1995   *ceptive Choice.* New York: Harper and Row; Boston: South End Press.
1987   Contraceptives: A Multitude of Meanings. In Helen Bequaert Holmes (ed.), *Issues in Reproductive Technology I: An Anthology,* 3–10. New York: Garland.

Heise, L. L., and C. Elias:
1995   Transforming AIDS Prevention to Meet Women's Needs: A Focus on Developing Countries. *Social Science and Medicine* 40(7): 931–43.

Hertz, Roy:
1984   A Quest for Better Contraception: The Ford Foundation's Contribution to Reproductive Science and Contraceptive Development, 1959–1983. *Contraception* 29(2): 287–319.

Hicks, Karen:
1994   *Surviving the Dalkon Shield IUD: Women vs. the Pharmaceutical Industry.* New York: Teachers College Press.

Himes, Norman E.:
1936   *Medical History of Contraception.* Baltimore: Williams and Wilkins.

Hodgson, Dennis:
1990   The Ideological Origins of the Population Association of America. *Population and Development Review* 17: 1–34.

Hogben, Lancelot:
1974   Francis Albert Eley Crew, 1886–1973. *Biographical Memoirs of Fellows of the Royal Society* 20: 134–53.

Holmes, Helen Bequaert (ed.):
1992   *Issues in Reproductive Technology I: An Anthology.* New York: Garland.

Holmes, Helen, Betty B. Hoskins, and Michael Gross (eds.):
1980   *Birth Control and Controlling Birth: Women-Centered Perspectives.* Clifton, N.J.: Humana Press.

Hughes, Everett C.:
1971   *The Sociological Eye.* Chicago: Aldine Atherton.

Hunt, Marcia:
1996   Implant Controversy Grows. *San Francisco Chronicle,* April 4: A4.

International Working Group on Vaginal Microbicides:
1996   Recommendations for the Development of Vaginal Microbicides. *AIDS* 10: UNAIDS1–UNAIDS6.

Kevles, Daniel J.:
1985   *In the Name of Eugenics: Genetics and the Uses of Human Heredity.* New York: Alfred A. Knopf.

Knaus, Hermann:
1934a   *Periodic Fertility and Sterility in Women.* Vienna: Wm. Maudrich.
1934b   *Periodic Fertility and Sterility in Woman: A Natural Method of Birth Control.* Chicago: Chicago Medical Book.

Koch, Ellen B.:
1995   Why the Development Process Should Be Part of Medical Technology Assessment: Examples from the Development of Medical Ultrasound. In Arie Rip, Thomas J.

Misa, and Johan Schot (eds.), *Managing Technology in Society: The Approach of Constructive Technology Assessment,* 231–63. London and New York: Pinter/St. Martin's Press.

Kopp, Marie E.:

1933   *Birth Control in Practice: Analysis of Ten Thousand Case Histories of the Birth Control Clinical Research Bureau.* New York: Robert M. McBride.

Kuiper, Heather, Suellen Miller, Elena Martinez, Lisa Loeb, and Philip Darney:

1997   Urban Adolescent Females' Views on the Implant and Contraceptive Decision-Making: A Double Paradox. *Family Planning Perspectives* 29(4): 167–72.

Kuo, Lenore:

1998   Secondary Discrimination as a Standard for Feminist Social Policy: Norplant and Probation, a Case Study. *Signs: Journal of Women in Culture and Society* 23(4): 907–44.

Langley, L. L. (ed.):

1973   *Contraception: Benchmark Papers in Human Physiology.* Stroudsburg, Penn.: Dowden, Hutchinson and Ross.

Latour, Bruno:

1991   *We Have Never Been Modern.* Translated by Catherine Porter. Cambridge: Harvard University Press.

Laughlin, Harry:

1976   Model Eugenical Sterilization Law of 1922. In Carl Bajema (ed.), *Eugenics Then and Now.* Benchmark Papers in Genetics/5. Stroudsburg, Penn.: Dowden, Hutchinson, and Ross, 1976.

Lillie, Frank R.:

1938   Zoological Sciences in the Future. *Science* 88 (July 22): 65–72.

Lissner, Elaine A.:

1992   Frontiers in Nonhormone Male Contraceptive Research. In Helen Bequaert Holmes (ed.), *Issues in Reproductive Technology I: An Anthology,* 53–70. New York: Garland.

Lock, Margaret, and Patricia A. Kaufert (eds.):

1998   *Pragmatic Women and Body Politics.* New York: Cambridge University Press.

Makepeace, A. W., C. L. Weinstein, and M. H. Freidman:

1937   The Effects of Progestin and Progesterone in Ovulation in the Rabbit. *American Journal of Physiology* 119: 512–16.

Marker, Russel E:

1986   The Early Production of Steroidal Hormones. *Center for the History of Chemistry News,* Spring, 3–6.

Marks, Lara:

1998   "A Cage of Ovulating Females": The History of the Early Oral Contraceptive Pill Clinical Trials, 1950–1959. In H. Kamminga and S. de Chardarevian (eds.), *Molecularising Biology and Medicine: New Practices and Alliances, 1910s–1970s.* Amsterdam: Harwood.

Marx, Preston A., A. Spira, A. Gettie, P. Dailey, R. Veazey, A. Lackner, C. J. Mahoney, C. Miller, L. Claypool, D. Ho, and N. Alexander:

1996   Progesterone Implants Enhance SIV Vaginal Transmission and Early Virus Load. *Nature Medicine* 2(10): 1084–89.

Mastroianni, Luigi Jr., Peter J. Donaldson, and Thomas T. Kane (eds.):

1990   Developing New Contraceptives: Obstacles and Opportunities. [NRC and IOM.] Washington, D.C.: National Academy Press.

McCabe, Michael:
  1998 Packard Foundation Gives $375 Million for Birth Control. *San Francisco Chronicle,* November 11: A8.
McCann, Carole R.:
  1994 *Birth Control Politics in the United States, 1916–1945.* Ithaca, N.Y.: Cornell University Press.
Meldrum, Marcia:
  1996 "Simple Methods" and "Determined Contraceptors": The Statistical Evaluation of Fertility Control, 1957–1968. *Bulletin of the History of Medicine* 70: 266–95.
Meyers, David W.:
  1970 *The Human Body and the Law: A Medico-Legal Study.* Chicago: Aldine.
Miller, Peter, and Nikolas Rose (eds.):
  1986 *The Power of Psychiatry.* Cambridge: Polity Press; New York: Blackwell.
Mintz, Morton:
  1985 *At Any Cost: Corporate Greed, Women, and the Dalkon Shield.* New York: Pantheon/Random House.
Mishell, Daniel R. Jr.:
  1998 Intrauterine Devices: Mechanisms of Action, Safety, and Efficacy. *Contraception* 58: 45S-53S.
Moench, Thomas R., Kevin J. Whaley, Timothy D. Mandrell, Barbara D. Bishop, Clara J. Witt, and Richard A. Cone:
  1993 The Cat/Feline Immunodeficiency Model for Transmucosal Transmission of AIDS: Nonoxynol-9 Contraceptive Jelly Blocks Transmission by an Infected Cell Inoculum. *AIDS* 7: 797–802.
Morsy, Soheir:
  1995 Maternal Mortality in Egypt: Selective Health Strategy and the Medicalization of Population Control. In Faye D. Ginsberg and Rayna Rapp (eds.), *Conceiving the New World Order: The Global Stratification of Reproduction,* 162–76. Berkeley: University of California Press.
Moskowitz, Ellen H., and Bruce Jennings (eds.):
  1996 *Coerced Contraception? Moral and Policy Challenges of Long-Acting Birth Control.* Washington, D.C.: Georgetown University Press.
National Science Foundation, Batelle Institute:
  1968/69 *Technology in Retrospect and Critical Events in Science* (*TRACES*) 1 (December 15, 1968) and 2 (January 30, 1969).
  1973 *Interactions of Science and Technology in the Innovative Process: Some Case Studies.* Final report/NSF-6667.
National Women's Health Network (NWHN):
  1985 *The Depo-Provera Debate: A Report by the National Women's Health Network.* Washington, D.C.: NWHN.
Notestein, Frank W.:
  1982 Demography in the United States: A Partial Account of the Development of the Field. *Population and Development Review* 8(4): 651–87.
Nye, Robert A.:
  1994 Love and Reproductive Biology in Fin-de-Siècle France: A Foucauldian Lacuna? In Jan Goldstein (ed.), *Foucault and the Writing of History,* 150–64. London: Blackwell.
Ogino, Kyusaku:
  1934 *Conception Period of Women.* Harrisburg, Penn.: Medical Arts Press.

Onorato, Suzanne:
    1991   The Population Council and the Development of Contraceptive Technologies. *Research Reports from the Rockefeller Archive Center* 1: 6–7.
Organizing Committee:
    1994   *Reproductive Health and Justice: International Women's Health Conference for Cairo '94, January 24–28, 1994, Rio De Janeiro.* New York: International Women's Health Coalition.
Oudshoorn, Nelly:
    1994   *Beyond the Natural Body: An Archeology of Sex Hormones.* London: Routledge.
    1995   Discourse Coalitions in Contraceptive Technologies: The Case of Male Contraceptives. Paper presented at meetings of the Society for Social Studies of Science, Charlottesville, Va.
    1996a The Decline of the One-Size-Fits-All Paradigm; or, How Reproductive Scientists Try to Cope with Postmodernity. In Nina Lyke and Rosi Braidotti (eds.), *Between Monsters, Goddesses, and Cyborgs: Feminist Confrontations with Science, Medicine, and Cyberspace,* 153–73. London: ZED Books.
    1996b A Natural Order of Things? Reproductive Sciences and the Politics of Othering. In George Robertson et al. (eds.), *Future Natural: Nature, Science, Culture,* 122–33. London: Routledge.
    1997a Shifting Boundaries between Industry and Science: The Role of the WHO in Contraceptive Development. In Jean-Paul Gaudiliere, Ilana Löwy, and D. Pestre (eds.), *The Invisible Industrialist: Manufacturers and the Construction of Scientific Knowledge.* London: Macmillan Press.
    1997b From Population Control Politics to Chemicals: The WHO as an Intermediary Organization in Contraceptive Development. *Social Studies of Science* 27: 41–72.
    1999   On Masculinities, Technologies, and Pain: The Testing of Male Contraceptive Technologies in the Clinic and the Media. *Science, Technology, and Human Values* 24(2): 265–89.
    2000   Drugs for Healthy People: The Culture of Testing and Approving Hormonal Contraceptives for Women and Men. London: Wellcome Institute.
 In prep. Bound by Culture: The Development of the Male Pill.
Parkes, A. S., and R. L. Noble:
    1938   Interruption of Early Pregnancy by Means of Orally Active Oestrogens. *British Medical Journal* 2: 557–59.
Paul, Julius:
    1973   State Eugenic Sterilization History: A Brief Overview. In Jonas Robitscher (ed.), *Eugenic Sterilization.* Springfield, Ill.: Charles Thomas.
Pauly, Philip J.:
    1987   *Controlling Life: Jacques Loeb and the Engineering Ideal in Biology.* New York: Oxford University Press.
    1993   Essay Review: The Eugenics Industry: Growth or Restructuring? *Journal of the History of Biology* 27: 131–45.
Perone, Nicola:
    1993   The History of Steroidal Contraceptive Development: The Progestins. *Perspectives in Biology and Medicine* 36(3): 347–62.
Petchesky, Rosalind Pollack, and Karen Judd (eds.):
    1998   *Negotiating Reproductive Rights: Women's Perspectives across Countries and Cultures.* In-

ternational Reproductive Rights Research Action Group (IRRRAG). London: Zed Books.

Piccinino, Linda J., and William D. Mosher:

1998 Trends in Contraceptive Use in the United States, 1982–1995. *Family Planning Perspectives* 30(1): 4–10, 46.

Pierpoint, Raymond:

1922 *Report of the Fifth International Neo-Malthusian and Birth Control Conference, London.* London: William Heinemann.

Pies, Cheri:

1997 The Ongoing Politics of Contraception: Norplant and Other Emerging Technologies. In Sheryl Burt Ruzek, Virginia L. Olesen, and Adele E. Clarke (eds.), *Women's Health: Complexities and Differences,* 520–46. Columbus: Ohio State University Press.

Pincus, Gregory:

1965 *The Control of Fertility.* New York: Academic.

Piotrow, Phyllis Tilson:

1973 *World Population Crisis: The United States' Response.* New York: Praeger.

Porter, Roy, and Lesley Hall:

1995 *The Facts of Life: The Creation of Sexual Knowledge in Britain, 1650–1950.* New Haven: Yale University Press.

Pramik, Mary Jean (ed.):

1978 *Norethindrone: The First Three Decades.* Palo Alto, Calif.: Syntex Laboratories.

Rakusen, Jill:

1981 Depo-Provera: The Extent of the Problem. In Helen Roberts (ed.), *Women, Health, and Reproduction,* 75–108. Boston: Routledge and Kegan Paul.

Ramirez de Arellano, Annette B., and Conrad Seipp:

1983 *Colonialism, Catholicism, and Contraception: A History of Birth Control in Puerto Rico.* Chapel Hill: University of North Carolina Press.

Randomsky, Michael L., Kevin J. Whaley, Richard A. Cone, and W. Mark Saltzman:

1992 Controlled Vaginal Delivery of Antibodies in the Mouse. *Biology of Reproduction* 47: 133–40.

Ravindran, T. K. Sundari, and Marge Berer:

1995 Contraceptive Safety and Effectiveness: Re-evaluating Women's Needs and Professional Criteria. *Reproductive Health Matters* 3: 6–12.

Reed, James:

1978 *From Private Vice to Public Virtue: The Birth Control Movement and American Society since 1830.* New York: Basic Books.

1984 *The Birth Control Movement and American Society: From Private Vice to Public Virtue.* 2d ed. Princeton: Princeton University Press.

Reilly, Philip R.:

1991 *The Surgical Solution: A History of Involuntary Sterilization in the United States.* Baltimore: Johns Hopkins University Press.

Reproductive Health Matters:

1993 Special Issue on Population and Family Planning Policies: Women-Centred Perspectives. *Reproductive Health Matters* 1 (May).

1995 Special Issue on Contraceptive Safety and Effectiveness: Re-Evaluating Women's Needs and Professional Criteria. *Reproductive Health Matters* 3 (May).

1996   *Beyond Acceptability: Users' Perspectives on Contraception.* London: Reproductive Health Matters for the World Health Organization.

Reynolds, Moira Davidson:

1994   *Women Advocates of Reproductive Rights.* Jefferson, N.C.: McFarland.

Richter, Judith:

1993   *Vaccination against Pregnancy: Miracle or Menace?* Amsterdam: Health Action International.

Riddle, John M.:

1992   *Contraception and Abortion from the Ancient World to the Renaissance.* Cambridge: Harvard University Press.

Riessman, Catherine Kohler:

1983   Women and Medicalization: A New Perspective. *Social Policy* 17(Summer): 3–18.

Ringheim, Karin:

1996   Whither Methods for Men? Emerging Gender Issues in Contraception. *Reproductive Health Matters* 7: 79–89.

Rip, Arie:

1986   Controversies as Informal Technology Assessment. *Knowledge* 8(2): 349–71.

Rip, Arie, Thomas J. Misa, and Johan Schot (eds.):

1995   *Managing Technology in Society: The Approach of Constructive Technology Assessment.* London and New York: Pinter/St. Martin's Press.

Robertson, A. F.:

1991   *Beyond the Family: The Social Organization of Human Reproduction.* Berkeley: University of California Press.

Robertson, William H.:

1989   *An Illustrated History of Contraception: A Concise Account of the Quest for Fertility Control.* Park Ridge, N.J.: Parthenon.

Robitscher, Jonas:

1973   *Eugenic Sterilization.* Springfield, Ill.: Charles Thomas.

Ruzek, Sheryl Burt:

1978   *The Women's Health Movement: Feminist Alternatives to Medical Control.* New York: Praeger.

Ruzek, Sheryl Burt, Virginia L. Olesen, and Adele E. Clarke (eds.):

1997   *Women's Health: Complexities and Differences.* Columbus: Ohio State University Press.

Saltzman, W. Mark, Michael L. Randomsky, Kevin J. Whaley, and Richard A. Cone:

1994   Antibody Diffusion in Human Cervical Mucus. *Biophysical Journal* 66 (February): 508–15.

Sanger, Margaret:

1919   Birth Control and Racial Betterment. *Birth Control Review* 3 (February): 11–12.

Sanger, Margaret (ed.):

1934   Biological and Medical Aspects of Contraception. American Conference on Birth Control and National Recovery. Washington, D.C.: National Committee on Federal Legislation for Birth Control.

Sanger, Margaret, and Hannah M. Stone (eds.):

1931   *The Practice of Contraception: An International Symposium and Survey.* Proceedings of the Seventh International Birth Control Conference, Zurich, 1930. Baltimore: Williams and Wilkins.

Schrater, Angeline Faye:
  1992 Contraceptive Vaccines: Promises and Problems. In Helen Bequaert Holmes (ed.), *Issues in Reproductive Technology I: An Anthology,* 31–52. New York. Garland.
Seaman, Barbara:
  1969 *The Doctors' Case against the Pill.* 2d ed. New York: Doubleday, 1980.
Seaman, Barbara, and Gideon Seaman:
  1977 *Women and the Crisis in Sex Hormones.* New York: Bantam.
Segal, Sheldon J.:
  1987 The Development of Modern Contraceptive Technology. *Technology in Society* 9: 277–82.
Sen, Gita, and Rachel C. Snow (eds.):
  1994 *Power and Decision: The Social Control of Reproduction.* Harvard Series on Population and International Health. Cambridge: Harvard School of Public Health/Harvard University Press.
Sen, Gita, Adrienne Germain, and Lincoln C. Chen (eds.):
  1994 *Population Policies Reconsidered: Health, Empowerment, and Rights.* Cambridge: Harvard University Press.
Setchell, Brian P. (ed.):
  1984 Male Reproduction. *Benchmark Papers in Human Physiology 17.* New York: Van Nostrand Reinhold.
Shapiro, Thomas M.:
  1985 *Population Control Politics: Women, Sterilization, and Reproductive Choice.* Philadelphia: Temple University Press.
Shelesnyak, M. C.:
  1963 Interdisciplinary Approaches to the Endocrinology of Reproduction. In Peter Eckstein and Frances Knowles (eds.), *Techniques in Endocrine Research,* 231–43. New York: Academic Press.
  1964 Exploration of Biological Bases for Fertility Control. In Selwyn Taylor (eds.), *Proceedings of the Second International Congress of Endocrinology, London.* Amsterdam and New York: Exerpta Medica Foundation.
  1966 Biodynamics and the Population Explosion. *Ariel* 13: 21–33.
  1974 Comments. In J. Meites, B. T. Donovan, and S. M. McCann (eds.), *Pioneers in Neuroendocrinology,* 269–78. New York: Plenum Press.
  1986 A History of Research on Nidation. *Annals of the New York Academy of Sciences* 476: 5–24.
Sherwood, Jill K., Larry Zeitlin, Kevin J. Whaley, Richard A. Cone, and Mark Saltzman:
  1996 Controlled Release of Antibodies for Long-Term Topical Passive Immunoprotection of Female Mice against Genital Herpes. *Nature Biotechnology* 14(4): 468–71.
Smith, M. G.:
  1926 On Interruption of Pregnancy by Injection of Ovarian Follicular Extract. *Bulletin of the Johns Hopkins Hospital* 39: 203–14.
Soloway, Richard A.:
  1995 The "Perfect Contraceptive": Eugenics and Birth Control Research in Britain and America in the Interwar Years. *Journal of Contemporary History* 30: 637–64.
Southam, Anna L.:
  1965 Historical Review of Intra-Uterine Devices. In S. J. Segal, A. Southam, and K. D.

Shafer (eds.), *Intra-Uterine Contraception: Proceedings of the Second International Conference.* International Congress Series no. 86. Amsterdam: Exerpta Medica Foundation.

Star, Susan Leigh, and James Griesemer:

1989   Institutional Ecology, "Translations," and Boundary Objects. *Social Studies of Science* 19: 387–420.

Stratton, Pamela, and Nancy Alexander:

1993   Prevention of Sexually Transmitted Infections: Physical and Chemical Barrier Methods. *Infectious Disease Clinics of North America* 7(4): 841–59.

Strauss, Anselm L.:

1993   *Continual Permutation of Action.* New York: Aldine de Gruyter.

Tietze, Christopher:

1962   Intra-Uterine Contraceptive Rings: History and Statistical Appraisal. In C. Tietze and S. Lewis (eds.), *Intra-Uterine Contraceptive Devices: Proceedings of the Conference,* 1–34. New York: Exerpta Medica Foundation.

1965a   *Bibliography of Fertility Control, 1950–1965.* Pub. no. 23. New York: National Committee on Maternal Health.

1965b   History and Statistical Evaluation of Intrauterine Contraceptive Devices. *Journal of Chronic Disease* 18: 1147–59.

Trussell, James:

1998   Contraceptive Efficacy of the Reality[R] Female Condom. *Contraception* 58: 147–48.

Tsing, Anna Lowenhaupt:

1993   *In the Realm of the Diamond Queen: Marginalities in Out-of-the-Way Places.* Princeton: Princeton University Press.

van Kammen, Jessica:

1999   Representing Users' Bodies: The Gendered Development of Anti-Fertility Vaccines. *Science, Technology, and Human Values* 24(3): 307–37.

Vaughan, Paul:

1970   *The Pill on Trial.* New York: Coward-McCann.

Voge, Cecil I. B.:

1933   *The Chemistry and Physics of Contraceptives.* London: Jonathan Cape.

Wajcman, Judy:

1991   *Feminism Confronts Technology.* University Park: Pennsylvania State University Press.

Walsh, Vivien:

1995   Social Criteria in the Commercialization of Human Reproductive Technology. In Arie Rip, Thomas J. Misa, and Johan Schot (eds.), *Managing Technology in Society: The Approach of Constructive Technology Assessment,* 261–83. London and New York: Pinter/St. Martin's Press.

Watkins, Elizabeth Siegel:

1998   *On the Pill: A Social History of Oral Contraceptives, 1950–1970.* Baltimore: Johns Hopkins University Press.

Weedman, Judith:

1998   The Structure of Incentives: Design and Client Roles in Application-Oriented Research. *Science, Technology, and Human Values* 23(3): 315–45.

Weingart, Peter:

1987   The Rationalization of Sexual Behavior: The Institutionalization of Eugenic Thought in Germany. *Journal of the History of Biology* 20(2): 159–93.

Weisman, Carol S.:
  1998   *Women's Health Care: Activist Traditions and Institutional Change.* Baltimore: Johns
         Hopkins University Press.
Westoff, Charles F.:
  1994   What's the World's Priority Task? Finally, Control Population. *New York Times Magazine,* February 6, 29–30.
Whaley, Kevin J., Ruth A. Barratt, Larry Zeitlin, Timothy E. Hoen, and Richard A. Cone:
  1993   Nonoxynol-9 Protects Mice against Vaginal Transmission of Genital Herpes Infections. *Journal of Infectious Diseases* 168: 1009–11.
Woolgar, Steve:
  1991   Configuring the User: The Case of Usability Trials. In John Law (ed.), *A Sociology of Monsters: Essays on Power, Technology, and Domination,* 57–102. New York: Routledge.
World Health Organization Task Force on Methods for the Regulation of Male Fertility:
  1995   Contraceptive Efficacy of Testosterone-Induced Azoospermia or Oligozoospermia in Normal Men. *Fertility and Sterility* 65: 821–29.
Wyatt, T. L., K. J. Whaley, R. A. Cone, and W. M. Saltzman:
  1998   Antigen Releasing Polymer Rings and Microspheres Stimulate Mucosal Immunity in the Vagina. *Journal of Controlled Release* 50(1): 93–102.
Zeitlin, L., K. J. Whaley, T. A. Hegarty, T. R. Moench, R. A. Cone, et al.:
  1997   Tests of Vaginal Microbicide in the Mouse Genital Herpes Model. *Contraception* 56(5): 329–35.
Zimmerman, Mary K.:
  1987   The Women's Health Movement: A Critique of Medical Enterprise and the Position of Women. In Beth B. Hess and Myra Marx Ferree (eds.), *Analyzing Gender: A Handbook of Social Science Research,* 442–73. Newbury Park: Sage.

3
Do Users Matter?

Jessika van Kammen

Most contraceptives have been developed for use by women. The methods available to women include diaphragms, the female condom, various intrauterine devices including some that release hormones, a variety of oral, injectable, and implantable hormone preparations, prolonged breastfeeding, periodical abstinence, sterilization, and various forms of emergency contraception. Men may choose periodical abstinence, coitus interruptus, or condoms, a technology first described some four hundred years ago.[1] More recently, different forms of male sterilization have become available.

Reproductive technologies profoundly affect women's lives. Therefore it is not surprising that the women's health movement studies them closely and that the involvement of users in the field of contraceptive development is especially important to them.[2] The development of modern contraceptive methods started to flourish after World War II and almost immediately became highly politicized (Clarke 1998). Most modern contraceptives have been developed within a framework of population control. Within this framework, the premises were that there is a problem of overpopulation, that contraceptives were a relevant technology to curtail population growth, and that especially the growth of poor populations in Third World countries should come to a stop. In the 1980s, women's health advocates documented recurrent instances of the coercive and/or misleading administration of contraceptive methods that had occurred in the context of population control programs, especially in Third World countries. These practices and the reactions of women's health advocates have been comprehensively reported and analyzed by Hartmann (1987). The other major concern of the women's health advocates has been the neglect of women's health and the biomedical standards for assessing safety and efficacy in contraceptive development (Mintzes 1992; Hardon 1992). Without equating female users with women's health advocates, the incessant critique of contraceptive development seems to indicate that women's experiences and perspectives were not sufficiently taken into account.

It seems to me that those who use a technology should have some say in its design. How, then, have female users been involved in the design of contraceptive methods? My claim is that if we wish to improve users' involvement in technological development, then we need to understand precisely how the involvement of users is constituted and sustained, from a technology's initial design to its eventual use. In this essay I study whether and how women have played a role in the incipient period of antifertility vaccine development.

Immunological contraceptives are still being developed.[3] Users do not matter only once a technology is in use. Users are involved from the inception of technology development. Madeleine Akrich (1992) argues that innovators "inscribe" their hypotheses about users into the technical content of the new technology. Technologies therefore contain a script: together with the actors and the settings in which they are supposed to act, technical objects define a framework of action. The projected users, according to the designers, are anticipated in the script. How were users involved in the design of antifertility vaccines? How did representations of users mediate in the designers' configuring of immunological contraceptives and their future users?[4]

The future end users of immunological contraceptives are the women who will be injected to regulate their fertility. Clearly, these potential users exist in an infinite variety of social, cultural, and personal settings. Moreover, as Akrich (1995, 174) signals, "'the user' is not a single entity taken on board when the project is launched, but a set of disparate characteristics which will not necessarily merge into a tight configuration ready to accommodate the definitive end user." Much work has to be done to represent users in such a way that they can guide innovators in developing new technologies.

By whom and how were different representations of end users of immunological contraceptives construed and what was their content? Akrich describes different *techniques* by which innovators generate representations of users. She distinguishes explicit techniques that are legitimized by a formal scientific and conceptual basis from implicit techniques of a more empirical kind, which lack such a legitimation. Explicit techniques include marketing surveys, consumer testing, and feedback on experience through after-sales services. The less formal techniques Akrich describes are the designers' reliance on personal experience, reliance on expert-consultants, and the adoption or rejection of representations present in products considered to have something in common with the innovation at hand. She then describes different strategies by which the divergent representations of users can be reconciled and integrated into the design. Akrich's study makes very clear that a range of different user representations are produced in designing a technology and that these representations have to be made compatible in the course of the developmental process. However, Akrich does not analyze how certain representations of users become more influential than others in certain circumstances. This last issue is important, since it could shed light on ways in which the involvement of users could be improved. In addition to Akrich's work, I will show how certain representations of users became embedded in the institutional context of contraceptive research and exerted a considerable influence on the development of new fertility regulating methods.

In order to further demonstrate how representations of users can accomplish the (implicit and explicit) guiding of researchers' work, I will call upon Joan Fujimura's (1987, 1992) concept of the *doability* of research. She describes the achievement of doability of research in terms of the alignment of three levels of work organization: the social world, the laboratory, and the experiment. Scientists make these levels fit together by a process of articulation: the organization and coordination of resources, the planning and allocation of tasks, the structuring and labeling of problems. Fujimura asserts that by the creation of packaged pieces of work (physical apparatus, standard procedures, and the like), the amount of articulation work between levels decreases, and this in turn facilitates the making of doable research problems. I will show that representations of users too are packageable and transferable and thereby condition the making of doable research problems. I will also explore other functions of representations of users.

Research on immunological methods to regulate fertility began in the early 1970s. Unlike hormonal methods, the immunological mechanism of action causes temporary infertility by provoking the production of antibodies against substances necessary to human reproduction, such as certain hormones and molecules of the sperm and the ovum. About 10 percent of the public funding available for research on new contraceptives is spent on antifertility vaccines (WHO/HRP 1993). The researchers involved are located in various contraceptive research institutions, predominantly in India and the United States. Their activities are coordinated by the World Health Organization (WHO), the Indian National Institute of Immunology, the American National Institute for Child Health and Development/National Institutes of Health (NICHD/ NIH), and the Population Council in the United States. The research is supported by public and private foundations (Richter 1996).

In the 1970s, nonprofit organizations were becoming important actors in the field of contraceptive development.[5] They directed their efforts mostly toward developing countries. One of them was the World Health Organization's

Human Reproduction Program (HRP). The WHO was the first institution to organize the research network for the development of immunological contraceptives, and it continues to be a main actor in this field. For this essay, I will concentrate on the creation of a research group at the WHO and its research program on immunological contraceptives.

First, I describe the actors that brought their users' representations into the setting up of the research program and show how some of these spokespersons became more solidly embedded within WHO than others. Then I will characterize what these representations looked like. I will conclude by analyzing the functions that representations of users accomplished in the emerging research on immunological contraceptives, and I will discuss some implications of my findings for the involvement of users in the design of new contraceptives.

WHO'S SETTING UP OF RESEARCH ON IMMUNOLOGICAL CONTRACEPTIVES

Criteria for Determining Priorities

The birth of the Special Program for Research, Development, and Research Training in Human Reproduction (HRP)[6] can be dated to November 1971, when its advisory group first met. Until then, WHO had been primarily a policy-oriented organization, and conducting research would be a new kind of activity. On the request of member states of the WHO, a feasibility project was conducted between November 1970 and April 1971 to look into the viability of an international agency like WHO undertaking research in the area of human reproduction. As Nelly Oudshoorn (1994, 114–17) describes in relating the story of the making of the Pill, the subject of family planning had been a controversial area of research. This was partly due to its relationship with the taboo-laden subject of sexuality.[7] In the 1960s, the status of family planning had begun to change. The governments of the United States and Europe came to consider population growth as a problem in itself and fertility regulating technologies as a possible solution (Clarke 1990, 21).[8] Research on fertility regulating methods therefore started to receive increasing support and legitimacy. The WHO also played an active part in achieving this transformation by defining the deficiencies in knowledge about human reproduction as a major public health problem and therefore as an appropriate area of attention for this organization (Oudshoorn 1998).

The feasibility project was financed by one of the member states, Sweden, and the Ford Foundation. For this project, staff and consultants to WHO met with scientists, research strategists, and administrators at seventy institutions in twenty-three countries (Kessler 1991, 47–48). Subsequently, the HRP was set up. There was a series of consultations on the design and function of the HRP by an advisory group consisting of representatives of member states, scientists, research administrators, and staff from WHO. Most of them had extensive experience in contraceptive-related research, both in academic and industrial settings. The eleven biomedical scientists clearly outnumbered the one sociologist/demographer in the advisory group.

Almost immediately after its foundation, the problem of determining priorities became acute for the HRP. The HRP advisory group specified the following factors to determine the suitability for inclusion in the HRP of any particular component or line of research:

1. Demand: explicit request from the WHO Member States, donors, intergovernmental agencies other than WHO;
2. Need and scientific rationale: as perceived by the scientific community;
3. Applicability: extent to which the results of the activity could be expected to have an impact on family planning;
4. Rationale for WHO being involved: distinctive contribution expected because of WHO's intergovernmental and impartial nature;
5. Feasibility: given available knowledge, manpower, and facilities and, for institution strengthening, the extent of governmental commitment;
6. Time and cost: financial investment and length of time needed to complete projects;
7. Duplication of work: whether research was also being conducted by other agencies, industry, etc. (Kessler 1991, 51)[9]

This is an intriguing list. It shows us which spokespersons were involved in HRP's decision making and which actors did not participate. The list indicates who was entitled to bring representations of users into the research on fertility regulation. Items 1 and 2 explicitly present to us some of the spokespersons whose needs and demands were to be taken into account: member states and the scientific community. Item 3 does not mention a specific actor; on the contrary, it explicitly leaves out who is going to speak for the impact on family planning. Will this be family planning organizations, health care providers, or other candidates? Items 4 through 7 are of a different order, reflecting the way in which WHO perceives its role as an intergovernmental organization acting as the directing and coordinating authority for international health matters and international health, with the HRP to support research and institutional strengthening in the area of fertility regulation. These items also point to HRP's positioning in the international field of research on fertility regulation.

I will now take a closer look at the two highest ranking criteria on this list.

I will also examine which other spokespersons HRP enrolled to bring users' representations to the stage and analyze which spokespersons became dominant.

HRP's Spokespersons

Demands of Member States

The most important criterion was the demands of member states. Member states made their wishes known through the World Health Assembly, directly to the HRP through WHO's regional committees and at ad hoc consultations at national and regional levels (WHO/HRP/AG 1979, 4). WHO is an intergovernmental organization. The request of member states was the raison d'être of the HRP. Some of the member states were also major donors to the HRP, which meant that their suggestions for areas of needed research required a response from the HRP. But to operationalize their demands was not an easy task. The member states differed widely in their requests. As the HRP stated in its specification of this first criterion: "In a sense this is a political criterion. The difficulty lies in rating the political importance to the Programme of requests from different sources, e.g., one request only, but from a large country such as India, or five requests from small African countries, or from the Vatican" (WHO/HRP/AG 1979, 6). There were considerable differences in the viewpoints of the member states. According to the introduction to the 1979 annual report:

> The hardware enthusiasts consider that the answer to the problems arising in family planning lies in better birth control technology. . . . The software advocates point out that, where motivation is high and the service infrastructure satisfactory, currently available methods are largely adequate. . . . The third group recognizes the shortcomings of both hardware and software, and their mutual interdependence. . . . All three viewpoints are represented among the Member States of WHO. (WHO/HRP 1979, 7–8).

This multiplicity of demands of member states had to be structured into a research program. Within the HRP, several task forces were set up by the advisory group. A task force consisted of an international, interdisciplinary group of scientists and clinicians collaborating in research oriented toward a specific set of predetermined goals and objectives (Griffin 1991, 166). When new demands from governments and donors arose, such as the assessment of currently available fertility regulating methods or problems in delivering family planning care, new task forces were set up (Kessler 1991, 50). In this way, consensus was maintained. As a consequence, separate task forces were created for the study of the safety and effectiveness of current methods of family planning and the development of new birth control technologies on the one side, and the acceptability of different methods of fertility regulation on the other. Meetings for the coordination of the research with other agencies involved in family planning (such as the UNFPA, the World Bank, and the Population Council) were convened along these same lines: one to deal with biomedical studies, and the other for psychosocial and service delivery research (Kessler 1991, 56).

To maintain its status as an apolitical agency, HRP had to practice an encompassing strategy at the policy-making level. Different voices from the member states were addressed through separate working areas in task forces so that confrontations between opposing forces could be avoided. The relationship between biomedical research and psychosocial and service research was not at all equal. For example, in 1976, within the US$10,000,000 available for research and development, HRP set aside only US$700,000 for psychosocial and service research (Kessler 1991, 56). The biomedical perspective of the hardware enthusiasts acquired a better equipped position than that of their psychosocially oriented counterparts.

Need According to the Scientific Community

The second item on the list of criteria for priority setting was the need and scientific rationale as conceived by members of the scientific community who sat on WHO's Advisory Committee on Medical Research[10] and the steering committees of the HRP's task forces (WHO/HRP/AG 1979, 4). Who was included in this scientific community, and what status did they procure vis-à-vis member states?

The research component of the HRP had been structured in three broad areas: the safety and effectiveness of current methods of fertility regulation, development of a variety of new methods, and psychosocial aspects of family planning. The scientific community took the lead in developing new methods. This is reflected in the HRP's 1979 annual report. The need for psychosocial and health service research was underscored in general terms by referring to the wide recognition of its importance. Similarly, research on available methods was reported to have been demanded by a whole range of actors, including the World Health Assembly, individual member states, multilateral organizations, and national agencies providing contraceptives to developing countries. Clinicians and scientists were mentioned at the end of the row. In the development of new methods, however, biomedical scientists pronouncedly manifested themselves: "The scientific community continues to be practically unanimous in pointing to the dangers and crudeness of presently available birth control technology, and of its failure to meet the wide range of individual needs, cultural requirements and service constraints. In the past year, this point of view has been expressed repeatedly and eloquently by such authorities as Diczfalusy, Djerassi, Segal and Short [references given]" (WHO/HRP 1979, 69).

The scientific community was represented by a number of authoritative biomedical scientists.[11] In contrast with the very general and dissenting demands of member states, these biomedical scientists readily agreed upon their far more specific needs. One of the scientists who became involved in the establishment of the HRP in 1972 was the physician Patrick Rowe. Rowe had previously been in charge of clinical research for the pharmaceutical firm G. D. Searle. In a 1995 interview, he told me, "The donor countries never dictated us to have these specific task forces formulated. They agreed on the overall objectives of the program. . . . We were looking at a number of different research leads. When you get into the more scientific and more sophisticated area, you have a committee that assesses these research lines. . . . The recommendations of the committee were then endorsed by the director of the program and by the director general of WHO" (Rowe 1995).

While the member states voiced the demand for new methods of fertility regulation, the scientific community provided the answer to the question of *which* methods should be developed. Therefore, they were in a favorable position to attune their interest in developing new methods to the needs that they perceived in the field of fertility regulation.

Immunological contraceptives were very attractive both to the WHO and to the scientists. In 1972 in Alma-Ata, the WHO had adopted Primary Health Care as a general approach to achieve Health for All in the Year 2000. The Primary Health Care strategy included family planning as a basic component (Alma-Ata Declaration 1972). Immunological contraceptives could be presented as low technology by emphasizing the method's ease of provision by paramedical personnel in family planning programs, its simplicity of use, and the low costs (WHO/HRP 1976, 6; WHO/HRP 1978, 3). This profile of immunological contraceptives fitted the features of a Primary Health Care strategy. At the same time, the immunological approach to family planning was totally new. Therefore, the scientists could argue that a large number of basic research questions needed answers (WHO/HRP 1974, 24; WHO/HRP 1975, 11). Scientists of the Task Force on Immunological Methods for Fertility Regulation pleaded for the inclusion of this basic research into their program. For example, at their first meeting in July 1973, they stated, "It is apparent that we need additional information on the immune response to a variety of antigens as it is evoked in various components of the female reproductive tract. . . . We propose a meeting of suitable workers and experts in the field to consider such topics . . . to consider the implementation of the crucial preliminary studies" (WHO/HRP/SC 1973, 24).

Subsequently, the HRP did convene a symposium. Here, the scientists discussed the issue of their need for more fundamental research. The veteran reproductive scientist and WHO consultant Egon Diczfalusy introduced the meeting and prudently addressed the importance of more basic research in the field of the two major disciplines involved, endocrinology and immunology. Diczfalusy said, "The role of these highly specific proteins in human endometrial function in general and in the process of implantation in particular remains to be established. Their continued study may perhaps offer a new lead for the development of an immunological method of fertility control" (Diczfalusy 1975, 22). "Indeed, a better understanding of the underlying immunological phenomena might offer a promising lead for the development of new methods for interfering with implantation" (25).[12]

The American sociologist Adele Clarke made a comprehensive analysis of strategies that researchers involved in contraceptive development use in order to go on doing what they think is scientifically most challenging. She also found that the involvement of reproductive scientists in the development of contraceptive technologies was based on a quid pro quo. "The driving force behind the development of 'scientific' means of contraception was and remains reproductive scientists' desire for professional autonomy as 'basic' scientists" (Clarke 1998, 48). The volatility of the nonexisting method, presented as low technology and yet requiring a lot of complex basic research, meant that immunological contraceptives could meet the wishes of both the scientists and the WHO. Moreover, doing research, especially biomedical research on a considerable scale, was a relatively new activity for the WHO (Kessler 1991, 50). This created the space in which biomedical scientists could become the backbone of the HRP, which came to depend on their notion of promising research leads.[13]

I will now move on to the third criterion for HRP's priority setting that the advisory group formulated: applicability. Who was in charge of assessing applicability?

Comparable Current Methods

The criterion of applicability that the advisory group formulated related the work of the HRP explicitly to the context of family planning programs. But HRP didn't specify who would elaborate this criterion. Strikingly, it was not organizations of family planning programs that would give a voice to the criterion of applicability within the HRP. The advisory group had clear ideas about what kind of studies could be expected to have an impact on family planning: "For example, for current methods, high rating would be given to safety and effectiveness studies of methods practiced on a wide scale or to studies removing fear from an otherwise highly acceptable method. For new methods, this rating reflects the extent to which the new method is an improvement over the most closely comparable current method and also the extent to which it would increase the number of family planning acceptors" (WHO/HRP/AG 1979, 8).

Thus, current fertility regulating methods were appointed to act as spokespersons for potential end users of a new method. Akrich (1995, 174) describes this implicit technique of representing users as "calling up the particular representation of the user incorporated in the comparable product." But current fertility regulating methods cannot speak. This spokesperson thus depended on actors entitled to call up users of products that could be defined as comparable.

By channeling the assessment of applicability through comparable existing products, the range of actors authorized to appraise this criterion was extended beyond family planning programs. Evaluating applicability no longer depended on experience in applying fertility regulating methods but on being able to call up a comparable product. In this way, the expertise of family planning programs was degraded and other actors could appropriate the assessment of applicability. The marginalizing of the expertise of family planning programs had another effect: the supply of products that could be declared comparable was extended beyond fertility regulating methods to include other products that could be defined as having something in common with the new method at hand, such as (antidisease) vaccines. I will show later that the biomedical scientists who were designing immunological contraceptives extensively relied on the technique of representing users by calling up the users implied in comparable products.

What happened with the other actors who could have claimed competence in assessing applicability: the social scientists?

Social Scientists: A Variety of Needs

The HRP also employed an explicit technique to generate representations of users. The initial HRP advisory group foresaw a role for social scientists: they were expected to indicate what characteristics would make a fertility regulating method acceptable. As HRP director Alexander Kessler wrote, "There was also to be a Task Force on the characteristics of different methods of fertility regulation that affect their acceptance in various sociocultural settings: social scientists were to provide specifications for desirable methods to be realized by their biomedical colleagues" (Kessler 1991, 48).

Two task forces involved social scientists. The Task Force on Psychosocial Research in Family Planning focused on the range of cultural, social, economic, and psychological factors that influence couples' decisions regarding the timing, spacing, and numbers of births and their use of family planning services (WHO/HRP 1979, 89). Meanwhile, the Task Force on Health Service Research in Family Planning was developing strategies and approaches to the delivery of family planning care and to the assessment of their efficacy and impact (WHO/HRP 1979, 98).

These task forces discovered that users' expressed needs and preferences for contraceptive methods varied widely among countries and specific settings.[14] This finding, acceptable to all parties, was readily adopted by the HRP:

> The Advisory Group reaffirmed the objectives of the program:
> —To provide Member States with a *variety* of safe, effective and acceptable fertility regulating methods to meet differing needs and different situations. (WHO/HRP 1976, 6)

The need for a variety of methods does not necessarily imply the development of new methods. But the discourse on variation in users' preferences in different settings legitimized the need for new methods. The biomedical scientists reasoned that a variety of methods was the appropriate solution to meet the diverse needs and preferences of users. They could therefore formulate the problem as the need for a wide variety of new fertility regulating methods (WHO/HRP 1977, 7).

To further legitimize the development of new methods, the biomedical scientists needed to define a product specification that would correspond to a demand. They therefore needed some clues about users' needs and preferences. If the explicit techniques of the social scientists were the only source of information on acceptability of contraceptive methods, biomedical scientists could have selected from among the preferences that social scientists were identifying. They could have left aside other users' preferences, as they were not developing the ideal contraceptive anyway. However, the biomedical scientists needed some reassurance that the new methods they envisioned indeed would be acceptable. Therefore, an additional implicit technique became articulated through another actor in the HRP: the clinicians in the task force steering committees.

Clinicians as Spokespersons for Users

Each task force had a steering committee,[15] which met approximately once a year to figure out what the precise research of that task force should be, generate research proposals, identify appropriate people, and discuss the results as they came in. The steering committee of the Task Force on Immunological Methods for Fertility Regulation included reproductive biologists, immunologists, and clinicians. The clinicians were needed to conduct clinical trials. They would advise the task force on the study design and the execution of the trial and interpret the results. But the clinicians on the steering committee had a dual task. David Griffin, manager of the Task Force on Immunological Methods for Fertility Regulation since 1975, told me:

> They were expected to provide their own expertise, and many of them were research clinicians who knew what the research process was about and they were engaged in the research and so on. But they were also looked to by the pure scientists, who are working in academic laboratories, who never come across patients in their work, as somebody who should be able to reflect the likely responses of people in their clinics if these methods were available. It was an interface, but it wasn't . . . based on any valid data. The sort of thing we would expect them to say is, "For God's sake, don't develop a vaccine that is going to inhibit ovulation or that is going to disrupt the menstrual cycle." This kind of very broad issues. But they were never recorded in there [in the minutes of Steering Committee meeting]. (Griffin 1995)

Thus, clinicians were expected by the other scientists to act as spokespersons for the users. Various authors have pointed to the "dual mission" of clinical practice in producing medical technologies and knowledge. Clinicians have both a professional and a scientific assignment: to care for their patients and to develop knowledge claims. They therefore can switch their framework and use scientific arguments as well as arguments based on clinical experience (Hiddinga 1995; Gelijns 1991). In the development of immunological contraceptives, clinicians became the embodiment of this reciprocal relationship between science and practice in the clinic. They alternated between their representations of users without making them explicit, without setting down their statements about users in minutes or other texts. Clinicians themselves were the packages by the means of which their representations of users became transferable.

■

In sum, I have described how member states, biomedical and social scientists, and clinicians were enrolled in the HRP. Organizations of family planning programs were put in the background. Within the organizational structure of the HRP, the biomedical scientists achieved an advantageous position to promote their perception of needs in the field of fertility regulation and to develop new methods. The clinicians enjoyed a special position in the Task Force on Immunological Methods for Fertility Regulation, thanks to their ability to predict whether a new method would be useful in the clinic. The representations of users of other candidate spokespersons became less well embedded in the institution. WHO member states and donors to the HRP, although formally at the top of the organization, in practice were too divided to direct the course of the research program. The social scientists were explicitly asked to examine the needs and preferences of users. But they were set aside in separate task forces, and their very general recommendation to offer a variety of methods did not give guidance to the biomedical scientists. On the contrary, the biomedical scientists mobilized this recommendation to account for the development of new methods.

Significantly, no representatives of contraceptive users in what Akrich (1995, 168) calls the "political sense" were present at the establishment of the HRP. The obvious candidates to act as political representatives of users would have been people involved in the women's health movement. But women's health advocates were not enlisted by the HRP.

Users were brought into the priority setting for research areas by various "cognitive representations," though. Here I will discuss the contents of these representations of future users that the various spokespersons to HRP had brought to the stage.

Representations of Users in Setting Up the HRP

Both the social and the biomedical scientists made use of the opportunity to define new products in terms of their relationship to comparable products. For the social scientists, studying the acceptability of a new method that did not yet exist presented a major methodological problem in that it was necessarily speculative.[16] Social scientists sidestepped this difficulty by studying the acceptability of *attributes* of existing methods. They issued questionnaires to the clients of family planning services. Their interviews dealt with attributes, such as the timing and duration of use, perceived effectiveness, probable effects on menstruation, and reliability of the methods (WHO/HRP 1979, 91–94). By focusing on such attributes of fertility regulating methods, the social scientists further specified the level on which products could be compared.

Studying these attributes of existing methods is not the only way to predict the acceptability of new methods. If women's health advocates had been enrolled, they might have proposed different ways to learn about users' needs and preferences. On the basis of their critique of the development and provision of contraceptives, they might have called attention to the importance of studying the contexts in which contraceptives are used in terms of women's health and rights. From the perspective of women's health advocates, other possibilities to generate representations of users might have emerged, such as to point out repeating mechanisms in contraceptive use or to indicate relevant categories of users. The social scientists did not examine the trade-offs between the attributes negotiated by users. As a result of the specific way in which the social scientists studied the users, the technical artifact itself was highlighted and not its uses or contexts or meanings. In contrast to any of the other possibilities, the decontextualized attributes that social scientists presented fitted nicely into the researchers' framework of concentrating on the artifact.

Not to specify for whom the method was meant or in which context it would be most useful had a number of advantages for the researchers. If they had specified that the method was meant for people of, for example, a certain sex, region of the world, stage in their reproductive life cycle, or socioeconomic stratum, the potential market would have diminished. In addition, to direct their endeavors explicitly toward people in less developed countries was politically risky. This had become very clear at the international government meeting on population in Bucharest in 1974. Here, the relationship between control of population growth and development was vigorously debated. If the researchers had started to mention contexts in which the method might be particularly useful, other circumstances could appear and turn out to be relevant.[17] Now it could be maintained that new methods would serve "the betterment of mankind" (Segal 1976, 126) or "individuals worldwide" (Griffin 1992, 111). Focusing on certain attributes of contraceptive methods and leaving out contexts in which these were to be used provided the researchers with the space to construct, and if necessary reconstruct, the universal acceptability of the new method.

Attributes were exactly the level of specification that the researchers required to conceive an appealing product profile for the nonexisting immunological contraceptives. The researchers announced that this novel method would be long-acting and easy to use (Diczfalusy 1975, 32; Talwar 1976, 129; Hearn 1976, 158). There was no need to specify to whom those attributes would be attractive.

The member states provided representations of users as well. The demands of member states were further specified in the HRP's 1978 annual report: Research "aims to meet the expressed needs of Member States for technology for family planning and infertility cure that is safer, more effective, better adapted for the needs of their populations" (3).

In this early stage, the demands that member states expressed were understood to be the needs of their *populations*. Some states have a compelling interest in regulating the rate of increase of their populations. From the perspective of these states, the population at large will benefit from measures to bring down demographic trends. The product profile that the researchers proposed, a method that would be long-acting and easy to administer, was therefore very attractive to them. Population policy programs are apt to be directed toward women of developing countries. Betsy Hartmann has pointed out that "emphasis on population control profoundly affects how family planning programs are organized and implemented in the field" (1987, 60). It also has a major impact on the way in which contraceptive technologies are developed.

There was one other representation of users that had to be articulated in this process of reconciling different definitions of users: that of the clinicians in the steering committee for the Task Force on Immunological Methods for Fertility Regulation and the clinicians on the HRP advisory board.

Significantly, they were gynecologists/obstetricians and not andrologists. That was not surprising for the time. Oudshoorn has demonstrated that the successful making of the Pill in the 1950s and 1960s had reinforced gynecologists' networks in the field of contraceptive development. This gynecological infrastructure—the availability of medical practices and institutions and professions in which contraceptive development takes place—is gendered (Oudshoorn 1994, 138–41). Traditionally, gynecologists have specialized in the reproductive functions of the female. Andrology, gynecology's counterpart for the male body, did not become an established profession until the 1970s and it has remained a marginal field. With obstetrics/gynecology taking charge of indicating the practicality of new methods in the clinic, the stage was set for the development of these new contraceptive methods on the female body.

In sum, there was no need to be explicit about the users for whom the new methods were intended. If they were too specific about for whom and in what settings new methods were meant to be used, scientists could lose their highly desired flexibility. Instead, it could be maintained that these methods would suit everybody in any context. The representations of users of the social scientists were adopters and rejecters of existing contraceptive methods. The member states envisioned subjects of population policy. And the representations of users of the clinicians were visitors of family planning clinics. These representations of users could be reconciled in a specific category of users: Third World women.

The number of task forces that HRP established in this initial period fluctuated around twenty. One was the Task Force on Immunological Methods for Fertility Regulation. Now I will analyze what functions representations of users accomplished in HRP. How did representations of users through this specific task force determine the organization of certain parts of the research and not others? And why did the task force concentrate on a certain type of immunological contraceptive?

THE TASK FORCE ON IMMUNOLOGICAL METHODS FOR FERTILITY REGULATION

Biomedical scientists played a key role in the establishment of the Task Force on Immunological Methods for Fertility Regulation. Who were these scientists who deposited the research on immunological methods at HRP? And what functions did their specific representations of users perform as HRP adopted a major segment of the development of immunological contraceptives?

In the early 1970s, two scientists contributed decisively to the progress of the research on immunological methods for fertility regulation: Vernon Stevens at Ohio State University in Columbus, Ohio, and Pran Talwar at the National Institute of Immunology in New Delhi. By comparing the representations of users of these two scientists, I will illustrate the role of representations of users in defining the institutional workspace in which the research was carried out.

An Alternative to the Pill

Vernon Stevens was trained as a reproductive biologist. In 1962, he received a grant from G. D. Searle to test compounds for an alternative contraceptive pill. The Food and Drug Administration had approved the first oral contraceptive, Searle's Enovid, in 1960 (Gelijns 1991, 166). The acceptance of Enovid did not mean that testing and developing had come to an end (Oudshoorn 1994, 134). Although initially Searle had the oral contraceptive market to itself, by the mid-1960s Syntex—through its two licensees, Ortho and Parke-Davis, as well as through its own sales force established in 1964—had gained the major share of the U.S. oral contraceptive market (Djerassi 1979, 252).[18]

In this context, Searle became interested in the use of contraceptive pills in other countries. In 1964 the company sent Stevens to visit clinics in Italy, Greece, Turkey, Lebanon, Pakistan, Egypt, Thailand, and Singapore. The trip ended in Sydney, Australia, at a symposium on the introduction of oral contraceptives. In a 1995 interview, Stevens told me: "I realized that the education and motivation of women in developing countries to take pills in the prescribed way was insufficient. Moreover, there were the costs; at that time they could cost the equivalent of a whole year's income. . . . At the symposium, the clinicians pointed out all the medical problems and the side effects. There were still a lot of problems at that time." As a result, Stevens said, he became involved in immunological methods.

From the clinical trials onward, the scientists had difficulty persuading women to take the Pill in the prescribed manner (Oudshoorn 1994, 125–32). The costs of the then available compound and the occurrence of side effects prompted further research as well (Pincus et al., quoted in Oudshoorn 1994, 112–37). Stevens conceived the immunological means of birth control as an alternative for oral contraceptives: requiring less discipline from the users, costing less, and producing fewer medical side effects. In the late 1960s, Stevens was trying out different ways to develop an immunological method to regulate fertility.

Oudshoorn pointed out that although the Pill was developed as a universal, context-independent contraceptive, it nevertheless contained a specific user: "A woman, medicalised enough to take medication regularly, who is accustomed to gynecological examinations and regular visits to the physician, and who does not have to hide contraception from her partner. It goes without saying that this portrait of the ideal user is more likely to be found in western industrialised countries with a well developed health care system" (Oudshoorn 1998, 161). By the same token, the less educated and motivated women with less purchasing power for whom Stevens conceived his alternative approach are more likely to be located in developing countries. This is in line with Akrich's (1995) finding that the technique of representing users by defining a comparable product seems to be particularly appropriate in situations where the innovators themselves have previously worked on the development of a comparable product.

Stevens's representation of the users nicely matched with WHO's mandate to direct its efforts especially to the needs of developing countries.[19] Immunological methods were attractive to HRP, because the users that these contraceptives promised to address were the poor and less motivated women in developing countries. WHO's HRP also became a first-rate option for Stevens. As Rowe remarked to me, "The company was uninterested. They were into hormonal contraception, and they didn't have any expertise in terms of immunology. . . . And it got at stages in Stevens's work that he needed to get some external funding because baboons are expensive animals" (Rowe 1995).

Like most pharmaceutical industries, the company concentrated on the safer strategy of improving oral contraceptives for the home market. The difficult FDA requirements, the litigious public climate, and the increased costs for research and liability insurance made this long-term, high-risk research particularly unattractive to them (Djerassi 1979, 67–89).[20] Additionally, nonprofit organizations such as Planned Parenthood United States and international agencies such as WHO[21] and Planned Parenthood International bargained that a lower price for contraceptives should be charged to family planning programs in developing countries. This diminished the pharmaceutical companies' prospects for vast profits (Mastroianni, Donaldson, and Kane 1990).

Other suitable partners would have been any of the other major nonprofit institutions that supported research on contraceptive methods especially for developing countries, like the Population Council,[22] the U.S. Agency for International Development, or the National Institutes of Health. However, these U.S. based and partly U.S. government–funded institutions refrained from supporting research in the United States that could be considered related to abortion. And this was the case with Stevens's immunological approach to human chorionic gonadotropin (hCG), a hormone released by the fertilized egg soon after fertilization. It continues to be produced by the placenta. It stimulates the corpus luteum on the surface of the ovary to produce the hormone progesterone, which is necessary to prepare the uterus for the implantation of the fertilized egg and for the maintenance of pregnancy. So this would be a postfertilization method (Stevens 1995, 1:2–3).[23]

Immunological Contraceptives Gain Access to the HRP

In 1971 and 1972, the HRP organized a series of meetings at which scientists defined the task forces and what kind of projects to support. The HRP convened a consultation in August 1972 in Boston, where the feasibility of contraception by interfering with specific placental proteins at the time of implantation was discussed by reproductive biologists (WHO/HRP/SC 1973, 6). Just before, Rowe had moved from G. D. Searle to WHO to set up the HRP, and he invited Stevens to this meeting (Rowe 1995; Stevens 1995). Here, Stevens presented his pioneering work on immunological interference with hCG.

Stevens's contribution to the development of potential human applications of immunological birth control consisted of coupling a hormone or other substance necessary for reproduction to another substance. The modified molecule appears foreign to the immune system and elicits an immune reaction, not only against itself but also against the nonaltered hormone or other substance necessary for reproduction (Stevens 1973).[24] In our interview, Stevens (1995) recalled: "In the mid-1960s I established the fact that by chemically altering substances that were part of yourself, you could make them so that your body would raise immunity against them. . . . And then for some years thereafter I was looking for a target to use this principle again. I studied a lot of antigenic materials that compose the reproductive system. . . . I was just starting to focus in on hCG when the WHO program began in 1972."

Stevens had generated some data that nobody else could equal. He had developed the theory and conducted early experimentation; he had done laboratory work and set up a baboon colony for testing. Additionally, Stevens presented the findings from a clinical trial.[25] "The main thing was that we had preliminary data from a clinical trial to suggest that it would work. . . . In 1972, I took to them some data that I had generated before, that convinced enough people who took part in the decisions that this was a viable approach to develop new methods" (Stevens 1995).

Stevens had conducted a clinical trial among female prisoners in the United States before he was invited by the WHO. The data obtained in this study had not been published (Stevens 1996). These results were presented at the consultation meetings where the HRP was set up. Stevens had demonstrated that injection with the altered hCG effectively induced the formation of antibodies against unaltered hCG. The hormone hCG is necessary to preserve early pregnancy. It could be expected that antibodies against hCG would dispose of the hormone and thereby interrupt the establishment of pregnancy. This first clinical study also revealed an unexpected and less desirable side effect. Subsequent studies showed that the clinical trial participants did not ovulate. This possibly could be the effect of the immunization with the altered whole hCG (Stevens 1975, 364–65). Next, a more carefully designed study with control data was conducted. This clinical study suggested for the first time the applicability of an immunological approach to interfere with human reproduction (Stevens and Crystle 1973).

Stevens's approach was not readily embraced by the HRP. Early in 1973, Stevens presented his data again, this time before a panel of expert immunologists at Rockefeller University in New York. In the audience were two Nobel laureates in immunology who were supportive of Stevens's idea. Alexander Kessler had been working at Rockefeller University before he moved to WHO to set up the HRP, so he knew and respected these scientists (Stevens 1995). After this presentation, a definite plan of action for the Task Force on Immunological Methods for Fertility Regulation was drawn up (WHO/HRP/SC 1973, 6). In July 1973, Stevens got his first funding from the HRP, and his work has continued to receive support.

Shortly before this, the HRP had agreed to place emphasis on research and development efforts likely to yield results within a reasonable period of time (Kessler 1991, 50). What was so special in this new approach to change the recently established plans to give priority to short-term and medium-term research?

The WHO expected that the projected immunological method would meet all the requirements of an alternative for the pill. According to HRP's 1976 annual report, "A vaccine for fertility regulation has long held great appeal: it could provide long-term protection, be relatively simply to administer by paramedical personnel and be manufactured probably at low cost" (18).

Moreover, the potential impact on family planning programs was invariably considered to be high: "Because of the large number of questions that requires to be resolved, this development effort may be considered high risk and fairly long term (10–15 years). However, the impact of a vaccine, to be used either by men or women, especially in developing countries, would be so great as to warrant this involvement" (WHO/HRP 1974, 24).[26]

Thus, WHO's change in philosophy to include long-term research was facilitated by the fortunate correspondence between the users' representation in Stevens's projected method and HRP's desire to provide its member states with the means to have an impact on family planning. By allying his laboratory work with the concerns of WHO, Stevens created a doable research problem. Convincing the HRP to engage in such a risky undertaking as developing a completely new method would have been far more difficult if it had not been possible to relate the new method with existing methods that were perceived to have the same use, particularly the Pill. In contrast with the Pill, this method was foreseen to be long-acting. Its impact would not, like the Pill, depend on users' willingness to take one every day, nor, like the IUD, would it require insertion by trained medical personnel. And, as distinct from hormonal contraceptives, its manufacture costs were estimated to be low. Thus, the representation of users projected into existing contraceptives facilitated the alignment between the laboratory and the social world of policy making and financing. Representations of users could accomplish this role because they were packaged in a comparable method. By contrasting the vaccine with the former method, the user representation was transferred. Most packages Fujimura (1987) discusses are useful for aligning tasks at the level of the experiment with the laboratory. Representations of users are, therefore, an important addition. These can articulate the work between the laboratory and the social world of policy making and financing in the field of contraceptive development.

The alignment between the representations of users of Stevens and those of HRP made the research on immunological contraceptives doable. In contrast, Pran Talwar's research could not join the Task Force on Immunological Methods for Fertility Regulation. Nor could there be convergence between the technical objects that both innovators in the field of immunological contraceptives were designing.

Mobilizing the Vaccine Principle

Immunological contraceptives were specified not only as opposed to the Pill, but also as comparable to vaccines against disease. This was possible only after the development of the new product had been partly detached from the context of family planning programs. The list in HRP's 1976 annual report of reasons why a vaccine for fertility regulation would hold a great appeal contained an additional item: "It might also have great acceptability in view of the positive association that most people have with immunization" (18).

Where did this specification of immunological contraceptives originate? From its inception in 1972 onward, institution strengthening had been part of HRP's mandate. Several locations were assigned the status of WHO research and training centers, among them the All Indian Institute of Medical Sciences in New Delhi.[27] There, first as head of the department of biochemistry and then as head of the RTC in immunology, Talwar was also advancing the development of immunological methods of contraception (WHO/HRP/SC 1973, 27; Diczfalusy 1975, 370; Talwar 1976, 129).

In January 1974, Talwar received some β-hCG from Stevens. (Talwar 1976, 130; Stevens 1995). By then it had become clear that the use of the whole hCG molecule could lead to potentially dangerous cross-reactions with other hormones. Stevens had abandoned the use of whole hCG and now used only the β-subunit of hCG.[28] Talwar was also seeking a product with minimal cross-reactivity with other hormones, and he therefore purified and processed the β-hCG.[29] Additionally, in order to render the processed β-hCG more antigenic, Talwar linked the preparation with tetanus toxoid (TT) (Talwar 1976, 131; Talwar, Sharma, et al. 1976, 218). Talwar reports

> The choice of tetanus toxoid as a carrier for the present purpose was based on a number of considerations: (1) it is one of the purest bacterial antigens available and has a very low incidence of local reactions, discomfort and fever; (2) it evokes immunity of a duration which is advantageous for health care programmes; (3) it is approved for human use, and (4) tetanus is an appreciable health hazard, especially in developing countries. The present studies show that processed β-hCG-TT elicits antibodies not only to hCG but also against tetanus. It has thus a double benefit (Talwar, Sharma, et al. 1976, 221).[30]

By linking β-hCG to tetanus toxoid, Talwar had coupled immunological contraceptives with the principle of vaccination against disease. Tetanus toxoid was an effective immunogenic carrier. Conjugated to tetanus toxoid, the β-hCG could be made antigenic at lower doses than Stevens's hapten conjugated antigens. This innovation of Talwar was adopted by the WHO's Task Force on Immunological Methods for Fertility Regulation,[31] which repeatedly described the new technology as a form of immunization. For example: "Immunization as a prophylactic measure is now so widely accepted that it has been suggested that one method of fertility regulation which might have wide appeal as well as great ease of service delivery would be an anti-fertility vaccine" (WHO/HRP 1978, 360).

This transfer of the definition of antidisease vaccines as highly acceptable to immunological contraceptives is an example of what Rakow and Navarro call "ideologically and technically bundling" technologies (1993, 148). As Akrich indicates, defining the technologies under consideration as comparable implies the existence of relationships between the type of users incorporated in the equivalent products (1995, 174). What sort of user representation could immunological contraceptives inherit from antidisease vaccines?

Vaccines against diseases are meant to be widely applied, long-acting, inexpensive, and easy to administer. None of these characteristics contradicted the idea of creating an alternative for the Pill that WHO and Stevens had envisioned. In addition, as a prophylactic measure against diseases, the vaccination principle is effective and intended to be effective, not only on an individual level but also on the level of populations.[32]

Population Control: More and Less Outspokenly

In contrast to Stevens's search for an alternative for the Pill, Talwar's representation of the future users of immunological contraceptive was too outspokenly linked with population policy to bring his research program into alignment with that of the HRP's Task Force on Immunological Methods for Fertility Regulation. For example, in July 1974, the second International Congress of Immunology was held at Brighton on the contribution that immunology could make to the solution of some of the health problems of developing countries. Here, Talwar pointed out that the most pressing of all problems facing his own and other developing countries was to stem the growth of their populations. And desperate situations justified desperate remedies, he said (Lancet 1974, 633).

Faced with these drastic standpoints, the consensus-seeking WHO had to do a delicate moderating job in finding a way to relate to the work of Talwar's team. And hence, in the section on Collaborative Centers of the HRP's annual report of 1975 it says: "All Indian Institute. Research in this line [anti-hCG vaccine] has been carried out in parallel with, but separate from, the Task Force" (66).

On March 12, 1974, only a few months after he received the β-hCG, Talwar and his team started a clinical trial to test the immunogenicity of the processed β-hCG conjugated to tetanus toxoid. Four women were injected with this conjugate (Talwar, Sharma, et al. 1976, 220; Talwar, Kumar, et al. 1976, 254). This limited interval obviously was not enough time for Talwar's team to have been able to conduct the minimal safety and toxicology experiments with this novel preparation in animals, as was required by international guidelines before proceeding with clinical trials for the development of any drug for human use.[33] Further, WHO had decided that the possibility of cross-reactions even between the β-subunit of hCG and LH was too high to risk studies in humans (Stevens 1975, 371).[34] After this episode, the HRP funding to Talwar's team was solely for animal studies to assess the immunogenicity, efficacy, and safety of the conjugate of processed β-hCG to tetanus toxoid in laboratory rodents and non-human primates (WHO/HRP 1976, 111; WHO/HRP 1978, 144).

Talwar sought and found other allies. In 1951, India had been the first member state to ask the WHO to conduct research in family planning (Kessler 1991, 43). Since that year, the Indian government adopted the policy of supporting biomedical research as an essential component of the high priority family planning program (Segal 1976, 125–26). India had been the first country in the world to adopt a population policy to reduce the rate of growth by reducing fertility, and this policy was implemented as part of the first five-year plan in 1950–55. In 1966, India's population policy was integrated in the Family

Planning Department within the Ministry of Health and the budget was substantially increased (UN/DIESA 1992). As a member state, India had frequently requested birth control vaccines from WHO/HRP (WHO/HRP/AG 1979, 101). Talwar's representation of users as populations that had to be controlled massively and quickly coincided with that of the Indian government. Talwar and his team were supported by the Family Planning Foundation of India and, from 1976 on, the Population Council (Talwar 1976, 130).

Two Different Prototypes

Stevens's and Talwar's representations of users could not be reconciled in terms of the technical objects they were designing. Their representations of users did indeed shape the technological development. Stevens and his team went on to prepare a synthetic peptide, depicting a small part of the β-subunit of hCG that is exclusive to the hormone's chemical structure (Stevens 1975, 375). Warned by the unforeseen side effects of cross-reactions in the hurried first clinical trial, this task force scientist now preferred to err on the side of prudence. To render the synthetic peptide-prototype sufficiently antigenic, Stevens's approach required a time-consuming and expensive research program to identify suitable adjuvants, vehicles, and delivery systems that then had to be tested for their antifertility effect in baboons (WHO/HRP 1979, 86).

In spite of Stevens's conclusion that the use of entire β-hCG as an antigen would not overcome the problem of cross-reactivity with other hormones, Talwar and his team chose the entire β-subunit as the antigen. Talwar stressed the chemical differences between the β-subunit of hCG and the β-subunit of the most closely related other hormone, human LH (Talwar 1978, 19). On the basis of their clinical trial in four women, the Indian group argued that there was no evidence of cross-reactivity with other hormones at physiological levels (Talwar, Kumar, et al. 1976, 261). And certainly, the immunological response and contraceptive efficacy of this larger antigen was more elevated (Talwar and Gaur 1987, 1075; Stevens 1995).

Both researchers claimed to develop an immunological method that would be safe and effective. But the technology they developed differed significantly, with Stevens's group pursuing utmost safety and Talwar's team striving after maximum efficacy.

CONCLUSIONS

In this essay I have demonstrated that representations of users were indeed involved in the development of immunological contraceptives from the incipient period on. This means that attempts to improve the involvement of users should take the agenda-setting stage into account.

In setting up the Task Force on Immunological Methods for Fertility Regulation and its initial research program, the HRP enrolled states, biomedical scientists, clinicians, and social scientists. The enrolled actors could perform as spokespersons for the potential end users of the contraceptive method to be developed. Users were thus involved in the technology development in a cognitive sense. Family planning organizations or women's health advocates were not enlisted at this stage, and their cognitive representations of users were not taken into account. One way to improve users' involvement might be to allow these "silent implicated actors" (Clarke and Montini 1993) to bring their perspectives on future users to the stage. The women's health movement had been critically following contraceptive developments since the 1960s, and women's health advocates could be considered political representatives of users.

To include the representations of users of these groups would have required a more contextualized and therefore more complex set of users' representations. Because of the institutional embeddedness of certain representations, and the many enabling functions that representations of users perform, this analysis suggests that including these political representatives might entail a lot of work for all the actors involved. The end users of the new method were represented in various ways by the spokespersons: as users of comparable methods, as populations, and as visitors of family planning clinics. It could go without saying that women in Third World countries were at stake. The representations of users were kept as implicit as possible without losing their function of enabling the researchers' work. I have described three ways in which representations of users accomplish this function.

First, the researchers needed representations of users to *anticipate* the use of the technology that they were designing. They did not need explicit and well-defined ideas of what the future users would look like. On the contrary, this would have constrained the researchers' license to direct the process of technological innovation. These representations of users should therefore preferably *not increase the complexity* of the definition of the problem to be addressed. Scientists could keep the complexity of the social, cultural, and personal contexts in which users do or don't plan their families out of view by only minimally specifying their representation of users. This was very useful. The outcome of a consensus-seeking process, the accompanying product specification as low cost, easy to administer, and long-acting proved quite stable. It was extended and elaborated in greater detail in the following years, but it was not changed.

Akrich (1995) found that implicit techniques for representing the user seemed to be more powerful than explicit ones. In this study, too, we saw that the only spokespersons who employed an explicit technique, social scientists with their surveys, had little impact on the direction of product development.

But social scientists were important in structuring the ways in which users could be thought of (as undefinable) and technology (as decontextualized things with definable attributes).

Second, representations of users were functional by *permitting alignment* among levels of work organization. Fujimura (1987, 1992) has argued that standardized packages contribute to the alignment of different levels of work organization. Representations of users are brought into action in the same way. Stevens constructed the representation of users of immunological contraceptives as the mirror image of Pill users, and this enabled the researchers to derive a product specification for the new method that they were designing. Talwar's representation of immunological contraceptive users as an extension of anti-disease-vaccine users further complemented this product specification. The resulting product specification could be detached from the specific practices of these scientists and thereby facilitated the alignment of the laboratory level with the level of policy making and financing in the field of contraceptive development.

Fujimura (1987) has described the alignment of three levels of work organization: the experiment, the laboratory, and the world of policy making and financing. In the case of medical technology development, a fourth level of work organization should be distinguished: clinical practice. Clinicians were appropriately staged to transfer their representations of users from clinical practice toward the meetings of the steering committee. The clinical practice level also had to be aligned in making the development of a new contraceptive technology doable, and representations of users established this link.

Moreover, representations of users had an impact on defining the institutional work space. HRP agreed with Talwar about the perceived urgency of reducing population growth. But unlike Talwar and his group, WHO did not adopt the representation of users derived from antidisease vaccines: populations as the level of intervention. HRP's ambiguity toward conceiving users of contraceptive methods as populations was relieved by concentrating their support on Stevens's work, while at the same time not abandoning Talwar's. Standardized packages, such as specific representations of users, not only enable but also condition the doability of research problems.

Finally, the scientific community's adherence to the *variety* of individual users' needs and of their settings was important in *legitimizing* their research toward the hardware and the software enthusiasts among the member states. When elaborating research needs, individual users and the variety of settings were not taken into account. The needs for research were phrased in terms of the attributes of methods to be developed and the basic research required to do so, and not in terms of users with specific needs and settings. The appeal to diversity could bridge political differences, but this type of diversity could only accomplish its role as long as the technology was perceived out of context.

NOTES

1. According to Carl Djerassi, "The use of a condom prototype was first documented in the sixteenth century when the Italian anatomist Gabrielle Fallopio . . . recommended a linen sheath as a prophylactic against syphilis. . . . By the late nineteenth century condoms . . . were used widely in Europe" (1979, 4).

2. Few studies have explored the involvement of users in technology development. Science and technology studies (STS) traditionally have focused on design and the designers, not on use and the users. Users have made their modest entry into STS at least in part due to attempts from a gender studies perspective to analyze women's contributions to technological development; see, e.g., Cowan 1987, Cockburn and Ormrod 1993, and Chabaud-Rychter 1994.

3. In 1993, women's health advocates called for a stop to this line of research. They demanded a reorientation of the research into contraceptives toward the development of methods that would enable users to exert greater control over their fertility and that would not affect women's health. They asked that contraceptive development be oriented toward local health care conditions and women's health and rights situation (Call for a Stop 1993, 4; Richter 1996).

4. The phrase "configuring the user" was introduced by Woolgar (1991) to indicate this process of defining the identities of potential users and setting constraints on their likely future actions.

5. Several nonprofit entities were formed at about the same time: the Contraceptive Development Branch of the National Institute of Child Health and Human Development in 1969, the International Committee for Contraceptive Research of the Population Council in 1970, Family Health International in 1971, and the WHO's Special Program of Research, Development, and Research Training in Human Reproduction in 1972. See Population Council 1990, 13.

6. The name of the program changed from Expanded Program of Research, Development, and Research Training in Human Reproduction from 1972 to 1976, to Special Program for Research, Development, and Research Training in 1977.

7. Other arguments put forward were that "family planning would result in aging of the population and cause a decrease in productivity," that overpopulation was "an economic and not a medical problem," and that "the duty of physicians is to preserve human life and not to stand in its way" (Work of the Fifth World Health Assembly, Population Problems: Chronicle of the World Health Organization 1952, quoted in Kessler 1991, 43).

8. In 1972, two influential documents emerged. An international group of industrialists and scientists known as the "Club of Rome" published their report "Limits to Growth," and an editorial called "Blueprint for Survival" appeared in the English journal *Ecologist*. Both publications promoted the achievement of worldwide balance by, among other things, limiting population growth.

9. In the HRP annual report from 1974, the criteria are formulated more loosely: "The choice of methods under development is determined by several criteria: potential demand for a method, probability of success in development, likely time and cost, extent of research by other groups and industry, potential for collaboration" (WHO/HRP 1974, 3). HRP criteria for setting priorities evolved and are formulated in detail in the document prepared for the meeting of the advisory group in September 1979 (Kessler 1996). See also WHO/HRP/ AG 1979, 6–8.

10. Later named the Scientific and Technical Advisory Group (STAG).

11. Egon Diczfalusy was head of the Reproductive Endocrinology Unit of the Karolinska Institute (one of the WHO research and training centers) and consultant to WHO. The chemist Carl Djerassi had been involved in the early development of the Pill and had just published *The Politics of Contraception* (1979), in which he discussed birth control from the triple perspective of science, industry, and public policy. The biomedical scientist Sheldon Segal was the director of the Rockefeller Foundation's Population Program and one of the originators of contraceptive implants (Population Council 1990, 12). Robert V. Short worked at the Medical Research Council Reproductive Biology Unit of the University of Edinburgh, United Kingdom, and in assessing scientists' attitudes toward WHO in his opening remarks to a symposium, he said, "Let us remember that WHO is us" (Short 1979, 221).

12. See also contributions to the general discussion of the Karolinska Symposium (Diczfalusy 1975) by G. J. V. Nossal on the need to know more about cellular and humoral sides of immunity in the female genital tract (436), O. Vyazov on the physiology and morphology of the blood-testis barrier (440), D. B. Amos on the causes of unexplained sterility (444), H. Goodman on the need for more fundamental research on the mechanisms of local immune responses and on sperm antigens (445), and C. A. Shivers on gaps in the knowledge on the surface of the egg and its accessibility (445).

13. See also Barzelatto 1991, 61.

14. See, e.g., the results of the comparative studies reported in WHO/HRP 1979, 89–91. See also Shah 1995.

15. In that time, the term used was "review group."

16. There seems to be little predictive value in users' statements about methods they have never used. As far as unavailable technologies are concerned, these are typically greeted with ambivalence (Concepcion, Mundigo, and Reeler 1991; Cottingham 1997).

17. Conversely, the continuity of research and development of immunological contraceptives was not affected by the HIV/AIDS pandemic in the 1980s.

18. In the late 1950s and early 1960s, four additional steroid oral contraceptives were synthesized and introduced into medical practice by Schering Laboratories in Germany, Organon in The Netherlands, and Wyeth Laboratories in Great Britain. And G. D. Searle developed an alternative steroid to replace its norethynodrel (Djerassi 1979, 253).

19. According to David Griffin, it is important to realize that WHO's focus on developing countries means acknowledging differences between service settings and cultural contexts in northern and southern countries and not allowing qualitatively inferior methods because of the perceived urgency of population growth in developing countries (Griffin 1995).

20. The development of the first modern method to regulate female fertility, the "Pill," became highly politicized when in the 1970s the U.S. Senate Select Committee on Small Business held a series of hearings to consider the Pill's safety and to determine whether users were adequately informed about side effects. These hearings received intensive press coverage (Djerassi 1979, 92; Gelijns 1991, 170). Since then, the nascent women's health advocacy movement raised concerns about the Dalkon Shield[R], the hormonal injectable Depo-Provera[R], and Norplant[R]. Gelijns (1991) points out how these events profoundly changed regulatory requirements for contraceptive development. In comparison with drugs taken for acute disease conditions, it is not surprising that regulatory requirements for contraceptives, meant to be used by healthy persons for about thirty years, are more stringent. Undesirable side effects that may be considered admissible in the case of drugs in life-threatening situations are not acceptable for contraceptives. As a consequence, developmental costs rose, while effective patent life decreased. Also, those opposing fertility control for reasons other than health (e.g., the right-to-life movement) became more vocal, rendering the public climate inhospitable to innovation (Bardin 1987). These factors resulted in the withdrawal of the pharmaceutical industry from this area (Djerassi 1979, 85).

21. As a result of the magnitude of its research and development, HRP changed its relations with industry. First, the rules for establishing the price of the method to the public sector were laid down in formal agreements with companies that were involved in collaboration with WHO. Second, WHO reviewed and revised its policy on patents. From December 1973 on, the HRP took out patent rights on inventions that were developed wholly or partly as a result of WHO funding. Until then, it had been WHO policy to ensure by means of publication the widest distribution of any patentable invention developed as a result of WHO-sponsored research (WHO/HRP 1975, 74–75). By these two measures HRP strengthened its position vis-à-vis pharmaceutical industry and reinforced its explicit aim of making available to family planning programs in developing countries the methods for fertility regulation that emerge from the research and development they support.

22. The Population Council was founded in 1952 and has portrayed itself as an international nonprofit organization "applying science and technology to the solution of population problems in developing countries" (Population Council 1990, 3).

23. The medical definition of abortion is the interruption of pregnancy, and pregnancy starts after implantation of the embryo. Other definitions of abortion appoint the moment of fertilization as the onset of pregnancy, and this definition has been adopted by the American pro-life movement. The political lobbying of this movement has been extremely influential over the years. The mechanism of action of the WHO prototype vaccine has not been elucidated (Dirnhofer et al. 1993), and it is not clear whether it is effective before or after implantation of the early embryo.

24. Until then, most studies had been done on the effects of injecting gonadotropins (LH and FSH) and hCG from one species into another to raise an antigenic effect (active heterologous immunization). This had resulted in cross-reaction with other endogenous hormones or in the attainment of high titers of antibodies against the antigen that did not neutralize the endogenous hormones. Stevens defined the problem differently. According to him, the problem was that isoantigens, that is, hormones or other body constituents from the same species, are rarely antigenic. Additionally, most adjuvants that could be used in animals to reinforce their antigenicity were unacceptable for human use. Therefore, he altered an isoantigen to render it more immunogenic. This was accomplished by hapten-coupling the hormone hCG with a diazonium salt (Stevens 1973, 496–505; Stevens 1975, 368).

25. Clinical trials form the core of the testing process for the development of new drugs. Clinical trials are customarily divided into three stages. Phase I trials concentrate on the testing of pharmacological properties and toxicity in a limited number of human subjects. Phase II trials test for effectiveness and appropriate dose level in a few hundred persons. Phase III trials test the new compound on a larger scale, thereby increasing the chance of discovering rare side effects. In this essay, only phase I clinical trials are at stake.

26. This expectation about the impact of antifertility vaccines on family planning

117

programs in developing countries is reiterated year after year. See, e.g., HRP annual reports for 1975, 1976, 1977, and 1978.

27. Other research and training centers were located in Stockholm (Karolinska Institute), Buenos Aires, Santiago, and Moscow (WHO/HRP 1979, 23).

28. For his first clinical trials in humans, Stevens had used altered whole hCG molecules. From fundamental research it appeared that the hormone hCG consisted of two subunits, denominated α-subunit and β-subunit (Canfield et al. 1971). The α-subunit of hCG is identical with the α-subunit of several other hormones, including luteinizing hormone (LH). LH is a hormone secreted by the pituitary gland at the base of the brain, which stimulates ovulation in women and production of testosterone in men. Therefore, antibodies against whole hCG did not discriminate between hCG and LH either biologically or immunologically. This is called cross-reactivity. In premenopausal women, cross-reactivity of the provoked antibodies with LH might cause them to stop ovulating and could result in amenorrhea and clinical symptoms of ovarian deficiency. Follow-up studies in four subjects of Stevens's clinical trial with whole hCG, approximately six months from the first immunization, suggested that these women actually stopped ovulating (Stevens 1975, 365).

29. β-hCG preparations displayed microheterogenicity when analyzed by electrophoresis on polyacrylamide gels. It resolved in about eight bands. These were cut into segments, and the reactivity of each of these bands was analyzed with anti-hCG serum and anti-hLH serum. The part with hLH reactivity was removed, partly chemically and partly by immunoabsorption with anti-ovine LH. Talwar found that the resulting preparation gave almost negligible cross-reaction with hLH (Diczfalusy 1975, 370; Talwar 1976, 131).

30. This "double benefit" is repeatedly stressed by Talwar. For example: "The conjugate has the additional merit of conferring protection against tetanus in the recipients" (Talwar 1976, 130). "In addition, the [birth control] vaccines impart simultaneous protection against tetanus" (interview with Talwar by Sunny and Shah 1994, 23).

31. When the HRP Task Force on Immunological Methods for Fertility Regulation came to the stage of clinical trials in 1986, they had changed to a vaccine based on a fraction of the hCG molecule coupled to another anti-disease vaccine, anti-diphtheria toxoid (Jones et al. 1988).

32. A microbe or virus cannot survive when more than 80 percent of the population has immunity against it. If a person has not been immunized or a person's immune system has not reacted strongly to the vaccine, that person is protected if most people around her or him are protected, because the person is less likely to be exposed to the virus or microbe. See also Richter 1993, 16.

33. The Task Force on Immunological Methods for Fertility Regulation published its first guidelines for the evaluation of the safety and efficacy of placental antigen vaccines for fertility regulation in 1978. It said: "Duration of the study before initiation of phase I trials in humans. It is proposed that these studies should have been conducted for a minimum of 6 months prior to initiation of phase I trials in humans" (370).

34. Also, Stevens had hoped that as pure as possible β-subunits of hCG might elicit antibody response to hCG but not to LH. When testing the β-subunit in baboons, the antibodies produced indeed reacted with baboon CG and not with baboon LH, and effectively reduced the baboons' fertility. These studies, therefore, indicated that in case an antigen could be prepared that elicited antibodies specific for hCG and not reacting with human LH, an immunological method for human fertility control might become feasible. However, the antibodies produced by injecting baboons with the β-subunit of hCG also reacted with human

CG and human LH (Stevens 1975, 368). This indicated that even with the β-subunit of the hCG molecule, cross-reaction was taking place in the test tube. Stevens then went on to prepare smaller parts of the β-subunit of hCG, which then could be tested for their specificity in eliciting antibodies exclusively against hCG (Stevens 1975, 368 and 375).

REFERENCES

Akrich, M.:
1992 The De-scription of Technical Objects. In W. Bijker and J. Law (eds.), *Shaping Technology/Building Society: Studies in Sociotechnical Change,* 205–24. Cambridge: MIT Press.
1995 User Representations: Practices, Methods, and Sociology. In A. Rip, T. J. Misa, and J. Schot (eds.), *Managing Technology in Society: The Approach of Constructive Technology Assessment,* 167–84. London: Pinter.

Alma-Ata Declaration:
1972 Alma-Ata: WHO.

Bardin, C. W.:
1987 Public Sector Contraceptive Development: History, Problems, and Prospects for the Future. *Technology in Society* 9: 289–305.

Barzelatto, J.:
1991 Continuity and Change: The Years 1984–1989. In J. Khanna, P. F. A. Van Look, and P. D. Griffin (eds.), *Biennial Report, 1990–1991,* 60–65. Geneva: WHO.

Canfield, R. E., F. J. Morgan, S. Kammerman, S. Bell, et al.:
1971 Studies of Human Gonadotropin. *Recent Progress in Hormone Research* 8: 121–56.

Chabaud-Rychter, D.:
1994 Women Users in the Design Process of a Food Robot. In C. Cockburn and R. Fürst-Dilić (eds.), *Bringing Technology Home: Gender and Technology in a Changing Europe,* 77–93. Buckingham, England: Open University Press.

Clarke, A. E.:
1990 Controversy and the Development of Reproductive Sciences. *Social Problems* 37: 18–37.
1998 Negotiating the Contraceptive Quid Pro Quo. Chapter 6 in Clarke, *Disciplining Reproduction: Modernity, American Life Sciences, and "the Problems of Sex."* Berkeley: University of California Press.

Clarke, A. E., and Montini T.:
1993 The Many Faces of RU486: Tales of Situated Knowledges and Technological Contestations. *Science, Technology, & Human Values* 18(1): 42–78.

Cockburn, C., and S. Ormrod:
1993 *Gender and Technology in the Making.* London: Polity Press.

Concepcion, M., A. Mundigo, and A. V. Reeler:
1991 Social Aspects Related to the Introduction of a Birth Control Vaccine. In G. L. Ada and P. D. Griffin (eds.), *Assessment of Safety and Efficacy of Vaccines to Regulate Fertility,* 233–45. Cambridge: Cambridge University Press.

Cottingham, J. (ed.):
1997 *Beyond Acceptability: Users' Perspectives on Contraception.* London: Reproductive Health Matters.

Cowan, R. S.:
  1987 The Consumption Junction: A Proposal for Research Strategies in the Sociology of Technology. In W. Bijker, T. Hughes, and T. Pinch (eds.), *The Social Construction of Technological Systems.* Cambridge: MIT Press, 261–80.

Diczfalusy, E.:
  1975 Steps in the Human Reproductive Process Susceptible to Immunological Interference. *Acta Endocrinologica Supplementum* 194: 13–36.
  1986 The First Fifteen Years: A Review. *Contraception* 34(1): 1–119.

Diczfalusy, E. (ed.):
  1975 Karolinska Symposium on Research in Reproductive Endocrinology. Seventh Symposium on Immunological Approaches to Fertility Control, July 29–31, 1974. *Acta Endocrinologica Supplementum* 194.

Dirnhofer, S., R. Klieber, R. De Leeuw, J. M. Bidart, et al.:
  1993 Functional and Immunological Relevance of the COOH-terminal Extension of Human Chorionic Gonadotropin β: Implications for the WHO Birth Control Vaccine. *FASEB Journal* 7: 1381–85.

Djerassi, C.:
  1979 *The Politics of Contraception.* New York: W. W. Norton.

Fujimura, J. H.:
  1987 Constructing "Doable" Research Problems in Cancer Research: Articulating Alignment. *Social Studies of Science* 17: 257- 93.
  1992 Crafting Science: Standardized Packages, Boundary Objects, and "Translation." In A. Pickering (ed.), *Science as Practice and Culture,* 168–211. Chicago: University of Chicago Press.

Gelijns, A. C.:
  1991 *Innovation in Medical Practice: The Dynamics of Medical Technology Development.* Washington, D.C.: National Academy Press.

Griffin, P. D.:
  1991 WHO Task Force on Vaccines for Fertility Regulation: Its Formation, Objectives, and Research Activities. *Human Reproduction* 6(1): 166–72.
  1992 Options for Immunocontraception and Issues to be Addressed in the Development of Birth Control Vaccines. *Scandinavian Journal of Immunology* 36 Suppl. 11: 111–17.
  1995 Personal interview with the author, October 19.

Hardon, A. P.:
  1992 The Needs of Women versus the Interests of Family Planning Personnel, Policymakers, and Researchers: Conflicting Views on Safety and Acceptability of Contraceptives. *Social Science and Medicine* 6(35): 753–66.

Hartmann, B.:
  1987 *Reproductive Rights and Wrongs: The Global Politics of Population Control and Contraceptive Choice.* New York: Harper and Row.

Hearn, J. P.:
  1976 Immunization against Pregnancy. *Proceedings of the Royal Society London* 195: 149–60.

Hiddinga, A.:
  1995 Changing Normality. Ph.D. dissertation, University of Amsterdam.

Jones, W. R., J. Bradley, S. J. Judd, E. H. Denholm, et al.:
  1988 Phase I Clinical Trial of World Health Organization's Birth Control Vaccine. *Lancet,* 1295–98.

Kessler, A.:

1991   Establishment and Early Development of the Programme. In J. Khanna, P. F. A. Van Look, and P. D. Griffin (eds.), *Biennial Report, 1990–1991*, 43–59. Geneva: WHO.

1996   Personal letter, February 14.

Lancet.

1974   Immunology and Developing Countries. Editorial. *Lancet,* Sept. 14, 632–33.

Mastroianni, L., P. Donaldson, and T. Kane (eds.).:

1990   *Developing New Contraceptives: Obstacles and Opportunities.* Washington, D.C.: National Academy Press.

Mintzes, B. (ed.):

1992   *A Question of Control: Women's Perspectives on the Development and Use of Contraceptive Technologies.* Amsterdam: Wemos Women and Pharmaceuticals Project and Health Action International.

Oudshoorn, N.:

1994   *Beyond the Natural Body: An Archaeology of Sex Hormones.* London: Routledge.

1998   Shifting Boundaries between Industry and Science: The Role of the WHO in Contraceptive R&D. In J. P. Gaudiliere, I. Löwy, and D. Pestre (eds.), *The Invisible Industrialist: Manufacturers and the Construction of Scientific Knowledge.* London: Macmillan Press.

Population Council:

1990   *Annual Report.* New York: Population Council.

Rakow, L. R., and V. Navarro:

1993   Remote Mothering and the Parallel Shift: Women Meet the Cellular Telephone. *Critical Studies in Mass Communication* 10: 144–57.

Richter, J.:

1993   *Vaccination against Pregnancy: Miracle or Menace?* Bielefeld: BUKO Pharma-Kampagne.

1996   *Vaccination against Pregnancy: Miracle or Menace?* London: Zed Books.

Rowe, P.:

1995   Personal interview with the author, October 20.

Segal, S. J.:

1976   Immunological Methods to Prevent Pregnancy: An Editorial Comment. *Contraception* 13(2): 125–27.

Shah, I.:

1995   Perspectives on Methods of Fertility Regulation: Setting a Research Agenda: A Background Paper. Unpublished paper.

Short, R. V.:

1979   Proceedings of a Symposium of the Society for the Study of Fertility and the WHO, Cambridge, July 1978. *Journal for Reproduction and Fertility* 55: 221.

Stevens, V. C.:

1973   Immunization of Female Baboons with Hapten-Coupled Gonadotropins. *Obstetrics and Gynecology* 42(4): 496–506.

1975   Fertility Control through Active Immunization Using Placenta Proteins. *Acta Endocrinologica Supplementum* 194: 357–75.

1995   Personal interview with the author, August 9.

1996   Personal letter, December 26.

Stevens, V. C., and C. D. Crystle:

1973 Effects of Immunization with Hapten-Coupled hCG on the Human Menstrual Cycle. *Obstetrics and Gynecology* 42(4): 484–95.

Sunny, S., and J. Shah:

1994 India's Birth Control Vaccine: New Hope or New Hazard? *Health and Nutrition,* 20–27.

Talwar, G. P.:

1976 Introduction. *Contraception* 13(2): 129–31.

1978 Anti-hCG Immunization. *Contraception* 18(1): 19–21.

Talwar, G. P., and A. Gaur:

1987 Recent Developments in Immunocontraception. *American Journal of Obstetrics and Gynecology,* 1075–78.

Talwar, G. P., S. Kumar, N. C. Sharma, J. S. Bajaj et al.:

1976 Clinical Profile and Toxicology Studies on Four Women Immunized with Pr-β-hCG-TT. *Contraception* 13(2): 253–68.

Talwar, G. P., N. C. Sharma, S. K. Dubey, M. Salahuddin et al.:

1976 Isoimmunization against human Chorionic Gonadotropin with Conjugates of Processed β-subunit of the Hormone and Tetanus Toxoid. *Proceedings of the National Academy of Science USA* 73(1): 218–22.

United Nations Department of International Economy and Social Affairs [UN/DIESA]:

1992 *Integrating Development and Population Planning in India.* New York: United Nations.

WHO/HRP:

1974 Annual Report. Geneva: WHO.

1975 Annual Report. Geneva: WHO.

1976 Annual Report. Geneva: WHO.

1977 Annual Report. Geneva: WHO.

1978 Annual Report. Geneva: WHO.

1979 Annual Report. Geneva: WHO.

1993 Fertility Regulating Vaccines. Report of a meeting between women's health advocates and scientists to review the current status of the development of fertility regulating vaccines, Geneva, August 17–18.

WHO/HRP/Advisory Group [WHO/HRP/AG]:

1979 Criteria and Priorities for Programme Strategy. Document prepared by the HRP Secretariat for the eleventh meeting of the Advisory Group, Geneva, September 24–27.

WHO/HRP Steering Committee of the Task Force on Immunological Methods for the Regulation of Fertility [WHO/HRP/SC]:

1973 Report of the Meeting of the Task Force on Immunological Methods for the Regulation of Fertility, Geneva, July 9–13.

WHO/HRP Task Force on Immunological Methods for Fertility Regulation:

1978 Evaluating the Safety and Efficacy of Placental Antigen Vaccines for Fertility Regulation. *Clinical and Experimental Immunology* 33: 360–75.

Woolgar, S.:

1991 Configuring the User: The Case of Usability Trials. In J. Law (ed.), *A Sociology of Monsters: Essays on Power, Technology, and Domination.* London: Routledge.

4

Imagined Men: Representations of Masculinities in Discourses on Male Contraceptive Technology

Nelly Oudshoorn

Birth control texts published before 1970 are intriguing. Anyone reading them without knowing more about reproduction would be tempted to conclude that there is only one sex involved in making babies: the female sex. Women have been the main focus of birth control technologies in the twentieth century. Since the Second World War, thirteen new contraceptives for women have been developed, including the contraceptive pill. The major methods of contraception available to men (the condom, withdrawal, and periodic abstinence) do not differ from those available to men over four hundred years ago (Davidson et al. 1985). Consequently, contraceptive technologies have a clear gender script: responsibility for contraception and its risks to health is delegated primarily to women, not to men. This chapter seeks to explore the role of different actors in rewriting this gender script. Special attention will be paid to how these actors configure the user of new contraceptive technologies, particularly contraceptives for men. Ever since the demand for new male contraceptives was first articulated, people have wondered whether men would be willing to use a contraceptive pill or injection if one were available. This is an intriguing debate because it enables us to study the mutual and simultaneous construction, or "co-construction," of a technology and its users. All the actors involved in the making of male contraceptives construed specific images of the prospective user.[1]

Recent studies in the sociology of science and technology have emphasized that users play an important role in technological development. Traditionally, users have been considered important actors in the diffusion and acceptance of new technologies. Technologies only work if they become accepted by users and embedded in society (Von Hippel 1976, 1988). More recently, the attention in STS has shifted from the analysis of users in the sociological sense (i.e., identifiable persons as such involved in the diffusion of technologies) toward users in the semiotic sense. As Akrich has suggested, "Innovators are from the very start constantly interested in their future users. They construct many different representations of these users, and objectify these representations in technological choices" (Akrich 1995, 168). In the development phase of a new technology, designers anticipate and define the preferences, motives, tastes, and competences of potential users and inscribe these views into the technical design of the new product (Akrich 1992, 208). This semiotic approach challenges the view that users only enter the picture once a new technology has been introduced on the market. Innovators actively draw users into the very heart of technological development.

Although Akrich tends to restrict her analysis of representations of users to the role of innovators, scientific experts are not the only actors who construct specific representations of the prospective user. In the case of male contraceptives, feminists and journalists have played an active role in articulating and demarcating the potential users of this technology in the making. Recent critics, particularly but not exclusively in cultural studies, have argued that the construction of cultural authority in science and technology can no longer be regarded as the exclusive domain of scientists.[2] These cultural studies extend the analysis of the production of knowledge to journalism and fiction discourse. Donna Haraway's *Primate Visions* (1989) and José Van Dyck's *Manufacturing Babies and Public Consent* (1995) are examples of the validity of this approach, showing how, in the fields of primatology and in vitro fertilization, the production of scientific facts and the construction of public consent are not restricted to scientific journals. In a similar vein, Greg Myers's *Writing Biology* (1990) demonstrates how the construction of biological facts is established as much in scientific journal texts as in popular texts and grant proposals.

Following these authors, I propose to extend the analysis of user representations to include feminist and journalistic texts. What types of representations of male users are dominant in feminist, scientific, and journalistic discourse? What role do these representations play in articulating and constructing the cultural feasibility of new male contraceptive technologies?

ARTICULATING THE NEED FOR MALE CONTRACEPTIVES

Innovation in the field of male contraceptive technology has been absent from the research agenda of scientists and industry for a long time. The introduction of men into contraceptive discourse may therefore be considered rather revolutionary. Like other revolutions, the revolution in the world of contraceptive technologies has its own heroes. The history of birth control reveals two illustrious protagonists: Chinese Premier Zhou Enlai and Indian Prime Minister Indira Gandhi. In the 1960s, Zhou ordered the development of new male contraceptives. In an interview with this author, Alvin Paulsen, a professor in reproductive physiology at the Medical School in Seattle and one of the pioneers in male contraceptive research, remembered this event: "If you have an authoritarian society like China and the second man in charge says, 'Let there be more work in the Male,' all of a sudden everyone started working on gossypol" (a male contraceptive agent introduced by Chinese scientists).

Population politics in India went one step further. In 1961 Gandhi attempted to introduce a law mandating a wide-scale forced sterilization for men (Stokes 1980, 31; Berelson 1969, 534–35). This was one step too far: protests against this proposal resulted in the fall of her cabinet. Notwithstanding this failure, Gandhi continued to promote the role of men in family planning, now putting her faith in the development of new contraceptives for women and men: "Family planning programs are awaiting a big breakthrough; without a safe, preferably oral drug which women and men can take, no amount of governmental commitment and political determination will avail" (Diczfalusy 1985, 5).

The fact that India and China entered the history of birth control technologies as advocates of male contraception is not just a coincidence. Both countries faced a rapidly growing population and, even more crucially, had strong authoritarian traditions. Governmental control over family planning fitted seamlessly into the dominant politics of state control. By the 1960s, India and China had well-established governmental birth control programs. India, a former British colony, had the first government-sponsored birth control clinic in the world, which opened as early as 1930 (Clarke 1999). The first articulation of the need to include men as a target for birth control technologies thus came from the eastern hemisphere: Men should no longer be neglected, because they are a necessary tool to reduce population growth.

In the early 1970s the western industrialized world witnessed the emergence of a similar discourse. The actors involved in promoting the idea of male-oriented birth control technologies are more heterogeneous than in the East. The absence of conspicuous protagonists makes it difficult to pinpoint the origins of this discourse to a specific time and place. In the United States, it was the feminist movement which first advocated putting the man on the contraceptive agenda. Feminists became advocates of birth control technologies for men following the first publicity about health risks associated with the female contraceptive pill, especially increased risks of cancer and diseases of the circulatory system. Women's health advocates criticized the introduction of the pill and suggested that reproductive scientists and industry had shown inadequate concern for the health of women (Seaman and Seaman 1977; Gelijns and Pannenborg 1993, 227). Feminist publications with telling titles such as "His Safety or Hers?" illustrate the feminists' major concern: The use of contraceptives is a risky business and should not be assigned exclusively to women (Seaman and Seaman 1977, 329). Consequently, they pleaded for the development of male contraceptives that would make it possible to share the health risks of using contraceptives.

The growing interest in male contraception is also reflected in the scientific literature on reproductive physiology and birth control methods. The first publication to signal interest on the part of the scientific community appeared in *Science* in 1970. In "Birth Control after 1984," Carl Djerassi, a leading chemist who had been involved in the production of the steroids that eventually became the components of the female contraceptive pill, discussed possible new leads in contraceptive technologies. Drawing on a WHO report on developments in fertility control, Djerassi suggested three approaches, including "a male contraceptive pill" (Djerassi 1970, 941). In 1974, *Nature* published a report that dealt explicitly with this new envisioned birth control method under the heading "Oral Contraceptive for Men" (Briggs 1974).

One of the most powerful actors in the world of birth control technologies remained remarkably silent: the pharmaceutical industry.[3]

The impetus to change the status quo in contraceptive research to include male methods thus came from a contrasting set of motives that entailed two types of discourse: population control discourse, which framed the need for male contraceptives in terms of the technology's contribution to limit the population growth, and emancipation discourse, which articulated the need for male contraceptives in terms of sharing the risks and responsibilities of contraception between the sexes. Remarkably, the need to develop male contraceptives was not articulated by its potential users—men. The advocates for male methods were governments, public sector agencies, and some feminists. As Roy Greep, one of the leading reproductive biologists in the United States, put it: "It is the need for male contraceptives and not the demand that is expanding exponentially" (Greep 1975, 2).

FEMINIST DISCOURSE: ADVOCACY AND AMBIVALENCE

Feminist advocacy for male contraception originated from severe criticism of the role of scientists (and industry) in promoting new contraceptives for women, most notably the oral hormonal contraceptive and the Dalkon shield, an intrauterine device. In the late 1960s, feminist health advocates campaigned against the side effects of the Pill and accused the scientific community of not taking seriously the many complaints of Pill users. In *The Doctor's Case against the Pill* (1969), Barbara Seaman, a leading American women's health expert, documented the experiences of women using the Pill. On January 23, 1970, feminist health advocates in the United States interrupted Senator Gaylord Nelson's hearings on the Pill with a protest in which they demanded, "Why is there no pill for men?" (Seaman and Seaman 1977, 325). The feminist health movement was very active and strong in the late 1960s and the 1970s. In the late 1960s they prevented the FDA from licensing a newly developed long-acting injectable contraceptive (medroxy-progesterone, MDPA) for women. Feminist health advocates took the view that this new contraceptive conflicted with women's rights, since injections might easily be abused in certain societies. The "ban the jab" political lobby was an important factor in discouraging industry from further research of this kind (Matlin 1994, 125). In 1972, Barbara Seaman continued her criticism of the Pill in *Free and Female,* in which she accused scientists of sex discrimination for developing contraceptives for women and not for men, and in 1977 she devoted a whole chapter of *Women and the Crisis in Sex Hormones* to the male pill (Seaman and Seaman 1977).

Advocacy for the development of new male contraceptives was among the issues in feminist campaigns leading up to the international United Nations Conference on Population and Development held in Cairo in 1994 and the UN's Fourth World Conference on Women held in Beijing in 1995 (Committee on Women, Population, and the Environment 1992; Anonymous 1994). Both before and during these conferences, international women's health organizations expressed the need for both sexes to share responsibilities for family planning. They opposed the idea that family planning is the woman's responsibility and emphasized that "men have a personal and social responsibility for their own sexual behavior and fertility" (Committee on Women, Population, and the Environment 1992). This advocacy was quite successful. The Program of Action of the International Conference on Population and Development organized by the United Nations Population Fund in Cairo in 1994 included male responsibility in family planning as one of the means to reach gender equality: "The objective is to promote gender equality in all spheres of life, including family and community life, and to encourage and enable men to take responsibility for their sexual and reproductive behavior and their social and family roles" (UN 1994, 4, 25).

A closer look at women's health advocates' texts in this period reveals a shift in emphasis in feminist discourse. In contrast to the 1970s, more attention is paid to ways of changing men's behavior toward contraception and rather less to the development of new male contraceptives. Whereas detailed descriptions of possible male contraceptives dominated feminist texts in the 1970s, in the 1990s these texts emphasized the need for the development of "reproductive health services and social programs that sensitize men to their parental responsibilities" (Committee on Women, Population, and the Environment 1992, 2).[4]

Feminist discourse thus shows an ambivalence toward the need for new male contraceptives. Some feminist health advocates have been, and still are, among the most prominent actors in demanding the development of new male contraceptives. In their view, the "pill for men" may be "the magic solution that many modern-thinking people of both sexes are waiting for" (Seaman and Seaman 1977, 302). They consider the development of new male contraceptives an important tool to improve women's reproductive health because it increases the contraceptive options available to women (Lissner 1992, 54). But other feminists have questioned the possible contribution of new male contraceptives to women's reproductive health and can be considered "anti-users."[5] These feminists have argued that women are not comfortable with the idea of being dependent on somebody else for their contraceptive needs and that most men cannot be trusted: "Men's hearts may be in the right place, but when dealing with sexual matters, men are often far less mature than women" (Stokes 1980, 9). Moreover, men themselves did not demand new contraceptives (Corea 1985). Feminists thus faced a dilemma. The women's movement, at least in industrial countries, had long struggled to give women control over their own fertility. Margaret Sanger, a women's rights activist and pioneer for birth control in the United States and "the mother" of the first oral contraceptive for women, suggested that the most important threat to women's independence came from unwanted and unanticipated pregnancies. As early as the 1920s, she advocated birth control as a basic condition for the liberation of women (Christian Johnson 1977, 63).[6] Sanger believed it was essential that birth control should be in women's hands. In line with Sanger's arguments, feminists of the second wave of the women's liberation movement that emerged in the 1970s formulated women's free choice in childbearing as "the center of women's autonomy" (Bruce 1987, 380). The availability of female contraceptives, including abortion, became a cornerstone of this movement.

In this context it can easily be understood that feminists considered the shift toward male contraceptives to be a threat to women's autonomy. Radical feminists suggested that the use of male contraceptives implied that women should "once again place their fate in a man's hands" (Stokes 1980, 41). Judy Norsigian, coauthor of *Our Bodies, Ourselves,* the bible of the women's health movement in the United States and Europe in the 1970s and 1980s, concluded at the hearings on contraceptive research before the Select Committee on Population of the U.S. House of Representatives in 1978 that the emphasis on research for female contraceptives was not inappropriate, "since women are the ones who ultimately become pregnant and give birth" (Norsigian 1979, 29). In this testimony, she criticized policymakers in private organizations such as the

Population Council for male bias in setting priorities for research, not because their research policy only included female methods, but because they had recommended the development of male contraceptive methods as the first priority in a list of ten policy recommendations for future research (28).

Feminist discourse on new male contraceptives thus presents two conflicting images of the prospective user. The advocates of male contraception construe the image of men who are willing to share health risks and responsibilities for contraception with their partners. The slogan "Be responsible for your own sperm," introduced by Dutch feminists to parallel "Boss in your own belly," the slogan used by feminists to campaign for free abortion in the 1970s, exemplifies this image of the responsible, caring man. The opponents of new male contraceptives see a completely different picture. They represent the users as men who cannot be trusted. These feminists depend upon, and reproduce, the hegemonical, cultural stereotypes of masculinity that emphasize men's unreliability and lack of interest in matters of birth control.

SCIENTIFIC DISCOURSE: THE CONSTRUCTION OF
THE CARING MAN

Feminist discourse has thus evolved two types of user representations: the Caring Man and the Unreliable Man. In contrast, scientific discourse is more univocal. Reproductive scientists who work on male contraceptives construe an image of the user very similar to feminists' image of the Caring Man. This similarity in discourse is not a coincidence. Over the last two decades, sociologists of science have debunked the "ivory tower" image of science as an autonomous, independent world that operates apart from the rest of society. Instead, sociologists suggest that scientific discourse should be viewed as the result of "collective work across worlds with different viewpoints and agendas" (Fujimura 1992, 169).[7] In the case of male contraceptive research, reproductive scientists were not operating in isolation from available ideas and sociopolitical arrangements. They built their field in dialogue with eastern governments and feminists in the western world.

The similarity of user representations in feminist and scientific discourse can thus be understood as the result of alliances between the worlds of feminists and scientists.[8] This is not to say that feminists and reproductive scientists were friends right from the start. The first encounters between these groups were characterized by criticism and distrust, and can best be portrayed as dangerous liaisons, particularly for the scientists.

Since the 1970s, scientists working in the area of male reproduction were increasingly confronted with critical questions voiced by feminists about the reasons for the discrepancy between the availability of contraceptives for women and men. In "Contraceptive Research: A Male Chauvinist Plot?" Sheldon Segal, vice president of the Population Council in the 1970s, complained: "I think that I have not attended a single nonscientific meeting in the last two years at which the progress of contraceptive development was discussed where someone—usually a woman—has not asked: What about the men? Why aren't scientists trying to develop a new male contraceptive?" (Segal 1972, 21).

In this paper Segal simply rejected the criticism of feminists, particularly the work of Barbara Seaman. In 1975, American reproductive scientists William Bremner and David de Kretser entered the lion's den, namely, the feminist journal *Signs,* to report similar experiences. They characterized their confrontations with feminists, while carefully avoiding pinning the blame on feminist activism, as follows:

> As a general comment on the history of research in fertility control, it is of interest that contraceptive techniques for men seem to have lagged somewhat behind those available for women, particularly in the area of oral preparations. Questions about the reasons for this discrepancy are often asked of workers in the area of male contraception. The questions are occasionally asked with a certain degree of hostility, with the implication that scientists in the area of reproduction research have been responsive to male opinion, which is held to regard the female as the sex responsible for contraception. (Bremner and de Kretser 1975, 395)

Except for these individual confrontations, there were no direct interactions between feminists and scientists. Feminists depended on the media, which played a major intermediary role between the worlds of feminists and scientists. In the 1970s and 1980s, newspapers regularly repeated the question first posed by feminists: What about the male pill?

These criticisms shaped the discourse on male contraception in the 1970s. Many papers published on the subject of male contraception in this period included a section that explained why there was as yet no male equivalent to the (female) Pill. The initial reaction of most reproductive scientists was to defend their field against the charges of male chauvinism. Sheldon Segal and other scientists defended their field by arguing that their work simply reflected fundamental biological differences between the sexes:

> What are the facts about male contraceptive research? Is the failure thus far to find a new male method comparable to the pill indicative of male disinterest in women's well-being? I don't think so. The simple fact is that the number of targets—spermatogenesis, sperm maturation, sperm transport, and possibly, the chemical constitution of the seminal fluid—is far more lim-

ited in males than females. It is not surprising, then, that the number of approaches under study is fewer for male than for female methods. Even the forces of women's liberation cannot change the fact that the reproductive analogies between male and female end with sperm transport and egg transport, and that all subsequent events potentially subject to controlled interference occur only in the female. (Segal 1972, 21–22)

Other scientists offered similar "natural" explanations, but they agreed with feminists that there was a prejudice. However, not all scientists shared these biological explanations. Roy Greep, a leading reproductive scientist at Harvard Medical School and project director and editor of *Reproduction and Human Welfare: A Challenge to Research,* in the first extensive review of the reproductive sciences and contraceptive development initiated and funded by the Ford Foundation in 1976, turned the tables by suggesting that if scientists had simply followed "nature," they would have developed male contraceptives rather than female methods:

> The paucity of contraceptives available to the male and the inexcusable delay in developing a research program to correct this deficiency is not a readily understandable circumstance since there are potent biological reasons why the burden of responsibility for conception control should rightfully fall on the male. Firstly, it is the male that plays the initiating role in the procreation process. Procreation involves the union of egg and sperm, but it is only the sperm that must be transferred between the sexes. There is another and much overlooked circumstance that makes the practice of conception control by the male an imperative matter. This is the fact that men have a much longer fertile life than that of their female counterparts. . . . Men, therefore, constitute a target population for the implementation of conception control that could be of unparalleled significance to the future welfare of the human species. (Greep, Koblinsky, and Jaffe 1976, 2–3)

Greep and other scientists ascribed the gap between female and male methods to a lack of fundamental knowledge of the male reproductive system caused by institutional reasons. In *Reproduction and Human Welfare,* the authors, reviewing the state of the art in male reproductive physiology, concluded: "The number of basic and clinical investigators interested in andrology as opposed to gynaecology is very small, and the investment in basic research on the male has been only a very small fraction of that devoted to the female. . . . The state of our knowledge of the male is now nearly comparable to that preceding the development of oral contraceptives for the female. If adequate research support can be sustained, there is every reason to expect that the next fifteen years will see the development of safe effective means of fertility control in the male" (Greep, Koblinsky, and Jaffe 1976, 251).

The ways in which feminist criticism shaped reproductive discourse thus evolved from a debate on whether there existed male bias to a debate in which scientists used feminist criticism as a resource to argue for more funding of male reproductive research. Since the mid-1970s, publications with titles explicitly referring to emancipation, such as *Equality for the Sexes?* or *Bridging the Gender Gap: Another Hurdle Cleared,* have become common (Aldhous 1990; Handelsman 1991). Reproductive scientists explicitly began to frame the relevance of male contraceptive research in feminist terms, which culminated in the organization of three workshops on male fertility control in 1975, the year declared by the UN as the Woman's Year. The foreword to one of these workshops exemplifies this emerging discourse coalition: "As one of our main practical concerns is the control of human fertility, the last part of the book is devoted to the still scarce knowledge gained in male fertility control in recent years. Actually it was the purpose of the entire meeting which would have culminated during the Woman's Year into the round table on 'Perspectives in male fertility control'—as a contribution to a shared responsibility in responsible parenthood" (Hubinont, L'Hermite, and Schwers 1976, xi–xii).

Although feminists and scientists disagreed about many things, there was one mutual concern: the health risks of contraceptive methods for women, particularly the Pill. The major impact of the interaction between feminists and scientists was that the discourse on the need to develop male methods became framed increasingly in terms of sharing health risks between the sexes (Segal 1971, 17). In the late 1970s, reproductive scientists also adopted the "equal sharing of responsibility" argument, as exemplified by Alvin Paulsen's description of male contraceptive research in *Frontiers in Reproduction and Fertility Control* (1977): "In the past several years there has been renewed interest in developing methods for male contraception. The impetus for this activity has come from the consumer, rather than from the scientific community, resulting partly from a sincere concern with possible adverse reactions associated with use of the 'pill' by women, partly from a definite social trend toward sharing of responsibility for family planning between partners, and partly from a desire expressed by many men to assume control over their own fertility" (Paulsen 1977, 458).

The dialogue between reproductive scientists and feminists in the 1970s thus resulted in a merging of user representations. In reaction to feminist criticism, reproductive scientists constructed the image of the Caring Man as the prospective user of their technologies.

The construction of this user representation was not just a passive reproduction of feminist discourse. By adopting the image of the Caring Man, an image that clearly conflicted with hegemonic cultural stereotypes of men, scientists increasingly faced disbelief in this user representation. Critics of male contraceptives suggested that there existed a resistance against the envisioned male pill because men would have the feeling that they lose their freedom if they take responsibility for contraception (Haspels 1985). Even scientists within the field of male contraceptive research seem to have had doubts about the existence of the Caring Man. It is not unusual for scientists to praise the endurance of volunteers in their acknowledgments, which illustrates that the expectation of scientists was rather low with respect to the motivation of men to practice fertility control (Soufir et al. 1983, 631; Foegh 1983, 7). Reproductive scientists working on male contraception thus actively had to defend the image of the Caring Man. In their texts, they rejected the idea that men were not willing to use a new contraceptive by arguing that men have always played a large role in family planning. Before the introduction of the Pill and intrauterine devices (IUDs), most contraception depended on male methods (condoms and coitus interruptus), so they argued, and they referred to the increased number of vasectomies in the United States in the 1970s as "the most concrete example of male interest and responsibility in family planning" (Diller and Hembree 1977, 1273; de Kretser 1978). Two American clinicians turned the tables by arguing that the problem was not the motivation of individual men but the attitude of family planners, drug companies, and scientists, whom they blamed for relying on stereotypical images of the potential user. They argued that these negative images of male attitudes told more about the attitude of the observer than the observed:

> The attitudes of men regarding birth control and the family were frequently
> mentioned by investigators and family planners as having a deterrent effect
> on research interest in male contraception. . . . The assumed prevailing
> notions were that (1) family planning was a woman's problem and responsibil-
> ity because men were neither concerned nor interested; and (2) the male was
> perceived as sexually capricious, at least prior to marriage. . . . These stereo-
> typic notions have had serious impact on the potential role of the male in
> family planning in the United States, so much so that scientific investigators
> questioned the demand for a male contraceptive even if one were available.
> Family planners ignored men as consumers; drug companies were reluctant
> to invest in projects that appeared to have little profit; and researchers were
> discouraged from entering the field because of lack of interest and funding.
> Recent analysis of male attitudes and perceptions has shown the earlier stereo-
> types to be false. (Diller and Hembree 1977, 1273)

Reproductive scientists working on male contraceptives thus actively began articulating and defending new images of masculinity, mostly in close cooperation with family planning organizations.

In the 1970s, family planning organizations began to initiate educational programs and services specifically focused on men—quite an exceptional practice because in previous years family planning programs had focused almost exclusively on women (Gallen, Liskin, and Kok 1986, 904; Stokes 1980, 25). *Population Reports,* the journal of the Population Information Program of Johns Hopkins University in Baltimore, devoted a special issue to these programs:

> Programs to encourage men's involvement in family planning are springing up throughout the world. In countries as varied as Hong Kong, Jamaica, Mauritania, Mexico, Nigeria, the Philippines, the UK, the US, and Zimbabwe, programs offer men discussion groups, lectures, drop-in centers, counseling, "Fathers Clubs," videos, and more. Some programs are going to the workplace to reach men. With the encouragement of a growing number of family planning programs around the world, men are showing a new concern over family size and child spacing. They also are recognizing the benefits that they as well as their wives and children can derive from family planning. (Gallen, Liskin, and Kok 1986, 889)

The special issue was illustrated with pictures of posters developed by family planning associations, portraying a pregnant man with the text: "Would you be more careful if it was you that got pregnant?" in five different languages (Gallen, Liskin, and Kok 1986, 904–5).

The Population Council, a nonprofit, nongovernmental research organization established in 1951 specializing in reproductive health, has, together with the WHO, been one of the main actors in male contraceptive research and development. Since 1995 it has been playing an active networking role in advocating cultural change by publishing *Men and Families* and *Toward a New Partnership: Encouraging the Positive Involvement of Men as Supportive Partners in Reproductive Health.* These newsletters are distributed through the United States and Europe. *Men and Families* is also published in Spanish for distribution in Latin America and the Caribbean region. This newsletter aims to "provide an opportunity for researchers, program planners and activists to reflect, debate and advocate regarding men's roles in the families . . . and to contribute to gender equality, family democratization and resource utilization for the well-being of all family members" (Population Council 1995a, 1).

The advocates of new male contraceptives have thus embraced a project that is potentially much broader than the development of a new technology.

The endeavor to making new male contraceptives includes the making of a New Man:

> A male contraceptive pill may be on the market by the end of the century. And male family planning programs have struck a responsive chord in the United States as well as in parts of the Third World. These changes hold the promise of men participating more actively in family planning. By using effective male contraceptives, by supporting women in their choice of birth control, and by taking on additional family and childrearing responsibilities, men can assume a larger share of the burdens of contraception and the joys of having children. This will create not only a new role for men in family planning, but also a new role for men in the family and society. (Stokes 1980, 6–7).

In this advocacy, reproductive scientists and family planning organizations have constructed a new image of the user. In answer to feminist criticism that men cannot be trusted in matters of contraception, reproductive scientists have specified the potential user as a couple (not a man!) with a stable relationship (Haspels 1985, 27; Stokes 1980, 41). To quote Alvin Paulsen, one of the pioneers in male contraceptive research: "A hormonal non-barrier method for the control of male fertility is not for everyone. You have to give it to a monogamous couple that know and understand and trust each other" (Interview Paulsen). This redefinition of the user responds to the growing concern about sexually transmitted diseases, particularly AIDs, and its implications for the use of contraceptive methods that could protect against these diseases (Wu 1988).

This specification of the user also implies a construction of the nonuser: men with casual sexual relationships.[9] Family planning organizations have also constructed a nonuser. In family planning discourse, the nonuser is a "macho man": a man who wants a large family to prove his masculinity. For these men, contraception threatens the male ego (Stokes 1980, 8; Davidson et al. 1985, 4). "The widespread belief in many societies that a man is not a man who cannot father children, has exacerbated the unwillingness of the male to practise contraception. It is almost as if the male enjoyment of sex is heightened by the potential risk of pregnancy" (Gombe 1983, 203).

Although the advocates of new male contraceptives have tried to accommodate the constraints of machismo in shaping male attitudes toward contraception by referring to surveys in southern countries which found that a substantial majority of men approved the use of contraceptives, most actors agreed that "the macho man is half myth and half reality."[10] The classification of the macho man as a nonuser does not imply that advocates of new male contraceptives have simply abandoned the idea that these men could become potential users. As exemplified by the launch of specific family planning programs and newsletters that focus on men, the nonuser is considered a challenge to family planning programs and is consequently used as major tool to change the negative male attitudes toward contraception.

JOURNALISTIC DISCOURSE: IN DEFENSE OF
HEGEMONIC MASCULINITIES

Whereas scientific discourse is characterized by user representations that break with traditional cultural stereotypes of men, journalistic discourse, at least in The Netherlands, reads primarily like a defense of hegemonic masculinities. The reactions of the Dutch news media to a press release of the results of a large-scale clinical trial on contraceptive hormonal injections for men, organized by the WHO and launched in April 1996, shows that the media did not join in scientists' attempts to rewrite gender scripts concerning contraception.[11] Dutch newspapers emphasized that it is very likely that both men and women will reject this new technology. Women are portrayed as opponents of male contraceptives because they don't trust men in matters of contraception. Under the headline "Where are the cheers for the buttock-injection?" a journalist in *Haagse Post/De Tijd* told his readers that the male injection may be as reliable as the female Pill, but he asked, "How reliable are men?" The journalist cited the results of a nine-year survey of female visitors to a Dutch family planning clinic to convince his readers that women will never accept this technology: 80 percent of the woman said no to the idea of a new male contraceptive because they did not trust their partners with contraceptives (Leclair 1996).[12] In *De Volkskrant,* a female writer concluded: "It is a great invention that will please feminists in theory and ideology. But the injection will be hardly used in practice, I think. Women don't trust men with this. They want to keep it in their own hands. Imagine that you have to control your partner: 'Darling, did you take your injection?' . . . I'm afraid that this is again a feminist victory that is good for nobody" (Vries 1996).

Most journalists are convinced that the majority of (Dutch) men will never use male contraceptive injections. Here the criterion is not trust but pain. Most journalists emphasize the painful nature of injections in the buttock. All three leading national Dutch newspapers (*De Telegraaf, Trouw,* and *De Volkskrant*) construct the image of a painful technology and overly sensitive men, using headlines such as "The Injection-Pill for Men Is Reliable but No Fun" (*Trouw*) and "No INJECTION in My Buttock" (*De Telegraaf*). The article in *De Telegraaf* includes a photo of a man trying to inject himself. Journalists construct this image by quoting the opinions of the "men/women in the street" (*Telegraaf*) or well-known Dutchmen (*De Volkskrant*):

They need a weekly injection in the buttock? Oh, you can forget it. There is no man who will do that. Men are very over-sensitive to injections. (a female writer in *De Volkskrant,* April 4, 1996)

Terrible. A hypodermic injection. I don't like to do that any more. . . . Imagine that I sit there in a waiting room with all these men who can already feel the pain in their buttocks. (a male actor in *De Volkskrant,* April 4, 1996)

An injection is painful and men are ten times more sensitive to pain than women, I have been told. So I don't see a breakthrough for a male contraceptive. (a male physician in *De Volkskrant,* April 4, 1996)

In *Haagse Post/De Tijd,* the journalist chose the role of participant observer of the discussions among his colleagues and fellow journalists. I quote again: "Although the male participants in the trial were enthusiastic about the buttock-injection, Dutch men don't seem to like the idea at all. Giggling, they discussed the side effects that the guinea pigs ('those poor guys') had to endure in the trial" (Leclair 1996).

The editors of *Algemeen Dagblad* even made their female colleagues believe that the new male contraceptive would have a negative impact on the national economy, because men would have to stop working for one hour a week to get their injections (Leclair 1996).

Journalistic discourse added yet another representation of male users: the image of overly sensitive men. Moreover, journalistic texts represent male users as unreliable, an image that is also present in feminist discourse.[13] Journalistic discourse thus confirms and legitimates the dominant gender script in which the responsibilities and risks of contraception are delegated to women. By constructing these images, journalists simultaneously reproduce and contest hegemonic, cultural representations of masculinity.[14] The portrayal of men as unreliable corresponds to hegemonic views of masculinity that emphasize the unreliability and disinterest of men toward contraception.[15] The image of overly sensitive men, however, does not resemble any hegemonic view of masculinity. To the contrary, dominant cultural representations of masculinity portray men as brave and strong (Connell 1995). By representing men as overly sensitive to pain, journalists embrace the incorporation of hegemonic feminine representations in which women rather than men are portrayed as the sensitive, weaker sex.

Two journals add images of men that go beyond hegemonic representations of masculinity. *De Volkskrant* presents two advocates of new male contraceptives, a football player on the Dutch national team and a physician. They suggest that weekly injections are no problem at all and that there are men who want to have control in matters of contraception (Vries 1996). In two cases, the journalists explicitly articulate new male identities. *De Volkskrant* chooses to illustrate the article about the opinions of well-known Dutch men and women with a photo of an electric razor next to a strip of pills. And the journalist in *Haagse Post/De Tijd* predicts (although with an ironical undertone): "Within a couple of years there will be contraception pills and plasters for sale at each drugstore. There is no doubt that the advertisement boys will find a nice marketing strategy: sexy black plasters taped on muscular upper arms or carelessly stuck on a shaggy stubbled chin" (Leclair 1996).

The media coverage of the WHO press bulletin in The Netherlands thus shows a conflicting set of representations of male users rather than an advocacy for new male contraceptives.[16]

CONCLUSIONS

My analysis of discourse on male contraceptives shows that gender identities and users are not stable, predetermined entities. Scientists, feminists, and journalists have constructed a variety of representations of masculinity and male users. Feminist texts are characterized by ambivalent feelings toward new male contraceptive technologies, and they present two conflicting user representations. Advocates of new male contraceptives represent the anticipated users as men who are willing to share health risks and responsibilities for contraception with their partners. Opponents of these technologies construct an image of men who cannot be trusted. Scientific discourse is dominated by the image of the Caring Man. In the media, users are primarily represented as overly sensitive, unreliable men who will never use a contraceptive injection.

I would like to suggest that representations of users are not innocent. On the contrary, they can function as tools in enhancing the cultural feasibility of a technology, as exemplified by the representations in scientific texts discussed above, or they can be used to denounce the viability of a new technology, as was seen in the journalistic texts. Journalists have used representations of masculinities to argue that new male contraceptives would never be accepted by men and women.

Quite remarkably, dissenting voices that refute commonly shared representations of male identity are not restricted to feminist discourse, as one might be inclined to think. Respectable and established organizations such as the WHO and the Population Council are active participants in the construction of new meanings for masculinity. The active role of scientists in articulating new images of maleness reveals an important feature of the role of scientists in society. By articulating and defending the image of the Caring Man, reproductive scientists have actively intervened in the cultural debate on masculinities. Scientists thus acted as cultural entrepreneurs. As has been described by sociologists of science and technology, the introduction of a new technology requires cultural intervention to create a demand for this technology. Consequently, there is a lot of cultural work to do for scientists who want to introduce a new technology, especially if the technology is a cultural novelty. The development of new male contraceptives is definitely a cultural novelty. Innovation in the field of male contraceptive technology has been absent from the R&D agenda of scientists and industry for a very long time. The fact that reproductive scientists working on male contraceptives have begun advocating new images of masculinity and new roles for men can thus be read in two ways. A cynical reading suggests that reproductive scientists have only adopted this role because they are committed to their research field. If they don't contribute to changing hegemonic representations of masculinity, their technology will ultimately become a failure. A more optimistic reading suggests that reproductive scientists have adopted the role of cultural entrepreneurs because they want to make a difference by contributing to gender equality in family planning. This reading gives hope for the future.

NOTES

A French version of this paper appeared in Cahiers du GEDISST in September 1999. I would like to thank Alvin Paulsen for granting me the interview I cite in this chapter.

1. For other studies on the construction of users by scientists and engineers, see Woolgar 1991 and Akrich 1992, 1995.

2. For an example of the cultural studies approach, see Van Dyck 1995. Similar arguments have been put forward by social interactionist scholars such as Clarke 1990, Fujimura 1988, 1992, and Star 1989.

3. For an analysis of the role of the pharmaceutical industry in male contraceptive research, see Oudshoorn 1998.

4. For an exception to this shift in feminist texts, see Lissner 1992.

5. I borrow the concept of anti-user from Pinch and Bijker 1987.

6. Margaret Sanger was arrested for opening the first birth control clinic in New York in 1916, and she founded the American Birth Control League in 1920. In 1951, she convinced Gregory Pincus of the need to develop "a simple, cheap contraceptive" for women, and she created the financial conditions for this research, which eventually resulted in the first oral contraceptive for women (Maisel 1965, 207).

7. For more discussion of the social worlds approach in science and technology studies, see Clarke 1990, Fujimura 1988, and Star 1989.

8. For an analysis of the impact of governments on male contraceptive research, particularly in southern countries, see Oudshoorn 1997.

9. The notion of the projected nonuser has been introduced by Madeleine Akrich (1992).

10. For surveys specifically focused on the acceptance of male methods in southern countries, see Davidson et al. 1985 and Gallen, Liskin, and Kok 1986.

11. On April 2, 1996, the WHO released the results of a clinical trial involving four hundred men in nine countries in Europe, Asia, and the United States. The WHO press release resulted in worldwide media coverage. Due to practical considerations, I have restricted my analysis to Dutch newspapers, including four of the five leading national dailies—*Algemeen Dagblad, De Volkskrant, Trouw,* and *De Telegraaf*—and one weekly journal, *Haagse Post/De Tijd.* These newspapers reach large audiences in all socioeconomic classes of the Dutch population and cover the major political currents in The Netherlands. *Trouw* and *De Volkskrant* traditionally aim at the more progressive, left-wing public, whereas *Algemeen Dagblad* and *De Telegraaf* target more conservative, right-wing audiences. *Haagse Post/De Tijd* attracts both progressive and conservative readers. All journals can be portrayed as "serious" newspapers; I have not included the tabloid press in my analysis. The media coverage of the WHO trial consisted of two types of texts. Most newspapers devoted a short article to the completion of the testing of the new male contraceptive. These texts basically summarize the main results of the test, as described in the WHO press release. The newspapers also included longer articles in their "background to the news" sections. I have decided to focus specifically on these background articles because they provide a much richer source to study the role of nonexperts in the construction of scientific claims. Such articles do not just repeat the news as it is formulated in scientific press releases or national or international news agencies; they relate the news to much broader contexts than indicated in these sources. Remarkably, the journalists were all women, except for *Haagse Post/De Tijd.*

12. The journalist might as well have used a more recent survey that showed 67 percent of Dutch women stressed the need for new male contraceptive methods (Vennix 1990).

13. This construction also includes a specific representation of male bodies. In journalistic texts, male bodies are represented as having a reproductive system that is much more complex than that of women. In women, so the argument goes, contraception requires interference with ovulation, which occurs "only once each month." In men, on the other hand, contraception requires intervention in the production of "tens of millions of spermatozoa each day throughout the adult's life" (Fawcett 1978). This representation strategy is used in newspapers as a tool to convince the reader that the "delay" in the development of male contraceptives is caused by the complex nature of male bodies and not by male bias (as has been claimed by feminist health advocates). Although this representation of male bodies is also present in scientific texts, reproductive biologists have criticized the use of the complex nature of the male reproductive system as an argument to justify the delay in the development of new male contraceptives: "There is no evidence that it is more difficult to prevent 'billions' of sperm from being produced, or acting, than one egg. The difference is not the numbers produced, but the discontinuity of egg production in the female and the continuity in the male. In many ways, it is easier to target a continuous process (where time of treatment may be unimportant) than a discontinuous process" (Schwartz 1976, 248).

14. Connell (1995, 79) describes hegemonic masculinity as a cultural construction that does not necessarily need to correspond to the actual personalities of most men: "The number of men rigorously practicing the hegemonic pattern in its entirety may be quite small." Moreover, hegemonic masculinity does not mean total cultural dominance of these representations; alternatives may exist, but they are subordinated. As Connell (1987, 186) has suggested, hegemonic masculinity is always constructed in relation to subordinated masculinities (and in relation to women).

15. See Gilmore 1993 and Stycos 1996 for a further analysis of cultural views of the relationships between masculinity, contraception, and fertility.

16. A browse through the media coverage of the press bulletin, as collected by the WHO (1996b), indicates that other national presses also voiced criticism on the acceptability of the hormonal contraceptive injection, although they seem to adopt a less critical attitude than the Dutch press. The *New York Times* (April 7, 1996, Sunday late edition) concluded that "men might not relish the discomfort" (WHO 1996b, 4). Criticism on the painful nature of the contraceptive injection was also voiced by the Associated Press (International News Section), which quoted two experts who described the technology as "a painful injection in the buttock" and "an effective contraceptive, the only drawback being the painful method" (WHO 1996b, 38). The *Times* also covered the WHO press bulletin and quoted the head of the Association of the British Pharmaceutical Industry: "Giving millions of men a high dose of a potent steroid strikes me as unacceptable" (WHO 1996b, 30). Several radio reports in the United States voiced a similar message. *Good Day Wake Up,* broadcast by WNYW in New York, quoted a spokesperson for Marie Stopes International, a major international family planning organization, who concluded: "This research still has a long way to go. . . . Getting men to take responsibility will be the real test" (WHO 1996b, 2). Finally, Cable News Networks (CNN) devoted a program to the results of the clinical trial. The highlight of this program ran as follows: "Officials at the World Health Organization say a pill form of a male contraceptive is unlikely in the near future. Experts believe cultures will have to change before men will take the hormones" (WHO 1996b, 40).

REFERENCES

Akrich, Madeleine:
  1992 The De-scription of Technical Objects. In Wiebe E. Bijker and John Law (eds.), *Shaping Technology/Building Society: Studies in Sociotechnical Change,* 205–44. Cambridge: MIT Press.
  1995 User Representations: Practices, Methods, and Sociology. In Arie Rip, Thomas J. Misa, and Johan Schot (eds.), *Managing Technology in Society: The Approach of Constructive Technology Assessment,* 167–84. London: Pinter.
Aldhous, Peter:
  1990 Equality for the Sexes? *Nature* 347 (October 25): 701.
Anonymous:
  1994 "Het Elfde Gebod." Utrecht en Heemstede: Stichting Rhea en Stichting Onderzoek Voorlichting Bevolkingspolitiek.
Berelson, Bernard:
  1969 Beyond Family Planning. *Science* 163(16): 533–43.
Bremner, William J., and David M. de Kretser:
  1975 Contraceptives for Male. *Signs: Journal of Women in Culture and Society* 1(21): 387–96.
Briggs, M.:
  1974 Oral Contraceptive for Men. *Nature* 252: 585–86.
Bruce, J.:
  1987 Users' Perspectives on Contraceptive Technology and Delivery Systems. *Technology in Society* 9: 359–83.

Christian Johnson, R.:

1977 Feminism, Philanthropy, and Science in the Development of the Oral Contraceptive Pill. *Pharmacy in History* 19(2): 63–79.

Clarke, Adele:

1990 Controversy and the Development of Reproductive Sciences. *Social Problems* 37(1): 18–37.

1999 *Disciplining Reproduction: Modernity, American Life and "the Problems of Sex."* Berkeley: University of California Press.

Committee on Women, Population, and the Environment:

1992 *Women, Population, and the Environment: Call for a New Approach.* Massachusetts: The Committee.

Connell, R. W.:

1987 *Gender and Power.* Cambridge: Polity Press.

1995 *Masculinities.* Cambridge: Polity Press.

Corea, Gena:

1985 *The Hidden Malpractice.* New York: Harper & Row.

Davidson, Andrew R., Kye Choon Ahn, Subhas Chandra, Rogelio Diaz-Guerro, D.C. Dubey, and Amir Mehryar:

1985 Contraceptive choices for men: Existing and potential male methods, Report prepared for presentation at the Seminar on Determinants of Contraceptive Method Choice, August 26–29, East-West Population Institute, Honolulu, Hawaii.

de Kretser, David M.:

1978 Fertility regulation in the male. *Bulletin of the World Health Organization* 56(3): 353–60.

Diczfalusy, E.:

1985 Contraceptive Futurology or 1984 in 1984. *Contraception* 31(1): 1–10.

Diller, Lawrence, and Wylie Hembree:

1977 Male contraception and family planning: A social and historical review. *Fertility and Sterility* 28(12): 1271–79.

Djerassi, Carl:

1970 Birth Control after 1984. *Science* 169: 941–51.

Fawcett, D. W.:

1978 Prospects for Fertility Control in the Male. In M. C. Diamond and C. C. Korenbrot (eds.), *Hormonal Contraceptives, Estrogens, and Human Welfare,* 57–75. New York: Academic Press.

Foegh, Marie:

1983 Evaluation of Steroids as Contraceptives for Men. *Acta Endocrinologica,* supplementum 260.

Fujimura, Joan H.:

1988 The Molecular Biological Bandwagon in Cancer Research: Where Social Worlds Meet. *Social Problems* 35: 261–83.

1992 Crafting Science: Standardized Packages, Boundary Objects, and Translation. In Andy Pickering (ed.), *Science as Practice and Culture,* 168–215. Chicago: University of Chicago Press.

Gallen, Moira E., Laurie Liskin, and Neenaj Kok:

1986 Men—New Focus for Family Planning Programs. *Population Reports* 1(33): 889–919.

Gelijns, Annetine C., and C. Ok. Pannenborg:
    1993   The Development of Contraceptive Technology: Case Studies of Incentives and Disincentives to Innovation. *International Journal of Technology Assessment in Health Care* 9(2): 210–32.

Gilmore, D.:
    1993   *De man als mythe: Mannelijkheid in verschillende culturen.* Amsterdam: Maarten Muntinga.

Gombe, S.:
    1983   A review of the current status in male contraceptive studies. *East African Medical Journal* 60(4): 203–11.

Greep, Roy O.:
    1975   Some Reflections on Male Reproductive Biology and Contraception. In C. H. Spilman, T. J. Lobl, and K. T. Kirton (eds.), *Regulatory Mechanisms of Male Reproductive Physiology: Sixth Brook Lodge Workshop on Problems of Reproductive Biology,* 1–10. Oxford: Excerpta Medica; New York: American Elsevier.

Greep, Roy O., Marjorie A. Koblinsky, and Frederick S. Jaffe (eds.):
    1976   *Reproduction and Human Welfare: A Challenge to Research.* Cambridge: MIT Press.

Greep, Roy O., and Marjorie A. Koblinsky:
    1977   *A Review of the Reproductive Sciences and Contraceptive Development.* Cambridge: MIT Press.

Handelsman, D. J.:
    1991   Bridging the Gender Gap in Contraception: Another Hurdle Cleared. *Medical Journal of Australia* 154(4): 230–33.

Haraway, Donna:
    1989   *Primate Visions: Gender, Race, and Nature in the World of Modern Science.* New York: Routledge.

Haspels, A. A.:
    1985   Hormonen en de pil. *Cahiers Bio-wetenschappen en Maatschappij* 10(1): 19–27.

Hubinont, P.O., M. L'Hermite, and J. Schwers (eds.):
    1976   Sperm Action. *Progress in Reproductive Biology.* Vol. 1. Basel: S. Karger.

International Women's Health Coalition:
    1994   Women's Voices '94: Women's Declaration on Population Policies. Report prepared for the 1994 International Conference on Population Policies.

Leclair, A.:
    1996   Waar blijft het gejuich om de bilprik? *Haagse Post/De Tijd,* April 12, pp. 8–10.

Lissner, Elaine A.:
    1992   Frontiers in Nonhormonal Male Contraceptive Research. In Helen B. Holmes (ed.), *Issues in Reproductive Technology: An Anthology,* 53–69. New York: Garland.

Maisel, A. Q.:
    1965   *The Hormone Quest.* New York: Random House.

Matlin, S.:
    1994   The Pill—40 years on. *Education in Chemistry,* September, 123–27.

Myers, Greg:
    1990   *Writing Biology: Texts in the Social Construction of Scientific Knowledge.* Madison: University of Wisconsin Press.

Norsigian, Judy:
    1979   Redirecting Contraceptive Research. *Science for the People,* January/February, 27–31.

Oudshoorn, Nelly:

1997   On Power and Discourse: Feminists and Reproductive Scientists in the Quest for New Male Contraceptives. Unpublished manuscript.

1998   Shifting Boundaries between Industry and Science: The Role of the WHO in Contraceptive R&D. In J.-P. Gaudillière and I. Löwy (eds.), *The Invisible Industrialist: Manufactures and the Production of Scientific Knowledge*, 345–68. London: Macmillan Press.

Paulsen, C. Alvin:

1994   Interview, October 18. Seattle.

1997   Regulation of Male Fertility. In R. O. Greep and M. A. Koblinsky (eds.), *Frontiers in Reproduction and Fertility Control: A Review of the Reproductive Sciences and Contraceptive Development*, 458–65. Cambridge: MIT Press.

Pinch, Trevor J., and Wiebe E. Bijker:

1987   The Social Construction of Facts and Artefacts; or, How the Sociology of Science and the Sociology of Technology Might Benefit Each Other. In W. E. Bijker, T. P. Hughes, and T. J. Pinch (eds.), *The Social Construction of Technological Systems: New Directions in the Sociology and History of Technology*. Cambridge: MIT Press.

Population Council:

1995a   *Men and Families,* no. 1, February.

1995b   *Men and Families,* no. 2, September.

Schwartz, Neena B.:

1995   Comment on Bremner and de Kretser's "Contraceptives for Males." *Signs: Journal of Women in Culture and Society* 2(1): 247–48.

Seaman, Barbara:

1969   *The Doctor's Case against the Pill.* New York: Peter H. Wyden.

Seaman, Barbara, and Gideon Seaman:

1977   A Pill for Men. In *Women and the Crisis in Sex Hormones: An Investigation of the Dangerous Uses of Hormones: From Birth Control to Menopause and the Safe Alternatives,* 301–35. Brighton, Sussex: Harvester.

Segal, Sheldon J.:

1971   Beyond the Laboratory: Recent Research Advances in Fertility Regulation. *Family Planning Perspectives* 3(3): 17–21.

1972   Contraceptive Research: A Male Chauvinist Plot? *Family Planning Perspectives* 4(3): 21–25.

Soufir, Jean-Claude, Pierre Jouannet, Jocelyne Marson, and Arlette Soumach:

1983   Reversible inhibition of sperm production and gonadotrophin secretion in men following combined oral medroxyprogesterone acetate and percutaneoustestosterone treatment. *Acta Endocrinologica* 102(4): 625–32.

Star, Susan Leigh:

1989   *Regions of the Mind: Brain Research and the Quest for Scientific Certainty.* Stanford: Stanford University Press.

Stokes, Bruce:

1980   Men and Family Planning. *Worldwatch Paper* 41 (December): 5–48.

Stycos, J. M.:

1996   Men, couples, and family planning: A retrospective look. Working paper no. 96. Ithaca: Department of Rural Sociology, Cornell University.

Trouw:

1996   Prikpil voor mannen is geen pretje, maar wel betrouwbaar. April 6.

United Nations Population Fund:

1994   *International Conference on Population and Development: Programme of Action.* New York: United Nations.

Van Dyck, José:

1995   *Manufacturing Babies and Public Consent: Debating the New Reproductive Technologies.* London: Macmillan Press.

Vennix, P.:

1990   De pil en haar alternatieven. *Nisso studies. Nieuwe reeks* 6. Utrecht: Eburon.

Von Hippel, E.:

1976   The Dominant Role of Users in the Scientific Instrument Innovation Process. *Research Policy* 5: 212–39.

1988   *The Sources of Innovation.* Oxford: Oxford University Press.

Vries, C. de:

1996   Mannenpil? *Volkskrant,* April 4, p. 17.

World Health Organization:

1996a WHO Completes International Trial of a Hormonal Contraceptive for Men. Press release, April 2. Geneva: WHO.

1996b Nexis/Lexis. A Collection of the Media Coverage of the WHO press bulletin released on April 2.

Woolgar, Steve:

1991   Configuring the User: The Case of Usability Trials. In John Law (ed.), *A Sociology of Monsters: Essays on Power, Technology, and Domination,* 58–99. London: Routledge.

Wu, F. C. W.:

1988   Male contraception: Current status and future prospects. *Clinical Endocrinology* 29: 443–65.

5

Parenting the Pill: Early Testing of the Contraceptive Pill

Lara Marks

The oral contraceptive, introduced during the same period as the space race for the moon and the rapid expansion in manufactured consumer goods, is widely considered a great milestone in the battle of science over nature. Such visions not only colored the image of the Pill when it first appeared but have influenced its subsequent history. This has generated many myths about the oral contraceptive. One such legend is that it was developed by three "fathers": Gregory Pincus (biologist), Carl Djerassi (chemist), and John Rock (obstetrician-gynecologist).[1] In a 1995 paper, Djerassi goes as far as to call himself "The Mother of the Pill."[2] Such mythology partly stems from the fact that much of the early history of the oral contraceptive was written by the scientists and medical experts involved in its initial development, who had an interest in promoting themselves as its inventors.[3] Scientists have not been the only ones to eulogize their efforts. In 1965, for instance, Dr. Anne Biezanek noted, "Of all the great works that men have undertaken for women, [the Pill] must surely rank amongst the noblest. The work was instigated at a time when financial reward was very slight and the risks considerable. It was done in the teeth of social disapproval and in the teeth of great apathy on the part of the medical profession at large. The first men who devised those things at such risk to themselves must one day be named and honoured by all women as 'the instigators of the revolution.'"

This enthusiasm was soon tempered. Since 1970, when the side effects of the Pill began to be publicly debated, there has been much disapproval of its development. Many critics have attacked the original investigators for inadequately testing the product before releasing it onto the market. In this context the Pill is seen as a product developed by primarily male scientists to control women. On the basis of this assumption, women are depicted as having been used as unwitting guinea pigs.[4] Such criticism not only ignores the historical context in which the Pill was developed, but reinforces the idea that it arose out of the work of individual scientists.[5] Yet the oral contraceptive cannot be seen as a pure triumph for science, nor should it be seen as solely the invention of male scientists. These perspectives miss the complex social context in which the Pill was developed, as well as the large network of people and skills that were needed for its emergence.

This chapter focuses on the role women played in the development of the Pill in a variety of ways ranging from them being initiators and sponsors of the research, to the technicians and doctors who supervised the day-to-day running of the project, and the women who participated in the trials. These women's contribution to the development of the drug not only challenges the many historical myths surrounding it but expands our overall understanding of expertise and knowledge in the making of scientific technology. As the case of oral contraception shows, expertise and knowledge cannot be judged solely on the basis of the work of key individual scientific experts nor should it be confined to the site of the laboratory. The making of the Pill was dependent on the expertise of people from a multitude of disciplines.

WOMEN AS SPONSORS

When hormones were discovered in 1905, few would have imagined that just fifty years later millions of women would swallow synthetic hormones for contraceptive purposes. In 1921 Ludwig Haberlandt, an Austrian physiologist, hypothesized that a hormonal contraceptive was possible on the basis of experiments with mice and rabbits. During the interwar years his idea became increasingly feasible with the expanding knowledge gathered from investigations into the physiology of reproduction in animals and humans and the isolation of sex hormones. Despite these advances, many barriers remained in the manufacturing of a contraceptive pill. One of the problems was the expense of the hormones and the fact that many of them were largely ineffective if ingested orally.

Contraception was also illegal in many countries, and this made scientists reluctant to pursue such research (Vaughan 1972; Borell 1987; Oudshoorn 1994, 113–15). The strength of the impediments facing researchers can be seen from the long and bitter struggle many campaigners, particularly women, had mounted since the late nineteenth century for the right to contraceptive knowledge and the means to control fertility. For many, contraception held the key to women's freedom. As one family planning campaigner put it in 1929, "The emancipation and acknowledgement of an equal status for women can never be realized until motherhood is by choice and not by chance."[6] Many birth control crusaders experienced legal prosecution and imprisonment as a result of their activities.

One of the most important figures in the contraceptive battle was Margaret Sanger. She had originally been galvanized into the campaign by the bad health and high rates of maternal mortality she witnessed while working as a nurse on the Lower East Side of New York at the turn of the century. By the 1920s Sanger had succeeded in establishing a number of American birth control clinics and an international organization and journals to promote and stimulate scientific contraceptive research (Sanger 1937, 3–4). In 1937 one of Sanger's journals re-printed articles indicating the possibility of hormonal sterilizing agents for contraception (Kuzrock 1937; Henle 1937). For Sanger this represented the potential for a great leap in contraception. As early as 1912 she had expressed the hope of finding a "magic pill" that could be used for contraception.[7]

Sanger held that it was vital to find a contraceptive technique that would allow women full control over their fertility without the cooperation of the male, as necessitated by barrier contraceptive methods. Ideally she was looking for something that could be taken by mouth and not at the moment of inter-course. Writing to a friend in 1946, she summed up the strength of her feelings on the matter when she admitted that she felt increasingly despondent when she "saw and realized more than ever the inadequacy of the diaphragm reaching millions of women who need and should have something as simple as a birth control pill" (Gray 1979, 396).[8] Part of Sanger's interest in finding an oral contraceptive may have resulted from her repeated gallbladder attacks for which she had been prescribed pills. This had perhaps made her realize how easily a pill could be integrated into a person's daily routine (Gray 1979, 371). For Sanger, finding an easier method of contraception also represented a key to resolving what she and many others saw as the ever-increasing problem of high birthrates among the more impoverished population of the world. As she stated, "I consider that the world and almost all our civilization for the next twenty-five years is going to depend on a simple, cheap, safe contraceptive to be used in poverty-stricken slums and jungles, and among the most ignorant people" (Vaughan 1972, 27).

By the 1940s, scientists seemed on the verge of finding a substance that could provide an oral contraceptive. The breakthrough in steroid chemistry as a result of the appearance of cortisone to treat arthritis had resulted in an abundance of the cheap steroid progesterone. Despite the potential opportunities this opened up for contraceptive research, few scientists, however, were willing to take on the project. Given public attitudes, any scientist who attempted such research faced the possibility of losing scientific recognition and access to government funding.[9]

In looking to boost contraceptive research, Sanger found a powerful ally in Katharine McCormick. The second woman to graduate from Massachusetts Institute of Technology, McCormick had met Sanger in 1917. Trained in biology, McCormick had the necessary scientific background for understanding the research needed to achieve such a pill. Her marriage to Stanley McCormick, whose father had invented the mechanical reaper and established the International Harvester Company, meant that she also had financial resources at her disposal to invest in such a cause. In the words of John Rock, who planned the first human trials of the Pill, McCormick was "as rich as Croesus. She had a *vast* fortune . . . she couldn't even spend the interest on her *interest*" (cited in Vaughan 1972, 26).

Like Sanger, McCormick saw contraception as the key to women's empowerment. Part of her desire for better contraceptive methods may have resulted from her own experiences: her husband had become schizophrenic within two years of their marriage, and because she believed schizophrenia to be hereditary, McCormick was reluctant to have children. She had to balance this decision against constant sexual demands from her husband.[10] Significantly, in 1958 McCormick remarked that she "didn't give a hoot for a male contraceptive" and all that concerned her was a female one.[11] She also saw a foolproof contraceptive as an important weapon in the fight against population growth.[12] For twenty years McCormick corresponded with Sanger about furthering contraceptive research, but she was unable to commit much money to the cause until her husband's death in 1947. Up to that time, most of her finances had been invested in neuropsychiatric research in an effort to find a cure for schizophrenia to help her husband.[13]

In 1950 McCormick began to consult Sanger in earnest about the best way to invest her money in contraception (Vaughan 1972, 27). Sanger recommended the distribution of $25,000 ($100,000 a year) to five or six university laboratories to promote contraceptive projects.[14] McCormick, however, was temporarily unable to commit her funds to this cause because of the bureaucratic procedures involved in settling her late husband's estate (Reed 1978, 338).

Ironically, it was the network of contacts McCormick had built up as a result of her sponsorship of research into schizophrenia that proved vital to the development of the Pill. One of the people she had met through this work was Hudson Hoagland. In 1944 Hoagland had helped found the Worcester Foundation for Experimental Biology (WF). A nonprofit, tax-privileged educational and research institution in Massachusetts, the WF specialized in steroidal research.[15] Much of the research undertaken by the WF during the 1940s was directed at issues concerning the influence of hormones in diseases such as cancer, arthritis, and certain nervous and mental conditions (Worcester Foundation 1949–50, 4). The WF also had a strong research interest in reproductive physiology, which was to be important in the development of the Pill. Heading this research was Hudson's codirector, Gregory Pincus, who was a leading expert in mammalian sexual physiology.[16] During the late 1940s he directed his work toward understanding the process of fertilization so as to enable medical experts to prevent spontaneous abortion and menstrual disorders (Reed 1978, 340). By the 1950s Pincus had become an international figure in hormone and steroid research, and he enjoyed close ties with a number of pharmaceutical companies. The WF had also become a key clearing center for testing the physiological effects of new steroidal compounds produced by pharmaceutical companies.[17] Pincus thus had access to many of the latest discoveries in steroid chemistry, making him ideal for hormonal contraceptive research.

Sanger had met Pincus through Abraham Stone, an associate of the Planned Parenthood Foundation of America (PPFA) and director of the Margaret Sanger Research Bureau in New York. It was she who proposed Pincus consider directing his research toward contraception (Pincus 1965, 5–6). Pincus saw Sanger's suggestion as a useful way of gaining more money for the WF. Spurred on by Sanger, in 1951–52 Pincus received $6,500 from the PPFA to study hormonal contraception.[18] In January 1952, Pincus reported that the oral administration of ten milligrams of progesterone prevented ovulation in rabbits. From his perspective this showed progesterone to have contraceptive properties.[19] Despite these promising results, the PPFA was unwilling to invest any more in the project, and it remained low on the list of priorities within the WF.[20]

In March 1952, Sanger alerted McCormick to the contraceptive potential of Pincus's work.[21] That May, McCormick, aged seventy-six, moved from Santa Barbara to Boston with the intention of furthering Pincus's efforts. In June 1953, she agreed to pay $10,000 a year to pursue the project.[22] She subsequently raised her sponsorship to meet whatever expenses Pincus needed, including $50,000 to build a new animal house. McCormick also funded extra building space to expedite the human trials.[23] McCormick's financial support was crucial in freeing Pincus and his colleagues from what she saw as the frustrating bureaucratic red tape of the PPFA.[24]

McCormick's sponsorship was critical to the development of the Pill (Reed 1978, 433). Without her, Pincus had little financial support for his contraceptive investigations. The PPFA, the main American sponsor of contraceptive research in those years, was unenthusiastic about his research. From its perspective, Pincus remained far from achieving a marketable drug. Many of the PPFA's personnel were "consistently stuffy" about Pincus's efforts, preferring to sponsor research that upheld the "accepted social code." Their funding was directed toward existing methods of birth control or projects undertaken by physicians in clinical settings. For the medical staff of the PPFA, the Pill was too risky in terms of its potential side effects and ineffectiveness. They feared that any flaw in the project would backfire on the organization and the family planning movement as a whole.[25] Pharmaceutical companies, with whom Pincus had close connections, were also not forthcoming with money for his contraceptive project (Vaughan 1972, 52; Reed 1978, 331–33 and 343–44).[26] As Pincus recalled in 1967, "In the search for an oral progestin we contacted a number of companies indicating that our objective was a contraceptive, and practically all of them refused to cooperate because this was considered a 'dangerous field.'"[27] Once it proved a success, pharmaceutical companies and PPFA members changed their tune. McCormick stood out in that she was willing to fund research that had practical applications. Much of the research prior to her involvement with Pincus had focused on basic science with little attention to its practical implications.[28]

McCormick's financial support became crucial when insufficient finances threatened to halt the Pill project in 1953.[29] One of the most pressing problems at this time was finding a sponsor for human clinical trials, which were costly to set up and run. The overall illegality of contraceptive research made this difficult. In 1953, for instance, a philanthropist withdrew previously promised money for human clinical trials upon discovering they were to be conducted in Massachusetts, where the laws forbade contraceptive research.[30] Such laws, however, did not stop McCormick.[31] For her the Pill represented a chance to overcome many of the legal and social obstacles in the promotion of contraception. By 1960 McCormick had provided over $1 million for clinically testing the Pill. This supported clinical trials in Massachusetts and New York as well as in Puerto Rico and Haiti. These trials provided the data on which the FDA based its approval of the drug.[32]

Writing in 1956, nine months after the launch of the first large-scale clinical trials, Sanger recognized the significance of McCormick's contribution. As she said,

> Dear Kay,
> You must, indeed, feel a certain pride in your judgement. Gregory Pincus had been working for at least ten years on the progesterone of reproductive process in animals. He had practically no money for this work. . . . Then you came along with your fine interest and enthusiasm—with your faith and wonderful directives—[and] things began to happen and at last the reports . . . are now out in the outstanding scientific magazine and the conspiracy of silence has been broken.[33]

McCormick took a highly active interest in the day-to-day running of the project. Her words "freezing in Boston for the Pill" in 1955 capture the essence of her commitment (Asbell 1995, 134).[34] McCormick was scrupulous in following the progress of the Pill. Her biological training meant that she could take an active interest in the laboratory work. She frequently paid visits to the WF to keep an eye on progress. In this she was merely repeating a pattern she had followed in all her previous charitable contributions. According to her lawyer, McCormick would only sponsor a project where she understood "each problem and all of its details. Details were all-important to Katharine. She welcomed advice, listened to the opinions of others, spent endless hours going over every aspect of each problem to make sure that the ultimate result, regardless of time and expense, would measure up" to her objectives. From her lawyer's perspective, "no professional trustee ever gave the tenacious and conscientious attention to his duties that Katharine gave to her own self-imposed rules" (cited in Reed 1978, 337–38). McCormick was not a figure who could be dismissed easily. As Pincus recalled, she was not an "insignificant nothing, she was tall and carried herself like a ramrod. Little old woman she was *not*. She was a grenadier" (cited in Vaughan 1972, 26). If a project did not meet her expectations, McCormick was quite capable of withdrawing her interest and financial support.[35]

From 1954, when Pincus began to set up the initial human trials, until 1960, when the Pill was officially marketed, McCormick was in regular contact with Pincus. McCormick's letters indicate that she understood the complicated scientific nature of the experiments and clinical trials. In addition to examining the minutiae of the scientific and clinical methodology to be used, she helped evaluate staff and the sites for the trials as well as the kinds of patients who were suitable.[36] The degree to which Pincus valued McCormick's scientific input can be judged by the fact that he dedicated his book "to Mrs. Stanley McCormick because of her steadfast faith in scientific inquiry and her unswerving encouragement of human dignity" (Pincus 1985). By contrast, Sanger did not always grasp the fine mechanics of the science involved in the research. For this she relied on McCormick.[37] Hoagland also asked McCormick to become a trustee of the WF in 1954. In requesting this, Hoagland made it clear that he regarded her as more than just a sponsor. As he stated, "We would value your advice and active participation in the affairs of the Foundation."[38]

Neither McCormick's nor Sanger's name appears in any of the scientific articles published on the Pill. Nonetheless, their contributions were vital to its development. Women of social status and wealth, they were among the elite of their time. As long-standing campaigners for birth control, they helped put contraception on the public agenda. They were used to taking initiatives and finding money to push forward research and family planning policies. Such skills were no less critical than scientific ones in producing the oral contraceptive.[39] Given the taboos surrounding contraception and the lack of funding for such research, it is unlikely that Pincus would have applied his reproductive research experience to the formulation of a pill without Sanger's vision and encouragement. Equally, his research could not have made such rapid progress without McCormick's financial and moral support.

WOMEN AS TECHNICIANS

Women from less powerful backgrounds, including women technicians, were just as important in the making of the Pill. Yet their names are frequently missing from the official history of the Pill. As is the case with many scientific and technological innovations, their role has often been ignored due to their status as technicians. So entrenched is the status of Pincus and his fellow scientists in the history of the Pill, the technicians themselves stress the importance of Pincus's work over their own. Yet while Pincus and his scientific and medical colleagues designed the overall project, the day-to-day mechanics of such work could not have been done without the expertise and knowledge of such technicians.

At the WF, the technician who conducted the bulk of the animal tests and laboratory tests for humans was Anne Merrill. Pincus acknowledged in his book that much of the animal experimentation for the Pill could not have been achieved without her "meticulous efforts." In later years, Merrill was joined by others, among them Mary Ellen Fitts Johnson. Their joint labor reveals the complex and patient nature of laboratory work and how results were not achieved overnight. Their job demanded an intricate knowledge of the reproductive cycle of the experimental animals as well as an adeptness at laboratory work. In the later stages of the Pill's development, their tasks demanded ingenuity because the testing was performed outside the laboratory and in places where even basic scientific facilities were poor.

Much of the early work undertaken by the technicians involved testing orally active chemical substances in animals.[40] In 1952 and 1953, various compounds, including synthetic progestins, were tried out on animals. The explicit purpose of these tests was to find a compound suitable for human consumption.[41] This was not a quick process, because the action of each compound was completely unknown until tested on animals. In each case a control group of animals had initially to be screened to determine the standard effect expected from different doses of pure hormones. This was then matched against results of synthetic compounds given to animals.[42]

Several types of animals were used for the experiments. Rabbits were used because they ovulate within ten hours of mating. They were thus easy subjects for monitoring the effects of the experimental substances. Rats were used because they exhibit spontaneous ovulation in the course of their oestrous cycle that is comparable with the human female (Pincus 1965, 57 and 67–68). Work with each of these animals involved a great deal of preparation. This was more the case with rats than rabbits because the ovulation of the former was not easily observable and thus necessitated more time-consuming and complicated procedures. Female rabbits merely needed isolating for a few weeks before being given the experimental drug, and then they were checked for ovulation suppression after mating. By contrast, female rats not only had to be isolated from the male but had to have daily vaginal smears to determine the exact stage of their reproductive cycle. Each of these smears had to be observed under a microscope to determine the stage of the rat's oestrus cycle. Only when they were deemed to be at the appropriate moment of their cycle were they given the progesterone substance. Then caged with the male, the female rat was given daily vaginal examinations to detect sperm or vaginal secretions.[43]

Pregnancies in rabbits and rats were determined by palpating each animal's abdomen. Checking for ovulation was a more complicated process. Rabbits had to be checked within forty-eight hours of mating by surgically opening the abdomen (laparotomy), and checking for ruptured follicles in their ovaries. All the rabbits, because they were expensive, were stitched up after each laparotomy and were reused for other experiments once the compound had worn off. Rats, by contrast, were cheaper and could be sacrificed. They were also more delicate and thus more susceptible to damage than rabbits. In each case the rat's uterus and ovaries were closely scrutinized and weighed for signs of ovulation and fertilization.[44]

All of these stages were time-consuming. Not only did the animals have to be closely monitored; each stage involved a great deal of cleaning and washing and making of solutions.[45] Each phase was fiddly. When examining the tissue of the uterus, for instance, Merrill had to take "a piece of uterus" and put it "through umpteen . . . solutions . . . to fix it like embalming." She then had "to get rid of the embalming supplies" and "get it into wax, into some firm thing" so that it could be cut. All this had to be done by hand, which involved doing "two hours here, and five hours here." She and Fitts Johnson often had to run into the laboratory "at midnight to change something."[46] From the 1960s this process was made easier by rigging up a blade to the foot pedal of a sewing machine. This freed up the technician's hands in slicing the tissue. Prior to this the technician had to crank the machine with one hand while deftly catching the tissue with the other. Not surprisingly the technicians were constantly inventing new machinery to make their work easier.[47]

Undertaking regular medical checkups and investigative examinations with women was also complicated. The main difficulty was working away from the enclosed environment of the WF's small and well-equipped laboratory. Facilities were very basic in Puerto Rico and Haiti, where the bulk of the first trials were conducted. This meant that everything had to be taken from the WF and set up in these countries. As Fitts Johnson explained,

> It was a major undertaking, taking all the stuff down there. I mean, you literally had to take the lab, a portable lab with you. . . . We would box everything up ahead of time, we'd take an inventory of the supplies, and we'd have great big numbers on the box, and every time we'd get on a plane, we'd count. . . . If we stopped anywhere, or they unloaded anything, someone would double-check to see if anything got off-loaded. And when we arrived there, we would take the inventory, make sure all the boxes were with us. It really was a major production, getting everything there.[48]

It was not uncommon for equipment to be lost along the way. This was a serious problem because replacements were not available in Puerto Rico and Haiti. In addition to this, none of the equipment was disposable. Everything had to be washed before it could be reused. This included the needles, syringes, and glass slides. Washing was not a straightforward process, because Haiti had no large amounts of distilled water. As Merrill admitted, it was like working out in the middle of nowhere.[49]

Given these problems, only the most basic of blood and urine tests were performed in Puerto Rico. Blood and other samples were preserved so that more elaborate tests could be done back in Worcester. Preserving these test samples was difficult due to the absence of storage and freezing.[50] One way round this was to import dry ice to help preserve the blood and other samples collected, but this was not foolproof. On one occasion in Haiti when they ran out of dry ice, Merrill spent hours hunting for a freezer to store the samples and finally used the one at the American embassy. Another problem confronting them in Haiti was the intermittent supply of electricity. This made it difficult to work with microscopes.[51]

Not only did technicians run the day-to-day routine of laboratory testing, but they were crucial to the analytical process. They were the ones who sorted out the hundreds of questionnaires and forms from the human trials. This involved taking a stack of reports and tallying them by hand. As Merrill and Fitts Johnson pointed out, "We didn't have computers back then. We had pens and paper. . . . [We were] inundated with papers. How many people had headaches, how many people had this, how many people had that. How many missed two pills during the month. I mean, you cross-referenced the data a zillion different ways by hand, and we would work all night."[52] This also demanded intricate mathematics.[53]

Such work took days and often involved staying up all night. The technicians got no extra pay for overtime. They received minimal salaries. As they recalled, the WF was "a non-profit place, and we were ladies, so we got minimum of everything!"[54] From their perspective they were willing to put in the hours for "the dedication to science, and learning."[55] They saw their work as helping women to have fewer children. Indeed, they had no idea that the outcome of their efforts was going "to turn the world upside down."[56]

Away from the WF, another technician who was vital to the development of the Pill was Miriam Menkin. Originally setting out to become a physician, Menkin, like many other women at her time, had been thwarted in her ambition by the demands of a husband and family. This had not stopped her from getting a bachelor's degree in science, specifically embryology and histology, and a master's degree in zoology with an emphasis in genetics. She had also twice completed the requirements for a Ph.D. at Harvard University but been denied the degree because she was unable to pay the course fees. Originally working with Pincus in the early 1930s on a project concerned with pituitary hormones that regulate ovulation, she had by 1938 joined the obstetrician John Rock at the Brookline Free Hospital for Women, where she became pivotal to his research into infertility and the emergence of in vitro fertilization. Menkin was no less important in Rock's work on the Pill in the 1950s (McLaughlin 1982, 72–89). She played a vital role not only in the necessary laboratory work but also in plotting the research and testing strategies proposed. Menkin also supervised the daily running of the clinical trials with the patients. This involved interviewing and checking that each patient had understood the instructions given by the doctors. Behind the scenes Menkin was also the "reference researcher and manuscript editor for scientific articles that reported the stage of [the Pill's] development." In later years she helped Rock write "popular pieces on the Pill and its role in curbing runaway birth rates" (McLaughlin 1982, 91).

WOMEN AS CLINICAL RESEARCHERS

Just as crucial as the technicians to the day-to-day running of the trials were the female physicians who organized and supervised the human clinical trials. Like Sanger and McCormick, women physicians brought a great deal of expertise from their fight for the contraceptive cause since the early years of the twentieth century. Many of them had turned to family planning work as a means of survival when unable to gain a foothold in more traditionally male medical domains. Considering it taboo, many male physicians by contrast were unwilling to take on contraceptive work.[57]

One of the most prominent physicians involved in the early large-scale clinical trials of the Pill was Dr. Edris Rice-Wray. She was an ideal ally for Pincus and his colleagues because she had an American training and approach to medical care that guaranteed them the collection of accurate data.[58] It was vital to have a person who could accurately assess the reproductive and menstrual patterns of patients and take vaginal smears.[59] At the time she met Pincus, Rice-Wray was on the faculty at the Puerto Rico Medical School and director of the Public Health Department's Field Training Center for nurses. She was also medical director of the Puerto Rican Family Planning Association, and she ran a contraceptive clinic where she trained medical students in contraceptive work. Rice-Wray conducted a number of trials with conventional barrier methods.[60] She had experience in organizing family planning programs and the necessary contacts for gaining access to possible test locations for the Pill (Reed 1978, 359; Oudshoorn 1994, 128). For her, the Pill project provided a financial opportunity to boost the poorly funded local Planned Parenthood Federation in San Juan.[61]

It was Rice-Wray's networks that decided the location of the first large-scale human trials. She proposed conducting the trial in Rio Piedras, a suburb of San Juan, where a new housing project had been set up as part of a slum-clearance campaign. Many of these families highly prized their new accommodations and were therefore unlikely to move away during the course of the trial. This would make them easy to monitor.[62] While Pincus and Rock were responsible for the overall research design of the Rio Piedras trial, Rice-Wray was in charge of the fieldwork. She was expected to recruit cases, distribute the Pill, monitor the reactions, and collect the necessary data (Ramirez de Arellano and Seipp 1983, 113).

Rice-Wray's supervision of the Rio Piedras trials was not easy. As had been the case in other trials, she found it difficult to ensure that the women stayed on the trial and adhered to the set regime of the Pill. Within the first month, thirty women dropped out of the trial when a local newspaper claimed the trial to be a "neomalthusian campaign" to sterilize and harm women.[63] Many women also left the trial on account of side effects such as nausea, dizziness, headaches, and vomiting.[64] Rice-Wray calculated that 17 percent of the subjects had these reactions during the first months of the trial. From her perspective, this phenomenon threatened the long-term viability of the Pill.[65] Some of these negative effects were overcome by diminishing the dose of oestrogen in the Pill and by supplying antacids. Many of the side effects also disappeared if women stayed on the medication for some time.[66] Side effects were not the only problem Rice-Wray faced. Some women were forced to abandon the trial because of objections from their husbands, others because they moved to another area. Some stopped because they wanted to become pregnant or to be sterilized.[67]

Finding replacements for these women, however, was easy. Women were continually begging to join the trial. A waiting list had to be drawn up to cope with the demand.[68]

Overall the dropout of patients was a trivial problem compared with the hostility toward the project from the secretary of health, who saw it as interfering with Rice-Wray's duties within the Public Health Department. In the end Rice-Wray was forced to resign her position and leave Puerto Rico.[69] Despite her resignation, she had furnished Pincus with a successful model for establishing other clinical trials elsewhere. Before her departure she had managed to collect data on 221 patients, none of whom had fallen pregnant due to method failure.[70]

Rice-Wray's involvement in the development of the Pill did not stop here. She soon became involved in trials elsewhere, setting up a trial in Haiti in 1957. Representing Pincus, Rice-Wray surveyed the types of women to be used in the Haiti trial and assessed the staff to conduct the project. She also took care of the financial side of the project and made regular checkups on the progress of the trial. This she combined with her frequent visits to Haiti to help in the reorganization of the medical school there. While responsible for the pill trials, Rice-Wray could not make this official for fear of disapproval from her new employer, the World Health Organization (WHO). Many of the member states of WHO were reluctant to be involved in anything to do with birth control. She was unable to even mention the words birth control in the organization.[71] In addition to the trials in Haiti, Rice-Wray set up the first trials of the Pill in Mexico. Employed as a technical consultant for the Association of Mexican Medical Schools, by December 1958 she had managed, at Pincus's suggestion, to set up trials in a gynecological clinic in collaboration with the Mexican pharmaceutical company, Syntex, which wanted to test its own pill, Norlutin. Rice-Wray also tested several other compounds produced by Syntex.[72]

Much of Rice-Wray's work in Mexico had to be conducted on a clandestine basis. She was unable to publicize any of the trial work she undertook at the gynecological clinic.[73] Rice-Wray outlined the difficulties she experienced to Pincus: "Of course you understand that we are not in any way known as a Planned Parenthood Clinic. We talk about everything *but* this service. Only to our most intimate friends do we give the information that over 75% of our patients have come for contraceptive advice."[74] The clinic itself was based in an apartment block so that it would be "less noticeable."[75] Opposition from the Roman Catholic Church as well as the government made the issue of contraception taboo in Mexico. Government officials were more interested in promoting population growth, which they saw as the key to industrialization, than in curbing the birthrate.[76]

Working conditions were thus not easy. Rice-Wray admitted to Pincus a year after starting the trial, "I have been working like mad and feel very worn out and exhausted." Not only did she have to conduct the work alongside her other professional duties, but she also campaigned for family planning in general.[77] Overall her efforts paid off. Within a year she had gained help from a number of Mexican doctors and other health professionals.[78] By January 1960, twenty-two doctors were paying regular visits to the clinic and taking an interest in the trials. In addition to this, a local Catholic priest had begun to support the work of the clinic and contraceptive trials.[79] By July 1961, a total of 2,073 patients had registered at the clinic, and 100 new patients were registering with the clinic every month. Of these, 76 percent were coming for contraceptive advice, many demanding the Pill. Indeed, many of the women refused to use any other method.[80]

Despite this success, the survival of the trials was constantly under threat. A major problem was the hostility Rice-Wray faced as an American.[81] By October 1961, she was experiencing problems on account of "envy and jealousy" on the part of four Mexican doctors. In the end their complaints reached the ears of the health minister, who closed the clinic on the pretext of the potential health hazards of hormonal steroids and the offense such work might cause the Catholic Church. The clinic was closed for three months. Ultimately, however, the episode won the clinic official recognition, which made it easier to conduct the trials.[82] Despite this, Rice-Wray had to scale down her involvement with the trials. As she wrote in the early 1970s to a British representative for Searle: "There is such a prejudice against Americans here in Mexico that in order for our clinic to collaborate with government in their family planning program, we had to get rid of the American image—meaning me—our clinic had been called Dr. Rice-Wray's clinic for too long. So I am out—retired—I remain as chief technical advisor. But the truth is that the less my American face is seen in the clinic, the better."[83]

In 1963 Rice-Wray also struggled to keep the clinic and the trials alive in the face of corruption from her clinic staff, who, behind her back, had begun to siphon away the funds provided by pharmaceutical companies to test pills. After a legal battle and moving the clinic to a new location, Rice-Wray managed to secure the future of the trials.[84] She went on to initiate pill programs in rural areas of Mexico.[85]

While instrumental in the setting up of the first large-scale human trials of the Pill and extending such trials to other locations, Rice-Wray was not the only one busy in this field. Another woman physician who played a vital role in the early testing of the Pill was the American-born Adaline Satterthwaite. Formerly a medical missionary in China, Satterthwaite had begun to work in 1952 for a small mission hospital in Puerto Rico. This hospital was based in

Humacao, a municipal district in a predominantly rural area in the eastern part of Puerto Rico, where much of the population was employed in sugar cane cutting. At the hospital Satterthwaite undertook obstetric deliveries and gynecological operations. She also ran her own family planning clinic in Humacao. In April 1957, she began a trial of the Pill with support from Pincus and financial assistance from the philanthropist Clarence Gamble.[86] As had been the case for Rice-Wray, Satterthwaite was particularly useful for conducting the trials because of her American training.[87] Working in a rural area, Satterthwaite was important to Pincus and his team because she could provide women from rural areas who were good comparative subjects for the more urban based trials in Rio Piedras.[88]

One of the reasons Satterthwaite decided to get involved in the trials was the desperation for contraception among her patients. Here the women were in worse health than in Rio Piedras. Most of them were anemic and suffered greatly from intestinal parasites as well as malnutrition. Many of these women walked miles in order to reach the hospital. For Satterthwaite the Pill project represented a major step forward in contraception. She had frequently encountered women who had been sterilized but were desperate to have more children. Sterilization was widespread in Puerto Rico. The despair of sterilized women who had changed husbands or lost a baby and could not have another child convinced her of the need for a reversible contraceptive method.[89] The Pill trials had no shortage of volunteers. Overall, Satterthwaite supervised 30 percent of the cases Pincus used as data for gaining official approval for the contraceptive pill in 1959.[90]

Fewer of the women in Humacao dropped out of the study than in Rio Piedras. Yet Satterthwaite encountered similar problems to those experienced by Rice-Wray, with negative reporting from local newspapers and opposition from local priests. She too was eventually forced to resign her position at the hospital as a result of antagonism to her trial work from the director of the hospital. Before resigning, however, she managed to enroll over a thousand women in trials to test different pills.[91]

Despite contending with hostility and anxiety, Satterthwaite and Rice-Wray accomplished work vital to the development of the Pill. They provided data to Pincus and his team as well as to a range of pharmaceutical companies. Their labors not only resulted in the success of the first Pill but also provided data for later variations of the Pill. The trials in Humacao and Mexico also provided comparative data to match against trials elsewhere. This was done independently of Pincus's research.[92]

In addition to the foundation work of Rice-Wray and Satterthwaite, the development of the Pill involved other women physicians. In 1958, for instance, Dr. Mary Calderone, medical director of the PPFA, helped launch trials of the

Pill in the United States. Her efforts in getting PPFA clinics to test the Pill provided one of the "largest testing group that any medication had ever had previously."[93] In Britain, female physicians also played a significant role in the launching of pill trials. These were conducted under the auspices of the Family Planning Association, the main tester and approver of the Pill in Britain (Marks forthcoming). Eleanor Mears, Aviva Wiseman, Margaret Jackson, Joan Nabarro, and Denise Pullen were just some of the many female physicians who were involved in testing the Pill in Britain. Wherever they were based, women physicians were key to the daily running and monitoring of the trials and the collection of accurate data. They were the ones who had the day-to-day contact with the patients and could observe their responses. As we have seen in the case of Rice-Wray and Satterthwaite, this was often conducted in environments in which they had to hide their activities and they rarely received full credit for their own work.

WOMEN AS RESEARCH SUBJECTS

Little of the work undertaken by the physicians could have been achieved without the cooperation and dedication of the female research subjects they worked with. The degree of cooperation expected of these women was particularly time-consuming in the very early stages of the trials.[94] This can be seen in the context of the first two small-scale trials conducted in 1954 among infertile women at the Free Hospital for Women and nurses at the Worcester State Hospital.[95] The aim of these trials was to calculate the length of time to continue the hormones as well as the dosage. All of this was very time-consuming. Women were observed for at least two of their normal menstrual cycles (labeled "control cycles") followed by two subsequent cycles with the oral administration of progesterone (supplied by Syntex). When taking the medication, the women were expected to swallow tablets every day (about one every six or eight hours) between the fifth and twenty-fifth day of their cycle. A number of the women also had to inject themselves with the compound or insert it as a vaginal suppository. Each woman had to take her own basal temperature readings and vaginal smears on a daily basis. All this data had to be marked on a chart. The women also had to collect urine over a forty-eight-hour period on the seventh and eighth postovulatory days for hormone analysis. Often the only way to collect urine over such a period would have confined women to their homes where they were near a toilet. The smell of the stored urine would not have been pleasant for these women. On top of this, the women had to have endometrial biopsies every month. A couple of the women also had laparotomies on the twenty-third day of their cycles. All of these procedures were to determine whether the compound had succeeded in suppressing ovulation and thereby had contraceptive potential. By June 1954, sixty women had participated in these two small-scale trials. Only half, however, had managed to provide the accurate information necessary for proving the contraceptive potential of hormonal steroids.[96]

Given these intensive procedures, women were clearly not just passive subjects. They had a very active role in investigative process. Women did not behave in the same way as laboratory animals. As McCormick pointed out, "Human females are not easy to investigate as are rabbits in cages. The latter can be intensively *controlled all the time,* whereas the human females leave town at unexpected times and so cannot be examined at a certain period; and they also forget to take the medicine sometimes;—in which case the whole experiment has to begin over again,—for scientific accuracy must be maintained or the resulting data are worthless."[97] The success of the Pill trials was therefore heavily dependent on the cooperation of women. The difficulties this caused was highlighted by McCormick:

> The *headache* of the tests is the co-operation necessary from the women patients.—There is so much of it and it must be accurate. I really do not know how it is obtained at all—for it *is* onerous—it really is—and requires intelligent attention, persistent attention for weeks. Rock says that he can get it only from women wishing to become fertile—: those who wish to be sterile are not ready to take so much trouble: I cannot see any way of overcoming this headache in the tests—unless one can furnish enough nurses to go around to their homes and see that the women patients do accomplish the tests regularly and correctly.[98]

For the investigators it was thus vital to find "intelligent enough" women who could "be relied upon to carry out" the procedures expected of them.[99] Infertile women participating in the trials were considered to have a higher degree of motivation to adhere to the instructions than other women because they hoped their participation would open up possibilities of a cure for their infertility.[100] Not all women, however, had such incentives, let alone the leisure or knowledge, to perform the intricate tests required. Women with families, for instance, were excluded from the early small-scale trials as they did not have the time considered imperative for undertaking the elaborate tests.[101]

Many of the small-scale trials found it difficult to keep the women compliant. This was most clearly illustrated in the case of a small-scale trial launched among female medical students (many of whom were American) at the School of Medicine at the University of Puerto Rico in San Juan in January 1955.[102] Despite threatening to fail the students in their exams should they not comply with the regulations of the trial, investigators had great difficulty in retaining them (Ramirez de Arellano and Seipp 1983, 111). Only thirteen out of the twenty-three women completed the trials. Some of the students dropped out to take up internships in the United States. One was forced to leave the school when she failed the course. Even students who completed the pilot study often did not adhere to the rules.[103] Alternatives were explored to see if student nurses from San Juan City Hospital and female prisoners from the Women's Correctional Institute at Vega Baja could be used instead. This, however, proved fruitless. Resentment on the part of the female prisoners toward the project proved enough to disrupt the discipline of the prison. In January 1956, investigators at the Medical School decided not to pursue any further work with the Pill because of the problem of obtaining suitable subjects.[104]

More success was achieved with a trial conducted among fifteen schizophrenic women studied at the Worcester State Hospital from 1956. These women were easier to monitor and control because they were within the confines of the hospital. The doctors were therefore less dependent on the women remembering to perform the necessary tests.[105] Although the investigators sought the consent of each patient's family to undertake the trials, the psychiatric patients themselves were far from being active subjects who had any choice about participating in the trial. By today's standards such trials would thus be regarded as unethical. During the 1950s, however, no official government guidelines existed about the use of humans as research subjects.[106] For those investigating the Pill, these psychiatric patients were not ideal subjects, because none of them were having sexual intercourse. This made it impossible to see if the administered hormones had contraceptive effects. Similarly, psychiatric problems can interfere with a woman's menstrual cycle. It was thus difficult to establish whether patterns of ovulation were affected by psychiatric causes or by the administered progesterone.[107]

The small-scale studies had the advantage in that they were mainly conducted among women within a hospital or institutional setting. Many of these women were also middle class, which meant they could read instructions. If the Pill was to be acceptable and as universal as the investigators intended, however, they needed to find women from a wider range of educational, cultural, geographic, and class backgrounds. Pincus and his team also needed a much larger group of women if they were to prove to scientific and lay communities the safety and effectiveness of such an oral contraceptive. This, however, was not going to be easy to find. A key question in launching larger-scale trials was whether women would continue to take pills faithfully outside a clinical setting.

Many of the women participating in the first large-scale trials in Rio Piedras were considered to have a high degree of motivation. Some of them were already visiting birth control clinics and had previously participated in short-term contraceptive trials (using conventional barrier methods). They were known to be desperate for an alternative means of contraception. Many were raising large families on a very small income and with little support from their husbands. Few of them were fully literate. These women therefore contrasted starkly with the more educated middle-class American women used in the previous small-scale trials. From the perspective of Pincus and his colleagues, if the women of Rio Piedras were willing to take the Pill and could understand how it worked, then the Pill could be used among other poor and illiterate women elsewhere (Vaughan 1972, 41; Reed 1978, 359).

All those included in the Rio Piedras study had to be under forty years old and to have already borne children to show they were fertile. They also had to be prepared to have another child if oral contraception failed. All the women had to guarantee long-term residence in the same area so that they would remain on the trial for a year.[108] Each woman was given a complete medical examination to ensure she was in good health before participating in the trial; this included gathering information on menstrual and pregnancy patterns.[109] Once on the trial, each woman was expected to take one pill a day from the fifth to the twenty-fourth day of her menstrual cycle.[110] She was expected to mark on a calendar the day she began taking the pills, the day she stopped, and the days on which she menstruated.[111]

Compliance with the instructions was ensured by the regular visit of a social worker to each woman at the end of each month's supply of pills. The social worker checked to see that the women had consumed the right number of pills on the appropriate days. She also asked detailed questions concerning side effects, length of menstrual cycle, and frequency of coitus.[112] Social workers were also deployed in other trials to monitor the progress of women.[113] Social worker observation, however, was not foolproof. One of the major difficulties the social workers encountered during the Rio Piedras project was that they did not always find the volunteers at home when they called. In addition, where too much time lapsed between visits, women often found it hard to recall crucial personal medical details, and this distorted the evidence collected. Problems also occurred in monitoring the number and time of the pills consumed. In order to make it easier for the women to know when to stop taking the medication, they were initially given only one month's supply of pills. These were supplemented by the social worker at the end of each month. This arrangement soon proved impractical, however, as the women were often absent when the social worker called. It thus became necessary to provide two bottles to ensure continuation of the regime. Even this system, however, was not guaranteed. When given two months' supply of pills, some women continued to take the pills without stopping for five days to allow for bleeding. Others feared that any gap in taking the medication would result in an immediate pregnancy, and they became agitated when the pills ran out and the social worker had not immediately replaced them. In order to combat such confusion, simple printed instructions were given out on the assumption that most women would be able to read or have a schoolchild read the instructions for them.[114]

Getting women to follow instructions was not a problem unique to the project launched in Rio Piedras. In Haiti, for instance, over 20 percent of the cases forgot to take the Pill and some stopped the medication whenever their husbands went away.[115] Some were illiterate and innumerate, which made instructions difficult to follow. Many could not remember when to take the Pills even when supplied with a calendar as a reminder. Even when they were given rosary beads, which they were to move individually each day on taking a pill, a number wore the beads in the belief that they alone provided protection against pregnancy without the need to take the Pill. Others ignored the instructions altogether, presuming that they should consume all the pills in one go.[116] Taking the pills was not always a case of merely swallowing just one pill a day. When women experienced breakthrough bleeding, they were expected to take an extra pill. These pills were supplied in an extra bottle marked with a cross, which was to be kept aside, but this directive was not always followed.[117] Some women found it easier to remember to take the pills than others. In Mexico City and Humacao, for instance, even the poorest illiterate women were faithful in taking the Pill.[118] Clearly much depended not only on the educational background of women but also on individual motivation and the skill of the instructor.

Besides taking a pill every day, women were asked to take part in other routine tests. As had been the case in the preliminary experiments, women taking part in the large-scale trials were expected to collect their urine for a twelve-hour period, from 7 a.m. to 7 p.m. on day 20 or 21 of the medication. Some patients who had discontinued the medication were also expected to collect their urine. Each woman was provided with a bottle and a set of instructions for the urine. These specimens were picked up from their homes. Given the basic accommodation and facilities, such a task would have been that much more difficult for these women than those involved in the earlier studies conducted in Massachusetts. The smell of collecting and storing the urine samples would also have been more off-putting in a hotter climate. In addition, patients had to agree to vaginal smears, endometrial biopsies, breast secretion smears, and cervical mucus tests. They also had to give blood samples for liver function tests and hemoglobin determinations. Women were also expected to have skin and cholesterol tests and endometrial smears. These tests became more elaborate as investigators learned more about possible side effects.[119] Some women who decided to come off the Pill in order to be sterilized were also asked to have ovarian biopsies.[120] Regular medical checkups were installed as part of the trials.[121] It was not always easy, however, to get women to come to these check-ups. In his 1958 publication on the Rio Piedras trial, Pincus admitted that they had only been able to collect blood samples from thirty-nine women and urine samples from forty-two. Endometrial biopsies had proven even harder to obtain (Pincus 1958).

The difficulty of getting women to undergo these tests underlines the fact that the women were active subjects. They could not be monitored twenty-four hours every day like animals. Yet their cooperation was vital if accuracy was to be achieved. Their ability to remember to take a pill and monitor the ways in which their bodies reacted to the medication was vital to the success of the Pill. Physicians working in Britain discovered that it was the women who were the most successful monitors of the effects of the Pill. As Margaret Jackson pointed out in 1960, "Greatly to my interest, I find that one of my best assessors of dose are the patients themselves. They settle their doses very often, and they settle them very well."[122] Once launched on the market, the success of the Pill continued to depend on women's faithfulness in keeping to its regime.

CONCLUSION

For many women swallowing the Pill today, the regime of the Pill could not appear simpler. It comes in a neatly labeled pack with a daily reminder of when to take the Pill and instructions on how to use it. Such simplicity, however, disguises the complexity of the technology and the expertise that went into its making and packaging. As this chapter shows, the Pill could not have been developed without a range of knowledge and expertise not only from scientists who drew up the plans for its creation but also from the technicians who followed this through and the physicians who supervised its clinical testing. It also could not have been achieved without the vision and insight of key women contraceptive campaigners and their financial support. Without Sanger and McCormick, it is debatable whether the Pill would have been produced so rapidly. And in the final analysis it could never have appeared without the dedication and commitment of the women who risked swallowing it. This not only involved taking a pill every day but intricate and time-consuming procedures to help monitor the impact of the drug on their bodies.

NOTES

I would like to thank Dorothy Hunt, Anne Merrill, Mary Ellen Fitts Johnson, Adaline Satterthwaite, and Celso Ramon Garcia for recalling their experiences with the development of the Pill. I am also grateful to Roger Short and John McCraken for their helpful comments on the development of endocrinology and to Shula Marks, Naomi Pfeffer, and Anne Summers for their comments on an earlier version of this chapter. Thanks are also due to Lynn Carson Lopez for sharing with me a tape of her mother and to Geoffrey Venning for letting me see his personal papers. I am also grateful for the help from the staff at the following archives: Library of Congress, Sophia Smith Library, Francis Countway Library, and the Contemporary Medical Archive Collection at the Wellcome Institute. Research for this paper was sponsored by the Wellcome Trust.

1. This attitude is captured in a statement by Oscar Hechter, who wrote shortly after the death of his friend Pincus: "Pincus for me represents the prototype of a *new* scientist, whose life and achievements merit critical examination and analysis. On a planet rapidly being irreversibly transformed by science and technology in ways not clearly foreseen, we desperately need information about the mechanisms by which individual scientists change the world. Pincus and his life merit a critical case study, because if new Pincuses arise in the future, they will have a powerful impact upon the world. . . . To oversimplify, some scientists become great by making important contributions to knowledge—discovery in the laboratory—and others become great as organizers and by making important applications of knowledge. Gregory Pincus, a scientist-statesman, was one of the latter" (Hechter 1968, quoted in B. Asbell 1995, 319). The importance of the word *father* is also epitomized by the gravestone of Pincus's coworker, Min Chueh Chang, which reads "M. C. Chang, The Father of the Birth Control Pill" (Asbell 1995, 324). Engraved on the instructions of his wife, this inscription could be seen as making up for the fact that during his lifetime Chang had felt his part in the development of the Pill had been underplayed. The idea of fathering the Pill has been used in many ways to describe these scientists' role. This is discussed in L. McLaughlin 1982, 93.

2. By calling himself mother rather than father of the Pill, Djerassi claims to be trying to challenge the patriarchal attitudes of society. For years Djerassi denied being the father of the Pill. But inside the dust jacket of one of his biographies he is described as the "Father of the Pill" (Djerassi 1992).

3. Subsequent scholars have adopted this approach. A survey undertaken by the National Science Foundation in 1967, for instance, summarizing the different scientific disciplines that went into the making of the Pill, asserts the importance of individual scientists. One of the diagrams accompanying the survey highlights the part of individual scientists involved in the physiology of reproduction, hormone research, and steroid chemistry that led to the development of the Pill. In this diagram the predominant names are male (National Science Foundation 1968).

4. For the ways journalists used this argument during the late 1960s and how subsequent writers took the same line, see Mintz 1969; Seaman 1969, 186; Statement by Washington Women's Liberation, cited in U.S. Senate 1970, pt. 16: 6470–71 and pt. 17: 7283–84; Boston Women's Health Collective (1984).

5. For the historical inaccuracy of such arguments, see L. Marks and S. White Junod (forthcoming).

6. Mrs. Walter Timme to Mrs. William K. Vanderbilt, 24 October 1929, accompanying mailing list for $1,000 letter, in Margaret Sanger's Papers, Library of Congress (henceforth MS-LC), cited in Chesler 1992, 325.

7. Sanger to Clarence J. Gamble, 1939, cited in G. Williams, unpublished "Manuscript Biography of Clarence Gamble," pp. 20–21, Research Materials for James Reed's Family Planning Oral History Project, MC 223, Schlesinger Archives.

8. See also Sanger to R. L. Dickinson, 28 May 1946, Margaret Sanger's Papers, Sophia Smith Library (henceforth MS-SS).

9. Reproductive science, a major component needed for the development of the Pill, was also considerably underfunded during this period: Clarke 1990, 27; Oudshoorn 1994, 114.

10. Interview with James Dean, Harvard University, in Gray 1979, 413 and 463.

11. McCormick to Sanger, 11 April 1958, MS-SS. Four years after the Pill was officially launched, McCormick reiterated her desire for a contraceptive that met the needs of women. As she wrote, "The oral contraceptive inaugurated and maintains a new era of sex relations for mankind,—fundamentally it is a sex revolution for human beings. . . . The oral contraceptive vitally concerns women and their bodies. I think that women do not care to have mechanical gadgets of one kind or another introduced into the innermost parts of their bodies, and that is solely a man's point of view that they do not object to this procedure." McCormick to Pincus, 8 August 1964, Gregory Pincus's Papers, Library of Congress (henceforth GP-LC), box 73.

12. McCormick to Sanger, 18 October 1951 and 22 January 1952; Sanger to McCormick, 26 February 1952, MS-SS.

13. In 1927, for instance, McCormick funded the establishment of a Neuroendocrine Research Foundation at Harvard University. This aimed to support the work of Roy G. Hoskins, an endocrinologist investigating the role of adrenal cortex malfunction in schizophrenia: Reed 1978, 338.

14. Sanger suggested laboratories in England and Germany. Germany was a surprising recommendation given the recent ending of World War II, but as Vaughan argues, "A cynic might suspect that Mrs. Sanger had in mind that country's ill-gotten experience of sterilizing undesirables." While Sanger was in favor of national sterilization, neither she nor McCormick pursued this as a serious option: Vaughan 1972, 27.

15. McCormick first met Hoagland when he was head of a small biology department at Clark University in Massachusetts: Worcester Foundation 1945, 9; Reed 1978, 338–39.

16. During the 1930s, Pincus had caused an uproar among scientific and lay communities as a result of his experiments with the in vitro fertilization of rabbit eggs and his claims to have produced fatherless (parthenogenetic) rabbits. According to Pincus, this scandal was a major factor leading to Harvard University's refusal to grant him tenure. For a more detailed description of Pincus's earlier work and the controversy it caused, see Reed 1978, 320–21 and 343–44. For more information on Pincus and the Worcester Foundation, see *Worcester Sunday Telegram,* 4 March 1951, p. 14. See also Vaughan 1972.

17. Pincus contacted Searle as early as 1939. Pincus to D. Wolfe, 28 June 1967, GP-LC, box 104.

18. Pincus had already received funds from the PPFA. In 1948–49, the PPFA awarded him $14,500 to investigate the early development of mammalian eggs: Reed 1978, 340.

19. Progress report to PPFA, 24 January 1952, GP-LC, box 12.

20. A. Stone to Pincus, 25 January 1952, Abraham Stone's Papers, Francis Countway Library (henceforth AS-FCL); Sanger to McCormick, 25 September 1952, MS-SS; Pincus 1965, 5. Pincus was not the only one to be doing contraceptive research at this time. Scientists at the National Drug Company in Philadelphia, for instance, were carrying out similar experiments on animals. See A. Stone to Sanger, 1 March 1952, MS-SS.

21. McCormick was not familiar with Pincus, despite her contact with Hoagland. McCormick to Sanger, 13 March 1952, MS-SS, correspondence files.

22. McCormick to Sanger, 4 June 1952, MS-SS, correspondence files.

23. McCormick to Pincus, 31 May 1954, GP-LC. See also McCormick to Crawford, 14 June 1956, GP-LC, box 21; minutes of a special meeting to the trustees of the WF, 6 December 1956, GP-LC, box 23.

24. McCormick to Sanger, 1 October 1952, 17 February 1954, and 31 May 1955, MS-SS; McCormick to Sanger, 13 November 1953, MS-LC. McCormick's funds were crucial to the WF's overall financial well-being. For the remainder of her life, McCormick donated between $150,000 and $180,000 annually to the WF. She also left the WF $1 million in her will. Reed 1978, 40.

25. Rock to Pincus, 26 June 1957, GP-LC, box 29; Pincus to McCormick, 18 July 1959, GP-LC; P. Henshaw, "Research Needs in Relation to Family Planning and Fertility Control," 10 August 1953, MS-LC; "PPFA Research Committee Papers," October 1951, MS-LC. See also Rock to McCormick, 26 September 1958, John Rock's Papers, Francis Countway Library (henceforth JR-FCL) and McCormick to Pincus, 14 July 1959, GP-LC, box 39.

26. See also McCormick to Sanger, 30 November 1956, and notes on McCormick's conversation with Dr. Rock, 2 April 1958, MS-SS.

27. Pincus to D. Wolfe, 28 June 1967, GP-LC, box 104.

28. McCormick to Sanger 8 May 1956, MS-SS, correspondence files.

29. Sanger to McCormick, 5 October 1953, MS-LC.

30. P. S. Henshaw to Pincus, 27 March 1953, GP-LC, box 14.

31. Pincus to McCormick, 5 March 1954, GP-LC; Ramirez de Arellano and Seipp 1983, 108–10.

32. "Grantors' Funds Balances January 31, 1956," and "Assets and Principal Accounts Balances: Grantors' Funds March 31, 1957," GP-LC; Johnson 1977, 71. For a detailed breakdown of how McCormick's funds were spent on the Pill project, see "Mrs. Stanley McCormick's grants, for the year ending December 31 1958," GP-LC, box 39. Most of the money was used to pay investigators' salaries.

33. Sanger to McCormick, 12 December 1956, MS-SS, cited in Reed 1978, 344, and in Chesler 1992, 435. Two years later, Sanger reiterated this line, stating, "I consider almost all, at least 90% of his [Pincus] recent scientific successes have been because of you, who have given him financial support as well as moral encouragement": Sanger to McCormick, 19 August 1958, MS-SS.

34. In 1956 McCormick wrote, "Everything is as slow as molasses, but both Rock and Pincus seem to be moving towards more extensive 'field tests' and I am most anxious to get these going as fast as we can." McCormick to Sanger, 30 June 1956, MS-SS.

35. Memorandum from H. Hoagland to Pincus and B. Crawford, 14 February 1957, GP-LC, box 27. See also Pincus to McCormick, 15 August 1960, GP-LC, box 45.

36. McCormick to Sanger, 23 July 1954; 21 October 1954, MS-SS; "Procedure for progesterone tests," (n.d, c. 1954), JR-FCL; and GP-LC, box 17. See also "Suitable Experimental Subjects," and "Objectives for Experimentation," November 1954, JR-FCL; McCormick to Sanger 19, 21, 23 July 1954; 31 May 1955; 9 January 1956; 30 January 1956; 11 February 1956, 7 June 1956, MS-SS; McCormick to Sanger, 6 February 1956, GP-LC, box 22; McCormick to Sanger, 13 November 1953, MS-LC; Pincus to McCormick, 5 March 1954, MS-SS; Pincus to McCormick, 13 December 1956, GP-LC, box 21.

37. McCormick to Sanger, 17 June 1954, 2 July 1954, 21 October 1954, 1 February 1955, 9 January 1956, and 13 December 1957; Sanger to Pincus, 18 July 1957, MS-SS; Sanger to McCormick, 25 Sept 1952 and 23 March 1953, McCormick to Sanger, 13 November 1953, MS-LC.

38. Hoagland to McCormick, 8 April 1954, GP-LC.

39. Their pressure and campaigning were not unique to this period. In 1952 the Ford Foundation, for instance, began to invest heavily in research around population issues because of the pressure from its leaders' wives, who were family planning enthusiasts: Harkavy 1995, 10.

40. McCormick to Sanger, 13 November 1953, MS-LC.

41. Worcester Foundation, progress report to PPFA, 23 January 1953, GP-LC, box 14; report to the Rockefeller Foundation of Research on the Physiology of Mammalian Eggs and Sperm, 12 March 1953, GP-LC, box 23.

42. Interview with A. Merrill and M. E. Fitts Johnson by L. Marks, 8 April 1995, transcript, p. 18; See also Pincus 1965, 67–68.

43. Interview with D. Hunt by L. Marks, 7 April 1995, transcript, p. 34.

44. Progress report to PPFA, 24 January 1952, GP-LC, boxes 12 and 14; interview with Merrill and Fitts Johnson, transcript, pp. 10, 11–12, 15–16; and interview with Hunt, p. 34.

45. Interview with Hunt, transcript, p. 33.

46. Interview with Merrill and Fitts Johnson, transcript, p. 41.

47. Ibid., p. 83.

48. Ibid., pp. 22, 29.

49. Ibid.

50. Ibid., pp. 24, 30–31.

51. Ibid., pp. 24, 46, 82.

52. Ibid., p. 37.

53. Ibid., p. 84.

54. Ibid., p. 38.

55. Ibid., p. 39.

56. Ibid., p. 47.

57. For some idea of the ways in which women physicians were involved in family planning, see interview with Mary S. Calderone by J. Reed, 7 August 1974, transcript, Schlesinger Archives. See also Evans 1983.

58. Edris Rice-Wray graduated from Vassar College and obtained her medical qualifications from the University of Michigan and Northwestern University. Before Puerto Rico, she had run her own private practice of medicine in Chicago and Evanston, Illinois, and worked for Planned Parenthood clinics there.

59. Pincus to Sanger, 31 March 1954; McCormick to Sanger, 21 July 1954, MS-SS. Other places considered for the Pill's trials had been dismissed because of the absence of appropriate medical staff to supervise such a project. The possibility of conducting trials in Japan had been rejected because it was assumed staff there would have a "jealousy and resentment of American doctors": notes on talk with Dr. Pincus, 1 February 1955, MS-SS. See also McCormick to Sanger, 21 July 1954, notes on conversation with Pincus, 5 March 1956, McCormick to Sanger, 17 June 1954, Sanger to N. Larsen, 10 September 1954, Pincus to G. J. Watumull, 3 April 1956, notes on conversation with Dr. Rock, 9 January 1956, MS-SS; McCormick to Sanger, 13 November 1953, MS-LC: Pincus to McCormick, 5 March 1954, Sanger to Pincus, 29 May 1954, Pincus to McCormick, 28 December 1955, GP-LC, box 17; P. Henshaw to Pincus, 6 August 1954, GP-LC, box 16; Pincus to McCormick, 14 March 1956, GP-LC, box 21.

60. "Report on Puerto Rico," n.d., p. 3, AS-FCL; notes on conversation with Pincus, 5 March 1956, MS-SS.

61. Pincus to Sanger, 23 March 1956, MS-SS.

62. The setting up of the trials in Rio Piedras also had the advantage that the housing project superintendent was enthusiastic about the contraceptive tests and made every possible effort to supply records of the families living in the new flats: E. Rice-Wray, "Study Project of SC-4642," January 1957, p. 1, Clarence Gamble's Papers, Francis Countway Library (henceforth CG-FCL), box 50. See also notes on conversation with Pincus, 5 March 1956, MS-SS.

63. Translation from *El Imparcial,* 21 April 1956, GP-LC, box 22; Pincus to McCormick, 11 October 1956, JR-FCL; I. Rodriguez Pla to Pincus, n.d, and Rice-Wray to Pincus, 10 May 1956, 11 June 1956, GP-LC, box 22; McCormick to Sanger, 12 May 1956; E. Rice-Wray, "Study Project of SC-4642," January 1957, p. 3, CG-FCL, box 50.

64. Several patients also discovered that they were pregnant before taking the tablet: Edris Rice-Wray to G. Pincus, 11 June 1956, GP-LC, box 23.

65. Interview with Edris Rice-Wray by J. Reed, 14 March 1974, Schlesinger Library; McLaughlin 1982, 134; Vaughan 1972, 50; Pincus to McCormick, 11 October 1956, JR-FCL. Modifications in the trials meant that by July the women stopped complaining of side effects: D. Tyler to Pincus, 2 July 1956, GP-LC, box 23.

66. Pincus to Sanger, 22 July 1957, GP-LC, box 29; Pincus to McCormick, 27 July 1957, GP-LC, box 27.

67. Pincus to McCormick, 11 October 1956, GP-LC, box 21; C. Tietze to M. Synder, 15 August 1957, GP-LC, box 28.

68. I. Rodriguez Pla to Pincus, May 1956 and Rice-Wray to Pincus, 10 May 1956, GP-LC, box 22; McCormick to Sanger, 12 May 1956; E. Rice-Wray, "Study Project of SC-4642," January 1957, CG-FCL, box 50.

69. Rice-Wray to Pincus, 20 December 1956, GP-LC, box 22.

70. E. Rice-Wray, "Study Project on SC-4642," January 1957, CG-FCL, box 50; Rice-Wray 1957, JR-FCL.

71. Rice-Wray to Pincus, 10 August 1958, GP-LC, box 26.

72. The gynecological clinic was run under the auspices of the Association for the Welfare of the Family, but it was funded by Syntex and the IPPF: Rice-Wray to Pincus, 10 August 1958 and 15 September 1958, box 34; Rice-Wray to Pincus, 6 April 1959, box 40; Annual Report of the Asociación Mexicana Pro-Bienestar de la Familia, c. 1959/60, GP-LC, box 45; Pincus to McCormick, 11 March 1956, box 27; Pincus to McCormick 18 June 1959, box 39. All material held in GP-LC. Syntex had already begun to test Norlutin in Japan: Pincus to Rice-Wray, 18 August 1958, GP-LC, box 34. See also Rice-Wray to Pincus, 9 September 1958 and 15 September 1958, GP-LC, box 34.

73. One letter concerning the Mexican trials stressed, "We beg that you treat this whole report as confidential information. If it should fall into the wrong hands, our Mexican associates are convinced that the Church could do us a great deal of harm, even to the extent of forcing us to close the clinic. Our Annual Report published in Spanish for Mexican consumption deletes all references to planned parenthood. Unless one actually lives in Mexico, one cannot fully appreciate the power and influence of the Church, and the great care we must exercise." Letter "For our close friends and sympathisers." Letter attached to Annual Report of the Asociación Mexicana Pro-Bienestar de la Familia, c. 1959/60, GP-LC, box 45. See also Rice-Wray to Pincus, 6 April 1959, GP-LC, box 40; Annual Report of the Asociación Mexicana Pro-Bienestar de la Familia, c. 1959/60, GP-LC, box 45.

74. Rice-Wray to Pincus, 25 January 1960, GP-LC, box 45.

75. Interview with E. Rice-Wray, n.d, transcript, p. 1. Interview tape provided by Lynn Carson Lopez. See also interview with Rice-Wray by J. Reed, Schlesinger Library.

76. O. Mendoza to T. O. Griessemer, 25 June–16 July 1958, CG-FCL, box 108, fol. 1786; Rice-Wray to C. J. Gamble, 2 July 1959, CG-FCL, box 108, fol. 1787; Rice-Wray to Pincus, 6 April 1959, GP-LC, box 40.

77. Rice-Wray to Pincus, 25 January 1960, GP-LC, box 45.

78. Rice-Wray to Pincus, 15 August 1959, GP-LC, box 40; Rice-Wray to C. J. Gamble, 15 August 1959, CG-FCL, box 108, fol. 1787.

79. Rice-Wray to Pincus, 25 January 1960, GP-LC, box 45.

80. Rice-Wray to Pincus, 6 July 1961, GP-LC, box 50. See also Rice-Wray 1963.

81. Rice-Wray to C. J. Gamble, 2 July 1959, CG-FCL, box 108, fol. 1787.

82. "Progress Report of the Difficulties of the Clinic of the Asociación Mexicana Pro-Bienestar de la Familia up to August 24th 1961," CG-FCL, box 108, fol. 1791. Recognition had partly been gained as a result of protests many of the clinic's patients had made to the government. One of these patients was the wife of a government minister who later became the president of Mexico. Interview with E. Rice-Wary, n.d., transcript, pp. 2–5.

83. In the end Rice-Wray directed her energies toward training health professionals in family planning: Rice-Wray to G. Venning, n.d., Venning's Papers, personal collection. Letter was probably written in 1974. Interview with E. Rice-Wray, n.d., transcript, pp. 13, 16.

84. Interview with E. Rice-Wray, transcript pp. 7–8.

85. Rice-Wray to G. Venning, n.d, Venning's Papers, personal collection.

86. Gamble used his inheritance from Procter and Gamble to sponsor contraceptive research around the world. Trained as a physician, he took an interest in making birth control medically and socially respectable. For more on Gamble see D. and G. Williams 1978.

87. Satterthwaite had undertaken her medical training at the University of California, San Francisco. After graduating, she had practiced obstetrics and gynecology in New Jersey. Before working in China, she gained surgical experience in Puerto Rico. At that time it was difficult for women physicians to get surgical placements. Interview with A. Satterthwaite by L. Marks, April 1995, transcript, pp. 1, 4, 7.

88. Pincus to McCormick, 11 March 1957, GP-LC, box 27.

89. Satterthwaite interviewed by Marks, transcript, pp. 9, 11, 12, 15.

90. Interview with Adaline Satterthwaite by James Reed, 19 June 1974, transcript, pp. 21, 27, Schlesinger Library, Family Oral History Project. See also Pincus, Rock, and Garcia 1959; Pincus, Rock, Garcia, Rice-Wray, and Rodriguez Pla 1958.

91. Interview with Satterthwaite by Reed, transcript, pp. 22, 29.

92. Ibid., p. 25; interview with E. Rice-Wray, n.d., transcript, pp. 6, 9–11, 14–15. See also Rice-Wray, Goldzieher, and Aranda-Rosell 1963; Rice-Wray, Cervantes, Gutterrez, Aranda-Rosell, and Goldzieher 1965.

93. Interview with Mary Calderone by Reed, 7 August 1974, transcript, p. 22, Schlesinger Library, Family Planning Oral History Project.

94. These tests were conducted among women in a variety of places, including Jerusalem and Japan. Zondek to Pincus, 27 June 1953, box 15, GP-LC. Few guidelines existed during the 1950s for the way in which trials had to be conducted. No distinction was made in this period between toxicity trials (known today as Phase I) and clinical efficacy trials (now known as Phase II). The procedures expected of the women participating in the Pill trials show there was some blurring of the boundaries between trials for toxicity and clinical efficacy. For more information on the history of human experimentation and clinical trials before the emergence of Phase I and Phase II trials in the 1960s, see Lederer 1995 and H. Marks 1997.

95. Pincus to Rock, 15 May 1953, JR-FCL.

96. McCormick to Sanger, 17 June 1954, MS-SS.

97. McCormick to Sanger, 13 November 1953, MS-LC.

98. McCormick to Sanger, 21 July 1954, MS-SS.

99. McCormick to Sanger, 21 October 1954, MS-SS.

100. This was known as the Rock rebound phenomenon, whereby women would become fertile by resting their ovaries for a period of time.

101. McCormick to Sanger, 19 July 1954, MS-SS.

102. D. Tyler to Pincus, 20 October 1954, M. F. Fuster to Pincus, 1 November 1954, box 17, GP-LC.

103. C. R. Garcia to Pincus, 18 June 1955, J. Diaz Carazo to Pincus, 16 September 1955, GP-LC, box 18.

104. J. Diaz Carazo to Pincus, 16 September 1955, and Pincus to D. Tyler, 30 September 1955, box 18, GP-LC; J. Diaz Carazo to Pincus, 31 January 1956, box 22, GP-LC; McCormick's notes on conversation with Pincus, 5 March 1956, MS-SS.

105. "Protocol on Progesterone Therapy in Psychotic Women," n.d, GP-LC, box 17; "Progress Report: Studies of the Effects of Progestational Compounds upon Psychotic Subjects," 22 July 1957, GP-LC, box 30.

106. Stringent guidelines for the use of humans as research subjects only emerged in the 1970s. For more information on this, see Lederer 1995.

107. Interview with Celso Ramon Garcia by L. Marks, April 1995, transcript, p. 8; Vaughan 1972, 39.

108. McCormick's notes on conversation with Pincus, 5 March 1956, MS-SS; Rice-Wray, "Study Project of SC-4642"; interview with Merrill and Fitts Johnson, transcript, p. 20; Pincus 1958; Oudshoorn 1994, 128–29.

109. Pincus to A. Fishberg, 28 February 1956, box 22, GP-LC.

110. E. Rice-Wray, "Study Project of SC-4642."

111. Untitled instructions, February 1958, GP-LC, box 34.

112. Pincus to A. Fishberg, 28 February 1956, box 22, GP-LC; McCormick's notes on conversation with Pincus, 5 March 1956, MS-SS; Pincus 1958.

113. "Study of Long-Term Administration of 17 Ethinyl-19 Nortesteorne in Fertility Control (Preliminary Report)," n.d, GP-LC, box 45.

114. Rice-Wray, "Study Project of SC-4642"; Pincus 1958; interview with Merrill and Fitts Johnson, transcript, p. 35.

115. F. Laraque to Pincus, 7 July 1958, GP-LC, box 32; L. Honorat to R. Crosier, 27 August 1958, GP-LC, box 32.

116. Interview with Merrill and Fitts Johnson, transcript, p. 35.

117. "Study of Long-Term Administration of 17 Ethinyl-19 Nortesterone in Fertility Control (Preliminary Report)," n.d, GP-LC, box 45.

118. "Study of the Long-term Administration of 17 Ethinyl-19 Nortestosterone in Fertility Control," box 109, fol. 1789 and A. P. Satterthwaite and C. J. Gamble, "Control of Ovulation with Norethynodrel," 1962, box 53, fol. 849, CG-FCL.

119. Pincus to I. Rodriguez Pla, 7 November 1956, Rice-Wray to Pincus, 20 December 1956, GP-LC, box 22; Pincus to Satterthwaite, 20 August 1958, and Pincus to Satterthwaite, 15 September 1958, GP-LC, box 34; Pincus to M. Paniagua, 11 August 1950, GP-LC, box 45; interview with Merrill and Fitts Johnson, transcript, p. 21.

120. Pincus to Rice-Wray, 6 August 1956, and Rice-Wray to Pincus, 20 December 1956, GP-LC, box 22.

121. Interview with Garcia, transcript, p. 32; Pincus to McCormick, 11 October 1956, JR-FCL.

122. M. Jackson at IPPF Press Conference, 30 March 1960, FPA/A5/161/4, Contemporary Medical Archive Collection, Wellcome Institute.

REFERENCES

Asbell, B.:
  1995　*The Pill: A Biography of the Drug that Changed the World.* New York: Random House.
Berg, S. M.:
  1989　Gregory Goodwin Pincus: From Reproductive Biology to the Birth Control Pill: Underlying Motivations and Professional Goals. B. A. thesis, Harvard University.
Biezanek, A.:
  1965　*All Things New.* New York: Harper and Row.
Borell, M.:
  1987　Biologists and Birth Control, 1918–1938. *Journal of the History of Biology* 20: 51–87.
Boston Women's Health Collective:
  1984　*Our Bodies, Ourselves.* New York: Penguin.
Chesler, E.:
  1992　*Woman of Valor: Margaret Sanger and the Birth Control Movement.* New York: Simon and Schuster.
Clarke, A.:
  1990　Controversy and the Development of Reproductive Sciences. *Social Problems* 37: 18–37.
Djerassi, C.:
  1992　*The Pill, Pygmy Chimps, and Degas' Horse.* New York: Basic Books.
  1995　The Mother of the Pill. *Recent Progress in Hormone Research* 50:1–17.
Evans, B.:
  1983　*Freedom to Choose: The Life and Work of Helena Wright.* London: Bodley Head.
Gray, M.:
  1979　*Margaret Sanger: A Biography of the Champion of Birth Control.* New York: R. Marek.
Harkavy, O.:
  1995　*Curbing Population Growth: An Insider's Perspective on the Population Movement.* New York: Plenum.
Hechter, O.:
  1968　Homage to Gregory Pincus. *Perspectives in Biology and Medicine* (Spring 1968). Cited in Asbell 1995: 319.
Henle, W.:
  1937　The Relation of Spermatoxic Immunity to Fertility. Reprinted in *Journal of Contraception* 2(3–4): 30–31.
Johnson, R. C.:
  1977　Feminism, Philanthropy, and Science in the Development of the Oral Contraceptive Pill. *Pharmacy in History* 19(2): 63–77.
Kuzrock, R.:
  1937　The Prospects for Hormonal Sterilization. Reprinted in *Journal of Contraception* 2(3–4): 27–29.
Lederer, S.:
  1995　*Subjected to Science: Human Experimentation in America before the Second World War.* Baltimore: Johns Hopkins University Press.

Marks, H.:
  1997   *The Progress of Experiment: Science and Therapeutic Reform in the United States, 1900–1990.* Cambridge: Cambridge University Press.
Marks, L.:
  Forth- "Public Spirited and Enterprising Volunteers": The Council for the Investigation
  coming of Fertility Control and the British Clinical Trials of the Oral Contraceptive Pill, 1950s–1960s. In T. Tansey, ed., *Remedies and Healing Cultures in Britain and The Netherlands in the Twentieth Century.* Amsterdam: Rodopi.
Marks, L., and S. White Junod:
  Forth- Women on Trial: Approval of the First Oral Contraceptive Pill in the United States
  coming and Great Britain.
McLaughlin, L.:
  1982   *The Pill, John Rock, and the Church: A Biography of a Revolution.* Boston: Little, Brown.
Mintz, M.:
  1969   The Pill, Press, and Public at the Experts' Mercy. *Columbia Journalism Review,* Winter 1968–69: 4–10.
National Science Foundation
  1968   *Technology in Retrospect and Critical Events in Science* 1 (15 December 1968) and 2 (30 January 1969).
Oudshoorn, N.:
  1994   *Beyond the Natural Body: An Archaeology of Sex Hormones.* London: Routledge.
Pincus, G.
  1958   Fertility Control with Oral Medication. *American Journal of Obstetrics and Gynecology* 75: 1335
  1965   *The Control of Fertility.* New York: Academic Press.
Pincus, G., J. Rock, and C. R. Garcia:
  1959   Field Trials with Norethynodrel as an Oral Contraceptive. In *Report of the Proceedings of the Sixth International Conference on Planned Parenthood,* 14–21 February 1959, New Delhi, India.
Pincus, G., J. Rock, C. R. Garcia, E. Rice-Wray, and I. Rodriguez Pla:
  1958   Fertility Control with Oral Medication. *American Journal of Obstetrics and Gynecology,* June 1958: 1333–46.
Ramirez de Arellano, A. B., and C. Seipp:
  1983   *Colonialism, Catholicism and Contraception: A History of Birth Control in Puerto Rico.* Chapel Hill, N.C.
Reed, James:
  1978   *The Birth Control Movement and American Society: From Private Vice to Public Virtue.* Princeton: Princeton University Press.
Rice-Wray, E.:
  1957   Field Study with Enovid as a Contraceptive Agent. *Proceedings of a Symposium on 19-Nor Progestational Steroids.* Chicago: Searle.
  1963   Oral Contraception in Latin America. In *Proceeding of the VIIth International Conference on Planned Parenthood,* Singapore, February 1963, reprinted from *Excerpta Medica International Congress,* series no. 72.
Rice-Wray, E., J. W. Goldzieher, and A. Aranda-Rosell:
  1963   Oral Progestins in Fertility Control: A Comparative Study. *Fertility and Sterility* 14(4): 402–9.

Rice-Wray, E., A. Cervantes, J. Gutterrez, A. Aranda-Rosell, and J. W. Goldzieher:
    1965   The Acceptability of Oral Progestins in Fertility Control. *Metabolism,* 14(3), pt. 2:
          451–56.

Sanger, M.:
    1937   The Future of Contraception. *Journal of Contraception* 2(3–4): 32–34.

Seaman, B.:
    1969   *Doctors' Case against the Pill.* Reprint, Alameda, Calif.: Hunter House, 1995.

U.S. Senate
    1970   *Competitive Problems in the Drug Industry: Hearings before the Subcommittee on*
          Monopoly of the Select Committee on Small Business. 91st Cong., pts. 15–17,
          January–March 1970.

Vaughan, P.:
    1972   *The Pill on Trial.* London: Penguin.

Williams, D., and G. Williams (edited by E. P. Flint):
    1978   *Every Child a Wanted Child: Clarence James Gamble, M.D., and His Work in the Birth*
          Control Movement. Cambridge: Harvard University Press.

Worcester Foundation:
    1945   *Annual Report.*
    1949–50 *Annual Report.*

■ PART TWO

USERS, VALUES, AND MARKETS: Shaping Users through the Cultural and Legal Appropriation of In Vitro Fertilization

Marta Kirejczyk

For more than two decades in many parts of the world, societies in general and feminists in particular have been trying to come to terms with in vitro fertilization (IVF). Controversies erupt frequently. Debates on how to regulate IVF continue, and the actual practice is far from standardized. So what is so special about IVF that makes its passage from the quasi-experimental stage to a socially uncontested clinical use so difficult?

To begin with, IVF practitioners have pursued a controversial route from experiment to routine practice. The history of IVF contradicts the widely held norm that medical technologies follow a standard trajectory from laboratory development through animal testing and clinical trials before gaining wider use. It also contradicts the belief that each stage in development is not only carefully designed but also thoroughly evaluated. IVF was largely developed in the context of the clinical treatment of infertile women. Often unaware of the experimental status of IVF, these women saw it as a promising novel therapy. The precautions required for experiments on human subjects were not observed. Data on efficacy and safety have not been systematically collected. And even now, clinical IVF practice continues to be the main site where new fertilization technologies are developed and tested.

Furthermore, although IVF was developed and introduced as a treatment for infertile women, the radical separation of fertilization from the woman's body in the IVF procedure has given rise to a situation in which a wide range of end users can lay claim to this technology. Not only infertile women but also infertile men can be treated—via a woman's body—with IVF. Heterosexuals and lesbians, young and old, rich and poor are candidates, to name but a few controversial dimensions of user categories. Such claims to user entitlement, even if not actually formulated, force societies to reconsider the cultural meaning of family, parenthood, and kinship.

Another important factor contributes to the view of IVF as more than just a medical treatment for infertility. In each course of IVF treatment, a large number of human ova and embryos are produced. Not all are actually used to facilitate procreation. For the first time available outside women's bodies, human ova and embryos have become desired objects for scientific experiments. This has prompted renewed debate on the origins of human life, on the moral status of embryos and fetuses, and on the amount of protection they should enjoy. Thus, discussion of IVF also invokes themes from debates on abortion and on human cloning.

In many ways, women are involved in all these aspects. Women appear as users seeking assistance but are not always able to get it, as access to IVF may be limited by formal or informal regulations. Women are also bearers of new risks and responsibilities, although they are not always informed of these. And women are involved, sometimes unknowingly, as subjects of medical experiments and providers of sensitive experimental material, the egg cells. Women are also active participants in public debates and regulatory processes, as well as being passive participants when other actors represent their needs, qualities, and interests. The chapters in this section will discuss women as (potential) users of IVF in all of these roles. However, unlike other sections of this collection, here we emphasize women as *aggregated categories* of (potential) users of a service subject to market forces and (sometimes) government regulations.

This section focuses, namely, on the processes that in different cultural and political contexts regulate the practice of IVF and, more broadly, of fertilization techniques. Whether these processes are formal or not, whether they are finalized or still ongoing, they display some common features: Negotiations (especially in the at-table sense) are a central activity. These negotiations are not limited to policy networks but are also carried out in the mass media and in specialized professional arenas. These locations are interconnected, notably in that clinicians and their professional organizations are important actors in nearly all these sites.

The outcome of these negotiations has the practical importance of defining who is eligible for the use of these technologies and under what conditions, that is, defining the space within which women seeking assistance make their choices. Also at stake are cultural notions of gender and gender relations. Negotiations about the form of regulation, about the organization of clinical practice, or about the further development of technologies of fertilization involve negotiations about the meanings of gender. The outcome of these negotiations may be very different in different cultural, social, and political settings, as the authors of the chapters in this section will illustrate.

In chapter 6, I provide a theoretical framework for the cross-cultural comparison of the processes of cultural appropriation of reproductive technologies. I argue that, because of the radical separation of fertilization from the bodies, scripts inscribed in IVF technology are socially ambiguous. As a key element of these scripts, roles are ascribed to imagined or "virtual" users. In order to make sense of IVF, these roles then need to be translated into culturally acceptable practices and relations between women, men, and their children. The characteristics that are considered necessary requisites for the legitimate users of IVF—that is, what constitutes an acceptable candidate for motherhood, fatherhood . . . or life—are not given a priori. They are negotiated in public debates, in the clinical practices, and in formal regulations of this technology. Such regulations may be introduced by governments or self-imposed as codes of practice. Discussing three cases taken from the Dutch debates, I analyze the role played by values related to gender in the representations of women and men as potential users of IVF. These diverse, often contradictory, representations are instrumental in the construction of different categories of legitimate users and in a selective recognition of health hazards. I demonstrate how over time a slow but clear erosion of heterosexuality as the absolute norm governing reproductive practices has taken place in The Netherlands.

In chapter 7, Federico Neresini and Franca Bimbi discuss the regulatory debates in Italy, where the Roman Catholic Church enjoys a strong political position. The authors present a comprehensive analysis of the strategic games played by physicians, representatives of the Catholic Church, the political parties, and feminists at different negotiation sites. The debates are ridden with conflicts, and the positions taken by the actors differ from one forum to another. Bimbi and Neresini argue that the main goal of the Italian debates is not so much the regulation of practices of assisted fertilization as the cultural reconstruction of a "new natural order of procreation." In this process, medical doctors play a prominent role. It is they who, on the one hand, stretch the definition of "family" beyond the narrow confines of the conjugal relationship sanctioned by the Catholic Church and the Constitution. Clinicians define both married and stable unmarried couples as legitimate users of fertilization techniques. On the other hand, where the space for research is at stake, spokesmen for reproductive medicine readily adopt much more conservative positions in negotiations with the representatives of pro-life Catholic culture. Although women's voices are weak in current negotiations, Neresini and Bimbi's analysis of tensions at different forums provides an insight necessary for the intensification of an effective feminist involvement in the regulatory debates.

The weakness of feminist voices is also characteristic of the situation in India, which is discussed by Jyotsna Gupta in chapter 8. The background, however, is very different here. The public debates in which feminists participate actively concern the impacts on women of the official policies of population control and the struggle against the widespread practice of sex selection in favor of male offspring. Although a serious social problem, infertility has not become a public issue. Gupta analyzes the interplay between patriarchal cultural values and the free market of fertilization services. She shows how the two reinforce each other to the detriment of infertile women. On the one hand, infertility is seen as a shameful condition for women, and recourse to assisted fertilization techniques is surrounded by utmost secrecy. On the other hand, information about the treatments is unreliable, and practices are not guided either by formal regulation or by a professional code of conduct. As Gupta shows, in this profit-oriented market only those infertile women who are well-to-do can afford a fertilization treatment, often of very dubious quality.

Reliance upon market mechanisms is also characteristic for the United Kingdom where, in contrast to India, IVF practice has formally been regulated. In chapter 9, Naomi Pfeffer proposes a model for analyzing different types of formal regulations of reproductive technologies. She argues that in liberal democracies, formal regulations interfering with the principle of the individual free choice are justified by the need to overcome the shortcomings of market mechanisms. Pfeffer points out several forms that such justification takes. How particular reproductive services are formally regulated and what positions are assigned to women as potential users depends largely upon the type of justification favored by the state in a given period. Pfeffer illustrates the analytic possibilities of her model by comparing the regulation of abortion under the Labour government with the regulation of assisted fertilization under the rule of the Conservative Party. The effects of these two forms of regulations on women as potential users were very different, indeed. Whereas Labour considered women to be citizens with a right to free abortion, infertile women seeking medical assistance were viewed by Conservatives primarily as consumers in the market for IVF services. As in India, the purchasing power of infertile women in the United Kingdom is the main factor in defining today whether or not they will be able to become actual users of IVF technology.

In chapter 10, Françoise Laborie explicitly addresses the question of the relationship between gender and the development and use of fertilization technologies. Medical journals and scientific conferences are important places where this mutual relationship is being negotiated. She analyzes the reasons offered in the French medical debate for concern about the safety of intracytoplasmic sperm injection. ICSI is a recent technological extension of IVF designed specifically for dealing with male infertility. Laborie poses a seemingly simple question: Why does this debate focus exclusively on the risks run by infertile men and their male offspring? In other words, why does the debate focus only on risks *additional* to those run by women undergoing any form of IVF (including ICSI) and by resulting children of *both* sexes? In a detailed analysis she demonstrates that many reasons for concern about the safety of ICSI are valid for IVF as well. What is more, already in the 1980s many feminists insisted on the rigorous assessment of the risks run by women undergoing IVF and by their offspring. Yet to this day IVF hazards have not received the degree of consideration from the community of clinicians as have those of ICSI. Laborie shows convincingly that the asymmetric treatment of risks that by nature are gender-symmetric forms an important factor in the ongoing process of the mutual shaping of gender and fertilization technologies.

The relationship between gender and fertilization technology established in the course of technology development is grounded in a cosmopolitan culture of reproductive medicine, as Laborie suggests. The authors in part two make clear, however, that this relationship undergoes significant changes in the processes of cultural appropriation of this technology—for instance, through political processes aimed at regulation of the technology. It is in these processes, full of tensions and culturally localized, that the aggregate categories of legitimate (accepted, sanctioned) and actual (including sometimes illegitimate) users are shaped.

6

Enculturation through Script Selection: Political Discourse and Practice of In Vitro Fertilization in The Netherlands

Marta Kirejczyk

Is it possible to talk about Dutch, Danish, Indian, or Italian in vitro fertilization? And if so, what are the processes that make an IVF practice typically Dutch or Italian? In other words, how are we to address the issue of tension between the global and local features of technology? In exploring this question I have found it useful to stretch the concept of script being written into technical objects, as originally proposed by Madeleine Akrich (1992), perhaps in a way she did not foresee.

1. I propose to use the concept of script in order to describe a technology that cannot be identified with a single artifact.
2. I argue that some technologies, as IVF in the discussed case, may contain not one but multiple scripts.
3. I propose to look at the processes of localization or *enculturation* of IVF in terms of societal selection and cultural interpretation of scripts.
4. I think that a significant part of the enculturation is being effectuated through public debates on the acceptability of scripts and through the political regulation of a socially acceptable practice, which is, needless to say, closely related to the cultural norms and values of that society. Therefore, one may expect that each society will select and modify scripts to fit in with its values. But since values are neither static nor necessarily universally shared in contemporary societies, enculturation of a technology may also involve adjustments in norms and values.

In this chapter I will further outline these propositions and illustrate them by discussing the evolving selection and interpretation of some scripts contained in IVF in the Dutch context. I will pay special attention to the representations of users in public debates and to the effects of these representations on shaping IVF practice in this country. This focus allows me to elucidate the role played by norms and values related to gender in the processes of enculturation.[1]

THE CONCEPT OF SCRIPTS AND THEIR MACRO-SELECTION
IN THE CASE OF COMPOSED TECHNOLOGY

Some years ago, Madeleine Akrich published an article in which she proposed to look at technological objects as having a script written into them. She argued that the views and expectations of the designers concerning the social, political, economic, and moral context into which the technological objects will be introduced are "inscribed" into the technical content of the objects they design. She saw these inscriptions as (not always conscious) attempts of the designers to predetermine the relationships between the technical object and future users. Both objects and their future users are given well-defined roles to play in a projected sociotechnical setting. Some competencies and responsibilities are delegated to the artifacts, whereas others remain within the domain of the users. Akrich stressed that the actual sociotechnical setting in which an artifact is being introduced can differ considerably from the projected one. Also, it is far from certain that the real users will actually perform the roles envisaged in the script. They may themselves conceive of and actually perform quite different roles and thereby also rewrite the role not only for themselves but also for the technical object. It is in the process of confrontation between the scripts written into technical objects and the roles played by the real users that the final shape of the objects is established and the competencies between the object and other actors are distributed. New relations between people and things may arise from this process. The idea of technical objects having scripts paved the way for inquiries about the nature of gender scripts (Oost 1995; Oudshoorn 1996) being written into technical objects. The images of the future users and the societal context projected by the designers include cultural presuppositions about the differences between men and women, between masculinity and femininity. When these presumptions are inscribed in the design of the artifact, one can speak of gender script.

This conceptualization of script has some shortcomings, however. To begin with, not every technology can be represented as a clearly delineated technical object. Take, for example, in vitro fertilization. It involves material objects (such as medical instruments, drugs, and chemical media), procedures (such as hormonal stimulation protocols, prescriptions for handling gametes and embryos), collective and individual judgments (such as who should be treated with IVF and on what grounds, when to begin and when to stop the treatment), and tacit knowledge of medical staff and clinical embryologists (which underpins decisions as to which of the available embryos and gametes are suitable for use during IVF). So, as far as the projected sociotechnical context is concerned, the use of IVF technology requires well-equipped laboratories, specialized medical staff, and a social acceptance of medical intervention in the process of conception. But if we look at the type of user that is inscribed in IVF, the picture is less clear. At first sight, women with blocked fallopian tubes are the most obvious candidates as users of IVF. The suffering of this category of infertile patients motivated gynecologist Patrick Steptoe, in collaboration with embryologist Robert Edwards, to develop IVF. However, if one considers more closely the presumptions about the virtual users inscribed in IVF, they quickly become abstract and boil down to the willingness of a woman and a man to make gametes available for fertilization in laboratory conditions and the willingness of a woman to have an embryo implanted. These users, stripped from body, personality, and social relations, are inscribed into the configuration of the elements constituting IVF, making this technology a carrier of a whole range of scripts.

The most innovative feature of IVF consists of the physical separation of the process of fertilization from women's bodies. In the context of IVF, fertilization is no longer a result of sexual intercourse between a woman and a man but the outcome of the interaction between the egg cell and the sperm, which is mediated by a set of medical and laboratory procedures. IVF creates new material artifacts: egg cells and embryos outside the woman's body which, if placed in a female body, may develop into babies. The major distinction that is relevant in the context of IVF technology exists between the female and male gametes, not between the personalized male and female bodies. Consequently, the number of women and men involved in any one IVF procedure is not necessarily limited to two. Some parts of the procedure, hormonal stimulation of ovulation and ovum extraction, may be performed with one woman, whereas the embryo may be placed into the womb of another. The possibility of distributing the procedure over different bodies means that the risks and the burdens involved in the procedure may be distributed as well.

The material configuration of IVF makes possible the enactment of not one but a whole spectrum of scripts. One can try to restore the original relationship between the personalized bodies by limiting the performance of the fertilization procedure to the egg cells of women in whose wombs the embryos will be placed and by using exclusively the sperm of their male partners for that purpose. But the egg cells and the sperm may also be donated. Embryos created from the donated gametes may be gestated by surrogate mothers for different contracting persons; single men or women, homosexual, lesbian or heterosexual couples. Lesbian couples may bodily share the procreation. Male inability to parent genetically related offspring may be overcome by performing IVF on their female partners. The age barrier limiting the procreative potential of women may now be transgressed, and the succession of the generations may be altered. Human embryos could be gestated by female animals[2] and, at least in theory, human egg cells could be fertilized by the sperm of other primates. And scientists forecast that cloning of humans will soon become a real possibility.

The existence of a large array of technically possible reproductive combinations in IVF does not automatically mean that all of them will be performed. Depending upon the sociotechnical context into which the technology is introduced and upon the creativity of the users, some scripts may be rejected, others modified. Contrary to Akrich's suggestion, the capacity to modify or even to radically change the script of technology is not always limited to the individual users alone. A new technology can easily become a subject of controversies if it carries scripts that are seen as not congruent with the norms and values of vocal social groups. In such cases, public debates may arise. In the course of these debates, the scripts inscribed in the technology and the relevant social norms and values are reinterpreted and attuned to each other. Not only may scripts be rejected and modified but also norms and values may undergo change. In order to distinguish between the processes of script modification by the individual users and those that take place in public debates and political regulation, I will use the term *macro-selection of scripts* for instances of the latter. It is on this level, where collective actors and their values play a dominant role, that some categories of potential users are labeled legitimate and the boundaries are drawn within which these users are allowed to make their choices. In the debates on IVF technology in this country, the organizations of clinicians, patients, several advisory committees, political parties, government, and spokespersons for different social groups played a prominent role. Hence, the final performance of the script depends not only on the willingness of the individual users to enact their roles but also on reaching a certain degree of social acceptance for some or all (modified) scripts inscribed in IVF.

The public and political debates on IVF can therefore be seen as a process of selection and modification of scripts, as a process of enculturation or localization of technology. In the course of these debates, different images of men and women as prospective users of IVF are being mobilized, and some scripts become articulated in terms of socially acceptable relations between women, men, and offspring. At the same time, the notions about socially acceptable relations are changing.

In the following sections I will discuss three examples of processes of the societal selection of scripts. My choice of examples was guided by the question about the role of cultural notions of gender in the processes of enculturation. First, I will discuss the role of lifestyle and sexual preferences in the construction of medical grounds for IVF. Then I will move to the issue of egg cell donation and surrogacy, which reflects a fascinating feature of IVF as a double-faced technology: on the one hand, promising the realization of motherhood and, on the other, challenging cultural notions of motherhood. In the last example I will take up the question of postmenopausal motherhood.

LIFESTYLE, SEXUAL PREFERENCES, AND MEDICAL GROUNDS FOR IVF

When IVF was introduced into medical practice in The Netherlands in 1982–83, it had already been a subject of public and political debate. In the early debates, ambivalent opinions on IVF were voiced. On the one hand, IVF was proposed as a potential blessing for infertile women, who could not become pregnant in conventional ways. On the other hand, considerable attention was given to the possible scenarios of cloning identical human beings, genetic manipulation and selection of embryos, development of ecto-genesis, and surrogacy arrangements in combination with embryo donation. These scenarios, which seemed imminent at that time, represented a threat to the process of social acceptance of other scripts of IVF and, consequently, to the emerging IVF practice. In response to parliamentary demands for a governmental policy on IVF, the minister of health asked the prestigious and politically influential Health Council in 1982 to prepare an advisory report on IVF (Terpstra 1982; Minister of Health 1982).

While the Health Council worked on a draft report, a remarkable development took place in the popular media. In women's magazines and in the daily press, articles were published in which involuntarily childless women narrated their painful experiences of infertility and conveyed to the reader their desperate wish for a child (Klinkhamer 1983; *Algemeen Dagblad Extra* 1983; Groenewold 1984). As it happened, all these women were living in heterosexual unions, but the feelings of their male partners were not spelled out with equal clarity and intensity. The image of infertile women desperately longing for a child was also invoked in public statements by gynecologists. And since other experiences of infertility and the ways of coping with them were not represented in the media, a one-sided image of potential users grew in significance. IVF could put an end to the misery of an infertile woman if other scripts were counteracted.

The publication of the preliminary IVF report by the Health Council and the subsequent governmental regulation to place IVF clinics under a licensing system seemed to limit the performance of multiple IVF scripts to a single one (Gezondheidsraad 1984; Staatscourant 1985). The government decided that female infertility as a result of the blockage of both fallopian tubes should be the only medical ground for a statutory IVF. This restriction helped to demarcate the first borderline between the socially acceptable and unacceptable scripts of IVF and thereby contributed to the shaping of a favorable context for the emerging IVF practice. The development of cloning techniques, of the genetic manipulation of embryos or transgressing the human/animal barrier, was rejected as socially unacceptable. IVF was to be considered a medical technology for infertile women who wished to become mothers. In the debate, no reference was made to men as a party in procreation. But the question of whether all women with blocked tubes were eligible for IVF remained unanswered.

The latter question became politically prominent following the publication of a second, far more comprehensive IVF report by the Health Council (Gezondheidsraad 1986). The Council recommended that lesbian and single women should be eligible for IVF or AID (artificial insemination by donor) in exceptional cases only. The necessary condition these women were supposed to meet was a pledge to the practitioners that they would allow "a father figure" to play an important role in the life of the eventual child. The presence of a father figure was seen as the best way of safeguarding the interests of the child. In the same report, the Health Council proposed extending the medical grounds for IVF to male infertility. This opinion of the Health Council was similar to the views held by the Christian Democrat Party and by the influential Association for Family and Juvenile Law. The IVF working party of the Association claimed that each child born with the aid of reproductive technologies should have a juridical mother and a juridical father (FJR 1985). According to Dutch law, a woman who gives birth to a child is automatically the juridical mother of the child, whereas only a man married to the mother is automatically considered the juridical father. The Association recommended the introduction of a link between the written consent of a man to the IVF treatment of his female partner (whether the two married or not) and the legal recognition of his fatherhood. The same rule would apply to married couples and unmarried couples using donor sperm. The requirement of a written consent to treatment by both woman and man constituted already a part of the IVF practice. The policy paper issued by the government in 1988 contained, in somewhat moderated form, many elements put forward in the above reports (CDA 1988; *Kabinetsnotitie* 1988). The government stated that IVF technology should not be employed as an alternative for "natural procreation," but it fell short of proposing legislation to this effect. In this context, "natural procreation" meant procreation within a heterosexual union, either medically assisted or not.

These attempts to exclude lesbian and single women from using IVF and to include male infertility as a medical indication for IVF may be interpreted as a translation of the reproductive possibilities embodied in IVF into a socially noncontroversial setting for procreation, that of the nuclear family. Yet the value which the Health Council, the Association for Family and Juvenile Law, the Christian Democrats, and the government attached to the nuclear family as the privileged site for the procreation and upbringing of children was not shared by other social groups, including the medical and managerial staff of some IVF clinics. The women's movement and the secular political parties launched a successful opposition to what was seen as the discrimination of women on the grounds of their sexual preferences or lifestyles (Raad voor het Jeugdbeleid 1988; Emancipatieraad 1989). It was argued that, in the absence of solid empirical evidence, the claim that family arrangements other than heterosexual had a detrimental influence on children's development was purely ideological. As a result, artificial insemination by donor and IVF services remained available to single and lesbian women in this country. Today, half of the IVF clinics accept lesbian couples for IVF, provided the medical grounds for treatment can be identified. In practice, a number of failed attempts at artificial insemination by donor is considered sufficient grounds for IVF. The same indication applies to single women, but only one of the twelve licensed IVF clinics in this country accepts single women as clients. The restrictive attitude of the clinics toward lesbian and single women stands in sharp contrast with their readiness to accept men as the rightful users of IVF. Not one IVF clinic refuses to treat a woman if her male partner turns out to be infertile.

A number of factors contributed to the outcome of this process of script selection in which nonheterosexual women are not categorically excluded from IVF treatment. The fact that in the 1980s the practice of providing AID to women with a nonheterosexual lifestyle was not only institutionalized in the system of health care but also culturally noncontroversial facilitated this course of events. The vocal part of the women's movement was united on the issue of keeping access to AID and IVF services open for lesbian and single women. But perhaps the most important factor was that the appeal to the value of nondiscrimination on grounds of sexual preference coincided in time with the growing acceptance of homosexual unions and of homosexual parenthood in this country. The most recent IVF report of the Health Council clearly reflects this cultural shift (Gezondheidsraad 1997). The authors admit that the available research on the development of children does not support a comprehensive exclusion of lesbian couples from IVF treatment. Religious beliefs are the main ground for arguing in favor of such an exclusion. However, these beliefs are no longer universally shared by the citizens of this country.

Recently, the minister of health responsible for governmental policy on IVF aired a rather liberal view on this issue. She publicly expressed her understanding and sympathy for the possible requests of lesbian couples to use IVF technology in order to physically share the motherhood of their eventual child.[3] In such cases the fertilized egg cell of one woman is implanted into the womb of her partner, who carries the baby to term. Yet it is not very likely that the IVF script of bodily shared lesbian motherhood will soon be put into practice. The right-wing confessional political parties were quick to voice their disapproval of the minister's statement. The IVF clinicians made it clear that they were not prepared to play their part in this script. They argued that facilitating shared lesbian motherhood would amount to submitting healthy women to a hazardous medical intervention of hormonal stimulation of ovulation and egg retrieval. Remarkably, such prominent attention was never given to the same risks run by healthy women in order to help overcome the infertility of their male partners. On the contrary, not only did the politicians and the clinicians readily accept the IVF scripts that privilege heterosexual relationships; the envisaged users, female partners of infertile men, seem to have few objections to playing their roles in this script, and quite a number of them demand IVF treatment. It remains unclear whether lesbian couples would be interested in the mentioned form of procreative assistance. But in view of the political opposition, the minister was quick to tone down her earlier statement.

The quasi-official attitude toward providing IVF to single women is somewhat different. Although the Health Council does not plead for an across-the-board exclusion of this group of women from access to IVF, it recommends a careful individual screening of the applicants for their motives. The Council motivates its caution by referring to the reports from some clinics providing artificial insemination by donor in which the psychosocial profile is given of single women seeking medical assistance in procreation. The clinics describe the majority of single women calling for assistance as emotionally neglected and socially isolated and as maintaining abnormal relationships. The requests of these women for artificial insemination by donor are viewed as desperate attempts to put an end to the loneliness by begetting a child. The Health Council concludes that the image arising from other studies of somewhat older, self-aware, emotionally balanced, and socially successful single women who give ample thought to the idea of autonomous motherhood before making a decision is not representative of single women seeking AID.

The negative reports from the AID clinics probably mirror the situation of some single women in our society. However, the fact that these apparently morally dubious motives are attributed to single women only—without allowing for the possibility that women living in a homosexual or heterosexual union may lead similar lives and may have similar motives for seeking a child—reflects the degree to which single women and their wish for motherhood are still culturally seen as abnormal. Given the political influence of the Health Council, one can reasonably expect that the mentioned recommendation, if not met by a strong opposition, will become part of the routine. This means that all single women applying for IVF will have to prove that they do not form a serious risk for the development of their eventual children.

EGG CELL DONATION AND SURROGACY

The second example of sociopolitical selection and modification of potential scripts embodied in the IVF technology is the controversy over the regulation of egg cell donation and surrogacy. These debates were largely framed in terms of the urgency of countering the imminent threat of the commercialization of procreation and the need to protect the interests of the parties involved in the procedure, notably those of the eventual children.

Although surrogacy may be accomplished with or without the use of IVF technology, in the debates and in the regulation a clear distinction was not always made between the two forms of surrogacy, that is, when the surrogate mother has or does not have genetic ties with the child. The fear that surrogacy will give rise to widespread commercial practices and a strong commitment to avert such possible developments were important motives in the public and political debates. These fears were fed by media reports on the growing surrogacy industry in the United States and by the actual attempts of foreign citizens—Ms. K. Cotton from the United Kingdom and Mr. F. Torch from the United States—to set up mediating agencies in this country.

The views expressed in the debates of the 1980s ranged from the total rejection of possible surrogacy practices and the call for a legal ban, on the one hand, to the elaboration of conditions under which the arrangements between the contracting couple and the surrogate mother could be considered morally acceptable, on the other hand. Some debaters were ready to accept surrogacy practice only if no payments whatsoever to the surrogate mother were made. Others considered that the reimbursement of extra costs incurred during pregnancy was morally justified. At the other end of the spectrum, one could find those who thought that the most effective way to impede a free market style commercialization of surrogacy was to place the practice under the control of the specialized state agencies equipped with regulating and controlling powers. The envisaged agencies would be responsible for securing the anonymity of the parties involved, for designing a standard surrogacy contract, for fixing a uniform price for surrogacy services, for supervising the handing over of the child, and for the conveyance of the legal parenthood rights from the surrogate mother to the contracting couple. However, even the proponents of state-regulated surrogacy practice admitted that the numerous legal problems were difficult to solve. Could surrogacy contracts include binding prescriptions concerning the lifestyle of the surrogate mother during pregnancy, compulsory prenatal tests, or demands of abortion in case the child might be handicapped? Could such eventual stipulations of the contract be attuned to the autonomous rights of the woman over her body? How to proceed in situations of conflict or breach of contract? Should adoption law be relaxed for cases in which surrogacy was involved?

The debates on permissibility and on eventual regulation of surrogacy practices were accompanied by a proliferation of representations of women who would be willing to engage in surrogacy. One of these was the familiar image of an infertile woman desperately longing for a child but unable to have one herself due to a missing womb or another obstacle. Her situation could clearly count on some public sympathy. Then there was the highly idealized figure of the potential surrogate. She was portrayed as a mother intensely enjoying her family life. Out of love for children and sheer compassion, she was prepared to carry a baby for her less fortunate sister or friend (CDA 1988). The message behind these images was clear: The future regulation should allow some space for such a compassionate gift from one woman to another. Yet the media projected also strikingly different images of women likely to be attracted to surrogacy. Physical inability to beget a child would not be the only motive for seeking surrogacy. Some would chase after success and comfort. The imagined self-centered, ambitious professional women who pursued the joy of having a child but were not prepared to compromise any part of their career and exciting social life for the burdens of pregnancy were obvious candidates for future contracting mothers. Usually references were made to actresses, ballerinas, or successful businesswomen. These women were seen as likely to seek docile surrogates, prone to exploitation because of their poor financial and social situation. This image of an egocentric contracting mother was complemented by an equally negative portrait of the would-be surrogate as a woman motivated by the possibility of financial reward and the wish to experience the "pleasures of the pregnancy" without assuming the burdens of raising the child (Dik 1985; Cramer 1985; Gruijter 1985; CDA 1988).[4]

In the course of the public and parliamentary debates, a broad feeling of agreement developed. In the early 1990s, surrogacy was seen as a socially undesirable phenomenon which by no means should be encouraged. Only exceptional cases of fully altruistic surrogacy could be tolerated. It also became evident that in many cases surrogacy could be arranged in private. Therefore, a comprehensive ban would be ineffective. Surrogacy could, however, be kept in check by discouraging measures. One of these measures was the governmental and parliamentary decision not to introduce any changes in the adoption law that would facilitate the conveyance of legal parenthood in cases of surrogacy. At the same time, the Penal Code was amended with the aim of preempting any initiatives toward the commercialization of surrogacy. Since 1993, all forms of mediation in surrogacy contracts have been prohibited. Until recently, the prohibition covered not only setting up specialized agencies or publicly soliciting and offering surrogacy services. The provision of medical assistance in case of surrogacy also was banned. Private arrangements, with all the uncertainties for the parties involved regarding the rights, the risks, and the handing over of the child, were, however, tolerated.

The debate on surrogacy was closely linked to that on egg cell donation. The relations between the two women involved in the donation procedure emerged as an important issue. As already mentioned, Dutch law considers a woman who gives birth to a child as the only legal mother of that child. Motherhood is a natural fact, as opposed to fatherhood, which is considered a juridical fiction. Consequently, according to law a woman cannot deny her motherhood. Only if she is unable to assume the care for her child may she put the child up for adoption. Egg cell donation, whether or not in combination with surrogacy arrangements, posed the question of who should be regarded as the mother of the child: the one who donates the egg cell or the one who gives birth to the child. The answer to this question was by no means self-evident in the 1980s. On the one hand, the majority of the government advisory bodies and political parties favored the perpetuation of the existing concept of motherhood. On the other hand, some outstanding female lawyers argued that, in view of the newly available technological possibilities, the traditional concept of motherhood should be revised (Meer 1986; Rood de Boer 1984). According to these lawyers, legal motherhood could no longer be regarded as a natural fact. Consequently, a woman from whom a child was born should be given the right to deny or renounce her motherhood. And any other woman should have a legal right to recognize a motherless child as her own, a right that men enjoyed for a long time. Yet these proposals did not gain sufficient public and political support. The idea that a child could be motherless, or that two women would be able to claim motherhood rights, represented a profound break with the deeply rooted concept of unique biological motherhood. Faced with the problem of translating the unprecedented motherhood scripts embodied in IVF into culturally acceptable relations, the legislators opted to preserve the traditional concept of motherhood. In The Netherlands, only the woman who gives birth is the legitimate mother of the child, regardless of whether egg cell donation or surrogacy arrangements are involved in the process of procreation. Consequently, a surrogate mother cannot be forced to hand over the baby to the contracting would-be parents.

In 1989, the wish to secure a biologically undivided motherhood underlined a politically controversial decision of the Christian Democrat minister of health to put a legal ban on any form of egg cell donation (*Staatscourant* 1989).

For our understanding of the dynamic interplay between cultural values surrounding gender relations and their bearing upon the societal selection of scripts, it is very instructive to look briefly at the public outcry that followed. In their arguments, opponents of the ban on egg cell donation appealed to two broadly shared values in Dutch society: that of the individual autonomy of the citizen and that of nondiscrimination. The imposition of the ban by ministerial decision, without parliamentary debate or approval, was perceived as an unacceptable infringement of the autonomous rights of women in the sphere of procreation. The opponents, including eminent lawyers, ethicists, IVF clinicians, journalists, and spokespersons for the association of IVF patients, argued that the government had no right to prescribe the way individual people wish to organize their procreation. Furthermore, banning egg cell donation while sperm donation was allowed formed an unacceptable violation of the rights of women with regard to their bodies and a flagrant act of discrimination against infertile women, who—in contrast to infertile men—were denied the possibility of begetting a child (*Volkskrant* 1989; *Vrije Volk* 1989; Stomp 1989; *Trouw* 1989). The public perception of the ban on egg cell donation in terms of a threatened autonomy and discrimination between women and men proved so powerful that within weeks the comprehensive ban was replaced by a far more limited ban on egg cell donation in combination with surrogacy arrangements.

One interesting feature of this commotion is that no significant meaning was attached to the technologies involved in donation or to the profound difference between the bodily involvement of men donating sperm and of women donating egg cells. Whereas sperm donation does not require any technological intervention in the male body, women donating egg cells have to undergo a hazardous hormonal treatment and the drastic procedure of egg cell retrieval. The social norm of equal treatment, of nondiscrimination, was applied to situations which are profoundly unequal, without any reflection on the meaning of such (in)equality for women. Meanwhile, practice has shown that only a small number of women are willing to donate egg cells. The few donations that take place are nearly always between women who are kin or friends.

For some time the issue of surrogacy seemed settled. The number of surrogacy cases reported to the Juvenile Courts was extremely low. Advertisements soliciting surrogate mothers or offering surrogacy services disappeared from the magazines and the daily press. On at least one occasion, an owner of a clandestine agency hunting for would-be surrogate mothers in East European countries was prosecuted, as was a woman who in spite of the legal ban offered her services as surrogate in a feminist magazine (*Volkskrant* 1997). Clearly, surrogacy was not a popular solution to the problems of childlessness in this country. In the meantime, hidden from the public eye, a few couples appealed to the

Ministry of Health for individual exemption from the law banning non-commercial surrogacy in combination with egg donation and IVF. In some of these few cases, the permit was granted. Recently the Health Council called the attention of the government to what it saw as inconsistent in the current regulation of surrogacy. It pointed out that noncommercial surrogacy in combination with artificial insemination was not banned. The child resulting from such an arrangement is genetically related to the surrogate mother and to the contracting father. However, from the perspective of the contracting couple, a more satisfactory form of surrogacy, when the child is genetically related to both envisaged parents, was still prohibited. In order to correct the unwarranted inequality, the Council pleaded for the lifting of the ban on surrogacy through IVF. The minister swiftly followed this advice (Minister of Health 1997).

LATE MOTHERHOOD: TECHNOLOGICAL FORCING OF CULTURAL CHANGE?

Another interesting script carried by IVF refers to crossing the age boundary limiting the procreative capacity of women. Unlike men, who up to an advanced age can beget a child, women are by nature unable to conceive after menopause. According to the insights of the biomedical science, the main reason for this natural inability is the rapid loss eventually leading to absence of egg cells in ovaries. IVF in combination with the donation of egg cells provides in principle an opportunity to extend the reproductive capacity of women beyond the menopause. Thus the technology carries a promise of erasing one aspect of the biological difference between men and women and of modeling women's reproductive life as a mirror image of male natural capacities. Although menopause is a natural barrier, the exact age at which it occurs in individual women varies a great deal. Some women will pass menopause in their mid-thirties, whereas others will continue to menstruate into their fifties. However, the statistical chance of spontaneously getting pregnant decreases rapidly after the age of thirty-eight.

Biology is not the only element defining the age at which women may get babies and become mothers. Social conditions, beliefs, norms, and values are as important as, or perhaps even more important than, a sheer biological capacity. The availability of IVF and the particular pattern of its regulation form a part of the social context in which individual choices are made. The age limit for women applying for IVF was not on the agenda of the debates that were carried out in the 1980s. In practice, however, women above the age of forty were usually not accepted for IVF by the clinics. Two considerations contributed to the imposition of this age limit by the clinics themselves. One of these was the observation that the chance of a forty-year-old woman becoming pregnant with the aid of IVF is rather slim and decreases sharply with every following year. The clinics were also confronted with the requirements of the governmental licensing system introduced in 1989. These included a stipulation that a clinic should achieve an average rate of success of 10 percent in order to be eligible for a license. Obviously, treating women older than forty years would pull down the rate of success and endanger the prospects of obtaining a license. But one was aware of this IVF script. Already in 1986 the Health Council observed that a premature menopause could be considered good medical grounds for an IVF treatment in combination with egg cell donation (Gezondheidsraad 1986). Following the relaxation of the ban on egg cell donation in 1989, young postmenopausal women could in principle make use of this opportunity.

The age at which women give birth became an issue in the public debates of the 1990s. A 1991 inaugural lecture by gynecologist E. te Velde, entitled "Pregnancy in the Twenty-first Century," caught the public imagination. In the lecture Dr. te Velde considered the consequences of the recent trend among women in this country to postpone their first pregnancies. At that time, the average age of a woman giving birth to her first child was twenty-seven and rising. He argued that social conditions made it impossible for many young women to reconcile their ambitions regarding education and a professional career with the wish for a child and the demands of motherhood. He warned that the demand for technologies like IVF would grow if no social solution were found. Consequently, the future mode of procreation would be affected. It was quite possible that in the twenty-first century an increasing number of young women would opt for the early removal and cryopreservation of their egg cells. Once having completed their education and established a professional career, they would have the egg cells fertilized, get them implanted, and at a very advanced age give birth to one or more children (Velde 1991).

At the same time that this rather disturbing future scenario was spelled out, the first notices about postmenopausal women becoming mothers appeared in the media. In the United States and in Italy, women between forty and fifty were taking advantage of IVF. The age of postmenopausal mothers increased at a steady pace. In 1993 the birth of twins to a fifty-nine-year-old English woman upset the media. A few months later, a sixty-two-year-old Italian woman became the oldest "young mother" in the world. All these women became pregnant thanks to the egg cells donated by younger women. The revelations from the private clinic of the Italian gynecologist Antinori fascinated the media. Soon the press revealed that Antinori's clients included Dutch women of advanced age. The Dutch clients were active in organizing "La Cicogna Laboriosa" (the industrious stork), an international society aiming at supporting women with the wish for a child, and one of them even became president of the society (*NRC* 1990, 1994a, 1994b; Heering 1992; Evenblij 1993; Kleijwegt and Scherphuis 1994). The debate in the media that followed these revelations displayed many traits of a controversy. Some participants voiced opinions in favor of relaxing the age limit; others argued against facilitating late motherhood. However, even those who advocated a liberal policy on the question of age showed no enthusiasm for the prospect of "grandma" mommies.

Those opposing the use of IVF by postmenopausal women evoked the image of an old, physically worn woman confronted with the demanding task of raising a baby to adulthood. They argued that the situation of a child growing up with an old mother could not be compared to that of a child of an old father. In that case, the mother is usually young enough to compensate for the advanced age of the father. Older women becoming mothers with the aid of reproductive technologies were very likely to have older men as partners. The child, therefore, would be growing up with two old parents. One or both parents would die before the child reached adulthood. Even in the case of long-lived parents, the child's prospects were rather grim, they argued. His or her whole childhood would be overshadowed by the fear of becoming an orphan. Old mothers would lack the energy to care adequately for the baby and to respond to the needs of a young child for active physical play. Later, her child would have to endure numerous embarrassing situations at school, since the mother would often be taken for the grandmother. Such confusions would provoke many investigative questions and even jokes by the schoolmates of the child. The big age difference between parents and child would inevitably result in an emotional gap and a mutual lack of understanding. The intergenerational conflicts usually accompanying the passage from childhood to adolescence would therefore be significantly aggravated. By then both parents, if still alive, would be approaching the age of seventy and displaying symptoms of aging. The unprepared adolescent would face the difficult task of caring for his or her old parents. The problems would be further aggravated by the absence of genetic ties between mother and child. In short, the opponents expected that in the long run, neither mother nor child would be able to cope successfully with the consequences of postmenopausal motherhood. In an effort to prevent such a gloomy future, the Christian Democratic Party urged the government to introduce a ban on treating postmenopausal women with IVF (Evenblij 1993; Baart and Feenstra 1994; Hoksbergen 1996).

The opposition to the prospect of banning older women from the treatment was eloquently voiced by some ethicists, jurists, and gynecologists, one of whom was involved in caring for Dr. Antinori's Dutch clients. They played down the potential problems in the mother-child relationship and pointed to the expected advantages of late motherhood. Contrary to the common image projected by the opponents, advocates of older motherhood maintained that women who actually ventured the IVF treatment at an advanced age were in excellent health and in a good mental condition. In the words of one gynecologist, these were "spirited ladies, who knew very well what they were doing and had their reasons for it; extraordinary women with an extraordinary request and extraordinary problem" (Dr. R. C. W. Vermeulen quoted in Kleijwegt and Scherphuis 1994). The pessimistic speculations about their future family life were grossly exaggerated. The life expectancy of women was already high and still increasing, so the risk that a young child would be orphaned was not that dramatic.

Far from being a risk factor, the advanced age of a mother could turn out to be an asset in the child's development. The older women wishing to beget children through IVF were likely to have emotionally stable relationships with their partners. With a nearly completed professional career and no financial worries, these women would be in a good position to devote much time and attention to child rearing. The fears of a profound emotional gap occurring during the adolescence were based on speculations not substantiated by systematic data. To the contrary, many children were successfully raised by their grandparents. In short, the opposition to postmenopausal motherhood was labeled as discriminatory against elderly women. Some debaters, such as gynecologist Honnebier, even believed that if this opposition were subdued, reproductive technology could be helpful in solving the pressing problems of aging Dutch society. In his view, the advances in medical technology would permit future women to retain well-functioning ovaries until a very advanced age. Both men and women would be free to spend the largest part of their lives on working. Only after retirement would they get children and devote themselves fully to their upbringing. The number of years to live after completing this task would be limited, and the young adults would no longer be burdened with the care for the old. The ideal future society of Dr. Honnebier was composed of two generations only (Honnebier 1994).

Remarkably, the IVF clinicians, whose cooperation is a necessary condition for the realization of this IVF script, had many reservations about the prospects of late postmenopausal motherhood. Their attitude resulted partly from fear that embracing this type of procreative assistance would not contribute to the improvement of the controversial public image of IVF. They focused their argument on the increased medical hazards of late pregnancies for women and children. In their eyes, IVF was a treatment for the illness of infertility, a pathological condition in women who otherwise would be fertile. The inability of a sixty-year-old women to become pregnant was not a pathological phenomenon. It was natural, and it was not the task of IVF clinicians to assist these women in getting pregnant. Restoring fertility in postmenopausal women was equal to creating a pathological situation. The only departure from this position should be made for young women who passed menopause too early (Baart and Feenstra 1994).[5]

For quite some time the debate seemed to be floating in the air. Neither the potential new users of reproductive technology—older women—nor any social organization—including political parties—publicly voiced any demands in this respect. It was the self-appointed spokespersons for the potential end users and for the eventual children who defined the nature of the interests and sketched the images of elder women as mothers. The unquestioned assumption underlying the debate was that some older postmenopausal women cherish a latent wish to become pregnant and to give birth to a child. The availability of a technological solution can bring this wish into the open, transform it into a problem, and consequently create a new demand for IVF.

The hypothetical character of the debate changed with the publication of the official reports by the Ethical Committee of the Royal Dutch Medical Society (KNMG) and by the Health Council in 1996 and 1997 (KNMG 1996; Gezondheidsraad 1997). Although medical doctors, including IVF clinicians, were on both committees, the reports diverged strongly from the restrained position of the IVF clinics. The committees argued that natural barriers could not serve as a ground for moral judgments leading to refraining from medical intervention. Basically, there was no difference between the natural infertility of postmenopausal women and other forms of infertility. Some of these are caused by illnesses that are natural phenomena as well. Many natural phenomena are perceived as undesirable, and a medical intervention is deemed appropriate. Correspondingly, from the fact that at a certain age the occurrence of the menopause is not only a natural but also a normal event, it does not follow that medical attempts to change this situation should be considered morally reprehensible—even less so when the woman herself requests the assistance and there are no medical objections against the treatment. Also, these committees made an appeal to the norm of equal treatment. The age of menopause varies strongly, and therefore it cannot serve as a standard for deciding which women may be treated and which may not, they argued. Otherwise, one might end up treating older women who had not passed menopause and refusing to treat much younger postmenopausal women. Both committees pleaded for the replacement of the rigid age barrier with a flexible system of selection based on the individual prediction of chances for success. But since the individual assessment of the applicants' chances is not yet feasible, age limits for IVF in combination with egg donation should be relaxed, and some experimenting should be allowed. Provided no negative effects of late pregnancies and postmenopausal motherhood are observed, the Royal Dutch Medical Society pleaded for the provisional extension of the age limit to fifty-five. The Health Council argued for fixing the age barrier at forty-four for regular egg cell donations and for allowing experimental treatment of women up to the age of forty-eight years. In reply to these reports, the minister of health decided to extend the age limit to forty-four for treating postmenopausal women using donated egg cells (Minister of Health 1997).

ACCULTURATION OF IVF: GIVING GENDERED BODIES TO THE SCRIPTS OF INTERACTING GAMETES

In the above cases of the societal selection of scripts, I focused on the question of representation of likely users in the public and political debates and on the interplay between these representations and regulatory processes. In the final section of the chapter, I want to call attention to the gender-specific effects of those representations and to reflect upon the value of the proposed concept of macroselection of script for analyzing the processes of acculturation of technology.

In the first part of this chapter I argued that the most innovative element of IVF consists of removing the process of fertilization from the woman's body into a laboratory dish. The virtual users "inscribed" into that technology are supposed to satisfy two basic conditions. They must be willing to furnish their gametes for fertilization in the laboratory, and a woman must be prepared to have an embryo implanted. These virtual users have no social or cultural identity, and the nature of the social relations between them is not defined. To a certain degree they are interchangeable: any man, even a dead one, can provide sperm, and any woman can relinquish her egg cells for IVF or have an embryo implanted, as long as she has a womb. However, in a given cultural context, not just any man or any woman is perceived as a legitimate user of IVF, but only those who possess certain social characteristics, including the relationships that are deemed appropriate for the procreation and upbringing of children. These characteristics are thus not given a priori. They are negotiated in public debates, in clinical practice, and in official regulations. In this process the mode of representing some women and men as rightful and others as inappropriate users plays an important role.

A number of distinctive features of user representation come to the fore in the presented cases. One of these is a remarkable asymmetry between the representations of women and of men. Potential female users were represented either in terms of their wish for a child (heterosexuals, older women, and contracting mothers) or in terms of their supposed qualities as prospective social mothers (lesbians, single and older women). With one exception, two contrasting images were projected simultaneously of the same categories of women (e.g., of postmenopausal women, single women, surrogates, contracting mothers, etc.). On the one hand, these women seemed to possess all the characteristics needed for being qualified as rightful users; on the other hand, they seemed to lack those characteristics. Only relatively young heterosexual women escaped this dichotomy in the assessment of the quality of their desire for a child and of their suitability for social motherhood.

In contrast, men as a party in the application of IVF emerged as a homogeneous group. They were introduced into the debate in their well-established capacity as legal fathers. Their suitability for the social role of fathers was not scrutinized. It was just taken for granted that their absence is detrimental to the normal development of prospective children. At the same time, more in the clinical practice than in the public debate, infertile men in their capacity as patients were defined as rightful users of the IVF technology. Although in theory any infertile man, whether heterosexual, single, or homosexual, could take advantage of IVF, the pursued policy of discouraging surrogacy effectively limited the group of male users of IVF to men living in a heterosexual union.

So, next to infertility, the heterosexual relationship emerges as a single important social characteristic of the legitimate IVF user, whether it is she or he. However, both these requirements are subject to a certain degree of erosion due to the changing social and medical norms. As many cases of childlessness cannot be explained by somatic conditions, infertility as a medical category becomes more and more elusive, and the failure of other fertilization techniques is now accepted as a good ground for trying IVF. Also, women who do not live in heterosexual unions are no longer directly disqualified as users but are expected to undergo additional queries before being accepted for IVF. So it is not so much the infertility but the anticipated qualities of women as mothers that now define them as proper IVF users. In defining men as proper users, the requirement of heterosexuality has a different meaning. The wish for a child that these men may or may not cherish, their social qualities as fathers and of their female partners as mothers are neither discussed nor assessed but simply assumed. What really counts—but remains unspoken—is that women's bodies are needed as a medium for men's use of IVF.

Another noteworthy feature of users' representation in the debates on IVF is its selectivity and the effects of it. As I mentioned before, the material configuration of the IVF technique does not presuppose that only one woman and one man will be involved in the whole procedure. Different constituent parts of IVF may be performed on different bodies. Each part of the procedure carries more and less serious hazards with it. To spread the performance of IVF over three or more persons means to distribute the hazards. The social selection of scripts for the performance carries with it the acceptance of a specific distribution of hazards. The discussed cases suggest that not all people involved physically in the IVF procedure are perceived as users. The selective visibility of certain categories of users and the invisibility of others facilitates the process of the acceptance of different scripts.

The most obvious example is the case of infertile men being defined as users. In this case, women on whose bodies the whole procedure is being carried out remain invisible. Consequently, no consideration is given to the question of whether it is acceptable that these healthy and usually fertile women run serious health risks in order to "cure" male infertility. In the case of egg cell donation, younger infertile and postmenopausal women are perceived as the users of IVF. Women who are supposed to provide the egg cells are described as donors, although it is they, and not the women receiving egg cells, who undergo the major risks of IVF. The invisibility of donor women as users of IVF goes hand in hand with the lack of social recognition of the health hazards they are expected to run. The lack of acknowledgment of these hazards significantly facilitated the relaxation of the ban on egg cell donation.

As in the case of male infertility, this form of differential visibility of the users also has a gender aspect to it. Although only women are involved in the egg cell donations, it is their social relationship to a man that legitimizes the procedure. Once again, the way in which lesbian unions feature in the debate reveals the hidden norm. In this case the attention shifts from the women receiving egg cells to her egg-donating partner. The hazards involved in donation are fully avowed and get a practical significance. Now they serve as the main medical reason for refusing to assist lesbian couples in realizing bodily shared motherhood.

The discussed cases of the macroselection of scripts suggest that in the cultural context of The Netherlands, the ease with which scripts become accepted for performance largely depends on the translation of the abstract users inscribed in the IVF in terms of heterosexual relationships. For many, but not for all, collective actors involved in the process of acculturation of IVF, heterosexual women and men stand as the model for legitimate users. Heterosexuality, however, no longer functions as an absolute norm, but only as a culturally privileged one. Each claim of lesbian or single women on the use of this technology further undermines the cultural importance of heterosexuality in this country, especially but not exclusively each successful claim.

NOTES

An earlier version of this chapter was published in Dutch in *Tijdschrift voor Genderstudies* 1, no. 1 (1998): 25–33.

1. Some examples to be discussed here are taken from a detailed study of the processes of entrenchment of IVF in the Dutch health care system that I completed in 1996.

2. This was attempted unsuccessfully by an Australian team at the Queen Victoria Medical Center, Melbourne. Wood and Westmore 1983.

3. Speech by Minister E. Borst-Eilers during the International Women's Day meeting organized by the feminist monthly *Opzij,* Amsterdam, 8 March 1997.

4. The cited articles are based on interviews with lawyer H. Roscam Abbing (Dik 1985), gynecologist M. Slot (Cramer 1985), and A. Rörsch (Gruijter 1985 and CDA 1988).

5. Baart and Feenstra in turn cite their interview interlocutor, Dr. C. A. M. Jansen.

REFERENCES

Akrich, M.:
  1992   The De-scription of Technological Objects. In W. Bijker and J. Law (eds.), *Shaping Technology/Building Society,* 205–18. Cambridge: MIT Press.
Algemeen Dagblad Extra:
  1983   Eindelijk moeder [Mother at last], 16 May.
Baart, S., and G. Feenstra:
  1994   Ik durf te verdedigen dat leeftijdgrens wat omhoog moet. Onvruchtbaarheid op zestigjarige leeftijd is geen afwijking [I dare to argue that the age limit should be somewhat raised. Infertility at the age of sixty is not a dysfunction]. *De Volkskrant,* 11 January.
CDA, Wetenschappelijk Instituut voor het [Scientific Institute of the Christian Democratic Party]:
  1988   *Zinvol leven. Een christen-democratische bijdrage aan de discussie over draagmoederschap, kunstmatige inseminatie, gift en in vitro fertilisatie* [Meaningful life: A Christian Democratic contribution to the debate regarding surrogate motherhood, artificial insemination, GIFT and in vitro fertilization]. Deventer: Van Loghum Slaterus.
Cramer, J.:
  1985   Draagmoeders nog niet toegestaan [Surrogate mothers not yet permitted]. *Opzij,* September.
Dik, H.:
  1985   Als je echt een kind wilt, en het lukt niet . . . [When you really wish for a child, and it does not succeed . . .]. *Margriet,* no. 18.
Emancipatieraad [Emancipation Council]:
  1989   *Advies kunstmatige bevruchting en draagmoederschap* [Advice regarding artificial fertilization and surrogacy]. The Hague.
  1996   *Het late ouderschap: over uitstel en afstel. Advies maatschappelijke consequenties uitgesteld ouderschap* [Late parenthood: About delay and renunciation. Advice regarding societal consequences of delayed parenthood]. The Hague.
Evenblij, M.:
  1993   Oma wordt zwanger [Grandmother gets pregnant]. *De Volkskrant,* 30 January.
FJR [Society for Family and Juvenile Law]:
  1985   *Bijzondere wijzen van voortplanting. Draagmoederschap en de juridische problematiek* [Unusual modes of procreation: Surrogate motherhood and the legal questions]. Report.

Gezondheidsraad [Health Council]:

1984   *Interimadvies inzake in vitro fertilisatie* [Interim advice re: in vitro fertilization]. The Hague.

1986   *Advies inzake kunstmatige voortplanting* [Advice re: artificial procreation]. The Hague.

1997   *Het planningsbesluit IVF* [Planning decision re: IVF]. The Hague.

Groenewold, J.:

1984   Geboren op 5 augustus 1984. De eerste reageerbuis-tweeling in Nederland [Born on 5 August 1984. The first test-tube twin in The Netherlands]. *Libelle,* November: 10–17.

Gruijter, J. de:

1985   Manipuleren met de erfelijkheid; mensen op bestelling, vader overbodig [Manipulations of heredity, people on delivery, superfluous father]. *Elseviers Magazine,* 4 May.

Heering, A.:

1992   Zwangerschap 62-jarige vrouw verdeelt Italië [Pregnancy of a 62-year-old woman divides Italy]. *Twentsche Courant,* 2 May.

Hoksbergen, R.:

1996   Kinderen krijgen is nu eenmaal geen universeel mensen recht [Begetting children is not a universal human right]. *NRC,* 10 May.

Honnebier, W.:

1994   "Bejaard" ouderschap heeft voordelen ["Aged" parenthood has its advantages]. *NRC,* 13 January.

Ietswaart, H. F. J.:

1994   Late kinderwens is niet te vergelijken met face-lift [Late wish for a child cannot be compared with a face-lift]. *NRC,* 13 January.

Kabinetsnotitie kunstmatige bevruchting en draagmoederschap [Government's paper re: artificial fertilization and surrogate motherhood]:

1988   HTK, 1987–1988, 20 706, nos. 1 and 2.

Kirejczyk, M.:

1996   *Met technologie gezegend? Gender en de omstreden invoering van in vitro fertilisatie in de Nederlandse gezondheidszorg* [Blessed with technology? Gender and the controversial introduction of in vitro fertilization in the health care in The Netherlands]. Utrecht: Jan van Arkel.

Kleijwegt, M., and A. Scherphuis:

1994   Oude moeders en het woelige baren [Old mothers and turbulent birthgiving]. *Vrij Nederland,* 15 January: 11–13.

Klinkhamer, G.:

1983   Hoe de natuur een handje geholpen wordt [How Mother Nature gets a helping hand]. *Margriet,* 10 June.

KNMG [Royal Dutch Medical Society]:

1996   IVF op latere leeftijd [IVF at a later age]. *Medisch Contact* 51: 620–27.

Meer, J. van der:

1986   *Nieuw leven—ander recht: in vitro fertilisatie. Ethische, medische en juridische aspecten rond bevruchtingstechnieken* [New life—different law: In vitro fertilization. Ethical, medical and legal aspects of fertilization techniques]. Uitgeverij Prins: Brielle.

Minister of Health:

1982   *Adviesaanvrage in zake IVF aan de Gezondheidsraad* [Request to the Health Council for advice on IVF], HTK, 1981–82, no. 1338.

1997   *Standpunt in-vitrofertilisatie.* Brief aan de voorzitter van de Tweede Kamer [Position re: in vitro fertilization. Letter to the Speaker of the Parliament], 5 March.
        NRC:

1990   Menopauzale vrouwen baarden kinderen uit gedoneerde eicellen [Menopausal women gave birth to children from donated egg cells]. 30 October.

1994a   Oudere moeders [Elder mothers]. 15 January.

1994b   "Oudste moeder" is in Italië bevallen van gezonde zoon ["The oldest mother" has given birth to a healthy son in Italy]. 19 July.

Oost van, E.:

1995   Over "vrouwelijke" en "mannelijke" dingen [About "feminine" and "masculine" things]. In M. Brouns and M. Grünell (eds.), *Vrouwenstudies in de jaren negentig. Een kennismaking vanuit verschillende disciplines* [Women's Studies in the 1990s: An introduction from the perspective of different disciplines], 289–313. Bussum: Coutinho.

Oudshoorn, N. E. J.:

1996   *Genderscripts in technologie: noodlot of uitdaging?* [Gender scripts in technology: A fate or a challenge?] Inaugural lecture. Enschede: University of Twente.

Raad voor het Jeugdbeleid [Council for Youth Policy]:

1988   *Ouderschap zonder onderscheid. Een beleidsadvies over belangen van kinderen bij verantwoord ouderschap en kunstmatige voortplanting* [Parenthood without distinction: Policy advice re: children's interest in responsible parenthood and artificial procreation]. Rijswijk: Ministry of Welfare, Health, and Culture.

Rood de Boer, M.:

1984   Rechtsvragen met betrekking tot moederschap [Legal questions concerning motherhood]. *Tijdschrift voor Familie- en Jeugdrecht* [Journal for family and juvenile law], nos. 6–8, 232–38.

Staatscourant [State Gazette]:

1985   *Besluit tijdelijke regeling in vitro fertilisatie* [Decision re: temporary regulation of in vitro fertilization], no. 141, 24 July.

1989   *Wet ziekenhuisvoorzieningen, Planningsbesluit in vitro fertilisatie* [Hospital facilities law, Planning decision re: in vitro fertilization], no. 147, 31 July.

Stomp, R.:

1989   Verbod op eiceldonatie in strijd met mensenrechten. Brinkman probeert ethische opvattingen door te drukken [Ban on egg cell donation in contravention of human rights. Brinkman tries to impose ethical views]. *Haagsche Courant*, 5 August.

Terpstra, E.:

1982   *Parliamentary question.* HTK, 1981–82, no. 688.

Trouw:

1989   Verbod eiceldonatie strijdig met grondwet [Ban on egg cell donation in contravention of constitution]. 4 August.

Velde, E. R. te:

1991   *Zwanger worden in de 21ste eeuw: steeds later, steeds kunstmatiger* [Getting pregnant in the twenty-first century: Still later, increasingly artificial]. Inaugural lecture. Utrecht: Rijksuniversiteit [State University].

Volkskrant, de:

1989   Bevruchting slechts toegestaan met eigen cellen [Fertilization only permitted with own egg cells]. 3 August.

1997 Vrouw veroordeeld voor advertentie draagmoeder [Woman sentenced for surrogacy advertisement]. 3 March.

1997 Borst wil IVF na menopauze niet vergoeden [Borst does not want to reimburse IVF after the menopause]. 10 March.

Vrije Volk, het:

1989 "Wie dit bedacht, heeft er niets van begrepen" ["One who thought this out has no understanding whatsoever"] and "Onzinnig verbod" ["Absurd ban"]. 3 and 4 August.

Wood, C., and A. Westmore:

1983 *Test-Tube Conception.* Melbourne: Hill of Content.

7

The Lack and the "Need" of Regulation for Assisted Fertilization: The Italian Case

Federico Neresini and Franca Bimbi

Italy has no laws regulating the practice of assisted fertilization (AF). Leaving aside all other possible judgments, this lack of norms means that the various social actors are relatively free to interact within the general frame and thus that the various processes are more clearly observable. We take the case of Italy to analyze the process of deconstruction and reconstruction of the "natural" order of procreation at present taking place within the debate on AF. We therefore focus on the overall practice of AF rather than specific types of intervention, and by so doing we also overcome the problem of the scarcity and fragmentary nature of currently available knowledge on what really takes place in an unregulated system.

To this end, we have analyzed the texts produced by the interaction of the various social actors within the various contexts—institutional, biomedical research, the media, and social research. The term *text* is used here in its widest sense to include official documents, laws, newspaper articles, and articles in specialist journals. Clearly, the choice of documents for analysis is based on their relevance to our working hypotheses.

Our exposition is in five parts. The first deals with the theoretical apparatus that we feel is most suitable. In the second we reconstruct, albeit partially, the process whereby infertility comes to be regarded as a disease as well as the consequences of this for AF. The third part takes the present situation of lack of legislation as the starting point for an analysis of the positions of the various social actors involved. In the fourth part, we delve deeper into the present situation as regards recourse to such practices in Italy and, in particular, we present and discuss the findings of a study carried out on a sample of doctors. The final part examines women's position with respect to AF.

THE THEORETICAL MODEL

Discourse, viewpoints, and considerations on the subject of AF over the past twenty years in Italy tend to converge on a recurrent model of description and phenomenon analysis. According to this widely held interpretation, the problems before us at present have developed along lines whose fundamental stages we can reconstruct as follows:

a. The progressive growth in the basic knowledge of the biological mechanisms of human reproduction has brought about the development of technology that allows us to act ever more incisively on those mechanisms.
b. The growing intrusive force of this technology and its diffusion has generally thrown into confusion the order which until recently had reigned within the so-called natural process of reproduction, and this has led to new problems.
c. The breakdown in the balance that ruled the "natural process of reproduction" has prompted various social actors to become active on the new scene either to defend the interests which the preexisting order guaranteed them or to affirm the interests which that order denied them.

In our opinion, a different reconstruction of the process that has led to the formulation of the crucial questions on the subject of AF today is also possible. We believe that this alternative reconstruction reveals some important aspects that otherwise remain concealed behind what is taken for granted in the current interpretation.

First, the effective possibility of technological intervention to change some stages of a process that was until recently considered beyond our control has shown how the supposed naturalness of the whole process was far from intrinsic. Rather, it was produced by the stability of an "order" upheld by the consensus of various social actors. One has only to think of the way in which the birth of Louise Brown led us gradually to discover the present lack of agreement on what should be considered "natural" or "artificial" as regards reproduction, the family, parenthood, and childhood.

However, this should not mislead us into believing that technological interference in the preestablished order of things and the consequent disintegration of that order have created "new problems." Many aspects are analogous to the controversial issues in the debates on contraception and abortion: Where do you draw the line between "life" and "nonlife"? When can we start speaking in terms of "human life" with all its ethical implications? These problems have come up again and again. In the past, they were never solved, that is, *eliminated once and for all,* but simply—this adverb is something of a euphemism since the process was far from simple—*composed* within a precarious equilibrium. This delicate balance was not based on a stable consensus and would in any case have shown its inconsistencies at the first occasion. One example is the case of research on embryos and the fate of surplus embryos. The many questions as to the legitimacy of embryo research would never have arisen in the same way if the limits established by the 1978 Abortion Law, which is still in force in Italy, had enjoyed a large degree of consensus. While the law provides for the possibility of abortion within the first twelve weeks, we are engaged in heated discussions on whether or not it is lawful to suppress surplus embryos or use them for experimentation within a time span well below this limit. Thus, the growing recourse to AF has not given birth to "new problems," as was maintained in point (b) of our reconstruction. On the contrary, it has revealed the fragility of the solutions previously adopted for preexisting problems.

Second, the numerous social actors involved in the theme of AF all pursue a common object, namely, to persuade their interlocutors that their point of view on the whole matter is capable of redressing the lost balance. But it is perhaps misleading to talk in terms of social actors moving in a particular scene to defend or affirm certain interests. Likewise, it would also be inappropriate, for example, to assume that each social actor is the bearer of interests that are determined and determinable on a stable basis. In fact, the interests may vary due to interaction with the other social actors and because of changes in the context that this very interaction produces. In the same way, the alliances and counterpositions that are set up at a given time and in a given context among the social actors are not always the same; they may vary considerably. Consequently, the context within which the interaction occurs should not be taken as a fixed framework. Precisely because it is a product of such interaction, it is subject to a precarious balance that some try to maintain and others seek to change.

We must also bear in mind that social actors may shift from one context to another, either because they believe it is to their advantage or because they are forced to do so by others. In the case of AF, we can identify at least five forums within which the various social actors interact: the institutional forum, the medical research forum, the social research forum, the mass media forum, and that of the practice of AF. The last is subject to very great variability because of the individual and social histories of the subjects involved (Ventimiglia 1988), and it may conveniently be called the contingency forum.[1] Each forum is a prestructured context within which actors move according to preestablished rules and which they help to maintain through their interaction, although with some possibility of introducing modifications of a slight or profound nature. It is quite a different thing to speak of the "context" of AF, at least in the way we sociologists generally use the term. This "context" has yet to be structured, and most of the clashes and alliances among the various actors may be read as attempts to build the context that each believes is "appropriate" to AF.

In any case, it is thus even more evident that the stakes are not merely the regulation of AF practices but also the determining of the context most appropriate for discussing it. Similarly, the moves made by each actor in the various forums are not only aimed at asserting their own point of view within that forum but should also be read as part of a more complex strategy whose objective is to decide the "appropriate" context in which to place AF.

THE SOCIAL CONSTRUCTION OF INFERTILITY

Within the sphere of AF practices and the discussion they have provoked, there is perhaps one single item on which all agree: whoever has the right of access to AF, however AF is practiced, whatever the consequences may be, always, in each and every case, it is a matter that concerns doctors. At the very least, it is a question of establishing whether the matter concerns them exclusively or which other actors have the right and the competence to intervene alongside them.

We need to take a closer look at the widespread acceptance this notion enjoys. Let us, first of all, take up again some earlier observations on this subject. From an analysis of the assumptions on which a good part of the debate on AF is based, the following hypothesis emerged: The idea that scientific and technological developments have raised problems of ethics and regulation vis-à-vis AF tends to obscure the effective interests of the social actors involved. This seems to be especially true of doctors, who tend to appear as the "victims" rather than the perpetrators of technological progress. In fact, doctors have organized their participation in the debate on AF as if they themselves had not helped to create the situation we are now discussing, as if technological progress had gone ahead ineluctably without the aid of anyone at all. In fact, it is not hard to see that it is doctors who made possible the practices whose legality is being hotly disputed and for which legislative measures are rightly demanded.

On the other hand, it is also true that, although doctors have played an important role in bringing about the present situation, they now find themselves wrong-footed. This is partly due to the way in which the new context immediately filled up with social actors (such as women, couples, the unborn, politicians, judges, and priests) whose explicit or implicit aim was to take away some of the doctors' power of action. It is also partly because the media-guaranteed publicity for the doctors' most daring enterprises left them somewhat at a loss when they were faced with the increasing pressure to justify themselves, which came from many quarters.

This is how it came about that doctors had to try to legitimize their presence and strengthen their position by seeking "allies" who could back them up. The strategy they adopted to this end was one that had assured them success on numerous previous occasions. They brought out their most formidable ally: disease. The quickest way and the one that was most likely to enable them to regain control in an area that was slipping from their grasp was to establish that infertility was a disease and should therefore be treated. The principle whereby the presence of a disease requires the intervention of a doctor still retains its persuasive force intact, although it has become somewhat tarnished in recent times due in part to the lackluster approach of the doctors themselves.

A Strange "Disease"

For the last hundred years, the entire reproductive process has been medically assisted (Shorter 1982). Nevertheless, experimentation and applications to do with AF are no longer exclusively medical acts, by which we mean the search for the causes of diseases and their treatment. Indeed, the practices that concern us here involve fundamental changes in the rules of kinship as well as considerable alteration to the biological and social confines of life and death (Kuhse 1987). Moreover, although the technology used is often simple, the targeting and social use of such technology take place within a context of complex relations between social actors in the field and rules for decision making.

Within this context, doctors try to legitimize their interventions simply as support for the biological function of reproduction. The term *assisted fertilization* (AF) has, in fact, tended to prevail over *artificial reproduction* in everyday language. This shift highlights the influence of medical language on common speech, but it also tends to lend force to the image of medical techniques as simple aids to support "natural" functions and maintain the image of medicine at the service of "normal" physiological functions.

In actual fact, the physiopathology of reproduction, which comprises research into AF, deals with medical intervention and biomedical research into a process that includes the quality of semen and ovocytes, physiological and "social compatibility"[2] between semen and ovocytes, experimental treatment of frozen embryos and the intrauterine care of embryos, as well as in vitro fertilization and mechanical substitution for the maternal womb (Largey 1978; Walters and Singer 1982). The way the physiopathology of reproduction has developed reveals that its chief scientific aim is to experiment on the embryo rather than to treat infertility. Thus, along these lines, AF increasingly appears to be a mere by-product.

Our hypothesis is that in the process that goes from conception to birth, the physiopathology of reproduction tends increasingly to replace maternal decisions with medical ones. This has been brought about by the importance that the medical definitions of infertility give to the couple and by the increasing centrality of experimentation on embryos in biomedical research.[3] This centrality, however, is more generally due to advances in biomedical research tending to give a more prominent role to the regulation of life and death, in most medical fields, rather than the traditional medical paradigm of curing illness.

Three social actors have contributed over the past thirty years to the meta-discourse on the social definitions of fertility, infertility, and motherhood. Alternately clashing or forming alliances, they are the system of institutionalized religion, the medical system, and the system of feminist culture. None of them seem to have seriously considered infertility to be a disease, but despite this, AF is now seen as the chosen treatment for infertility. Our task is to explain this paradox.

For centuries, infertility was regarded as a moral illness of the female body in a context in which reproduction had nothing to do with a woman's right to choose, since it was the husband's property and a gift from God. In the second half of this century, the alliance between medicine and women as a social group on the subject of childbirth has brought to the fore the mother's decision as the criterion for medical intervention on women's bodies and their choices as regards reproduction.

In this context, the meaning of infertility has undergone two changes: it has shifted from being a moral illness to forming the limits to women's decisions and choices regarding childbirth, and it has gone from being a moral fault to being a possible disease of the reproductive organs of both women and men. Thus, through the alliance of women and the medical profession, two important changes came about: infertility moved from the ethical and religious sphere to that of medical research; virility lost its role of guarantor in patriarchal gender relations and became a site of possible disease.

In the 1970s, medical and surgical interventions for the treatment of female infertility did not enjoy a great deal of social legitimacy. We are not in a position to know whether the "failure" of traditional cures for infertility was due to the technical limitations of the treatment available or the very low demand by women. At that time, at least in Italy, the debate on childbirth focused above all on the need to limit births and on adoption as a response to the actual or assumed infertility of the couple.

Only since births have become rarer has there been an increase in the demand by women for the right to bear a child under conditions other than those generally considered optimal, that is, relatively young and married. Over the same period, the techniques of AF have begun to develop and establish themselves. So we can say that the desire for motherhood and the importance given to women's choice—but not the demand for treatment for infertility—have socially legitimized the development of fertilization techniques.

Despite this, however, in the new phase, the alliance between women and the medical profession has developed along lines which have, in the end, weakened women's influence on childbirth (Arditti, Duelli Klein, and Minden 1984). This process appears to be inscribed in the social construction of the medical definitions of infertility. If we analyze them, we may observe the shift of attention from the treatment of infertility to successful conception and, finally, to a marked interest in the embryo.

The medical definitions of infertility, which have been adopted internationally, are based not on medical paradigms regarding the pathology or dysfunction of the reproductive apparatus of male or female bodies but on a particular social paradigm: the heterosexual couple, sexually monogamous at least over a certain time span. In fact, the current medical definitions identify the pathology of infertility as all cases in which no children are born, although no specific cause emerges from individual examinations that may attribute infertility to one spouse or the other (Cittadini 1976). The definition that is generally adopted now is the involuntary absence of conception for a couple after a certain number of months (usually twenty-four but sometimes even twelve) of unprotected sexual intercourse.

We should note that infertility is defined without reference to a pathology of the biological apparatus or a dysfunction of the organism. Rather, the definition refers to the failed outcome of a social relationship and an action which depends on that particular relationship, defined according to specific criteria that have social connotations. In fact, in social contexts where sexual intercourse is no longer necessarily linked, even for women, either to marriage or to the stable couple, it would be possible to define infertility as a woman's inability to conceive or, independently, a man's inability to produce conception, despite, individually, having had unprotected sexual intercourse fairly regularly with one or more partners (Bimbi 1989).

The definition that has been adopted has obtained for the medical profession some highly important effects:

■ The separation between the possible pathology of the organism or physiological dysfunction and the definition of infertility weakens the confines of the knowledge of the causes of infertility, making the diagnosis provisional from a strictly medical point of view, but certain as regards the application of AF.

■ AF is more readily seen as a cure because, although it does not remove an often unknown pathology, it eliminates the cause of suffering for the woman or the couple, that is, the absence of offspring.

■ Reference to the couple permits a comprehensive definition of the disease called infertility, which also includes nonsterile bodies and infertility not stemming from the physiological apparatus of reproduction. This is shown by the fact that doctors count "sexual disturbances," clearly not of physiological origin, among the causes of infertility. These account for 6 percent of cases (SIFES 1991).

■ Reference to the couple gives greater social acceptability to the techniques of AF because it backs up two complementary beliefs to do with procreation: the couple's unselfish motives and the individual's selfish ones.

■ The importance given to the couple makes it more likely that AF will be accepted even in cultural contexts where the ideology of the family based on the married couple prevails. Reference to the joint desire of the couple makes recourse to donors of semen or ovocytes and even surrogate motherhood more acceptable. It is no accident that medicine has introduced the concepts of "homologous fertilization" and "heterologous fertilization."[4] Latour (1984) would have it that these are "hybrid" concepts, in that they confuse nature and society. The ovum and the spermatozoon have no affinity whatsoever and should therefore be regarded as heterologous. But the adopted definition considers their affinity on the basis of a recognized social tie, that is, the stable or married couple.

■ Finally, the importance given to the couple shifts attention from the treatment of the reproductive apparatus and the individual desire for motherhood or fatherhood to the practical solution to the problem of infertility, that is, conception.

The shift of focus first from the woman's desire to have a baby to that of the couple, and later from the couple's desire to the quality of conception, constitutes the greatest change that has taken place in the medical field of reproduction in recent years. The unborn child—as the result of successful conception and in the form of an embryo maintained outside the mother's body—has become the most important social object in the research into AF. Consequently, the conflict as to legal regulation of the techniques of procreation has also moved increasingly onto this terrain.

The medical profession expresses its demands for experimentation on embryos and greater freedom of action for medical decisions in respect of women's desire for motherhood by disproportionately broadening its claims for the legitimization of research into "the products of conception." This type of research aims to improve the health prospects for the embryo undergoing experimentation, any brothers or sisters who will thus have the chance to be born, as well as future human beings in general.

The recent results of biomedical research, including cloning, make it virtually impossible to interpret the paradigm of the infertility of the couple as simply a form of alliance between the patriarchal model of gender relations and the medical profession. Indeed, the woman's desire for motherhood, as well as the man's desire for fatherhood, are evoked in the legal, ethical, and political debate but tend to disappear from the scene when it comes to medical decisions. Even the notion of "informed consent" becomes a tenuous constraint within a framework of technical solutions predetermined by the system of health and research organizations.

Really, the only decision that women and men are allowed to make is whether or not to enter one sector or another of the medical system. Once they have entered, the decisions are preconstituted by scientific type reasoning, or rather constructed for the use of techniques that suit the type of experiment adopted. Therapeutic medicine tends to give way to experimentation and research, resulting in a decline in traditional medical paradigms on the ethics of the doctor-patient relationship (Shorter 1985).

Thus we can see that the medical profession offers interventions of great social significance; they choose the patients (the eugenic function), family models (social regulation of gender relations), and sexuality models (regulation of the individual's inclinations).

However, these functions are not expressed in a way that entirely conforms to the dominant norms, as many feminist authors have argued (Steinberg 1997). In Italy, the cultural influence of Catholic sexual and matrimonial morality on the behavior of individuals is declining, as demonstrated by the fact that the fertility rate is among the lowest in the world. At the same time, the influence of the Catholic Church on the political system is still very strong. In this context, medicine—by which we mean both research and the health care system—is trying to stretch the limits of the Catholic definition of the family, sexuality, and reproduction in order to assert its metasystem of meaning, which brings it, if not freedom of action, at least the possibility of negotiating.

Clearly, the way is anything but straightforward. The passage from experimentation to the acceptance of its application, in particular, requires many types of mediation. The mass media have been crucial for the transposition of medical language into common speech; the political and juridical system has produced both the formal legitimization for medical interventions and, to an extent, their cultural acceptance; bioethics has produced the scientific discourse on which to build social agreement (Overall 1987; Guizzardi 1996). Meanwhile, the epidemiological discourse is transforming the disease of infertility into a real epidemic.

The Resistible Rise of Infertility

To carry out the task that doctors have set, infertility must not only be a disease; it must be a continually expanding disease. Thus, the quantification of the spread of the "disease" in epidemiological terms becomes so crucial that the statistics are influenced—probably involuntarily—to move in the "right" direction. Reading the data on the diffusion of infertility, one often gets the impression that it is constructed in such a way as to produce an artificial increase.

The two documents that tackle the problem in the institutional forum[5] take as their starting point an article by Polly A. Marchbanks and colleagues, "Research on Infertility: Definition makes difference," which appeared in the *American Journal of Epidemiology* in 1989. The same reference was taken up by the social research forum (EURISPES 1995), using as a source the documents produced in the institutional forum and in the media forum,[6] although the source is never cited.

The first thing to note is the misuse made of Marchbanks et al.'s article outside the context in which it was produced, that is, the biomedical research forum. Indeed, the article points out, in the title itself, that when dealing with infertility, the definition makes the difference and that, consequently, great care is required. But the official Italian documents make somewhat rash use of the authors' estimates, eliminate all traces of uncertainty, and arbitrarily choose only one of the four estimates put forward in the original article. Thus despite the fact that the document produced by the Commission on Medically Assisted Procreation (1995) reports all four definitions proposed by Marchbanks et al., whose definitions and data the commission summed up as a table (see table 7.1), the spread of infertility is then calculated, without any justification, using the second definition ("no conception after two years of unprotected sexual intercourse"). It is also noteworthy that the assumption that the couple is the patient comes about without the problem being posed.

Both the National Committee on Bioethics (1995a) and the Commission on Medically Assisted Procreation (1995) go on to estimate the number of infertile Italian couples in a similar way. The calculation is based on the 300,000 marriages that take place in Italy every year, thereby excluding cohabiting couples.[7] It is then assumed that 20 percent of these are sterile (i.e., 60,000 couples).[8]

One could reasonably ask at this point why they decided to use the percentage that refers to the generally accepted definition whose limitations are well

Table 7.1 Estimated percentage of sterile couples in the population according to different definitions of sterility (%)

a. No conception after twelve months of unprotected sexual intercourse	32.6
b. No conception after two years of unprotected sexual intercourse	20.6
c. Couples who consult a specialist after two years of trying to conceive	8.6
d. Couples in whom a cause of sterility has been diagnosed after at least two years of trying to conceive	6.1

Source: Commission on Medically Assisted Procreation (1995).

known, instead of adopting a more cautious definition, since estimates were involved. The answer is all too easy to see: A more cautious definition would have considerably reduced the importance of the spread of the disease.

But perhaps the real point is this: By defining infertility as a disease of the couple, all the estimates are carried out on the assumption that all 300,000 couples who married in the year in question decided to have children within the first two years of marriage. This assumption is obviously false, but it serves to inflate the statistics for the spread of this disease. Let us for a moment imagine that, in fact, only two-thirds of these 300,000 newlywed couples decide to have a child within the first two years of marriage. Even with such a cautious limitation, the estimate for sterile couples would fall to 40,000 and the figure for couples consulting a specialist would drop to just over 17,000.

The way Marchbanks et al.'s article has been used brings to the fore other important considerations. First of all, it is assumed acritically that data regarding the United States may be used as a valid indicator of what occurs in Italy. This should not be overlooked, especially if one considers the very different demographic growth of the two countries. It should at least have raised the suspicion that the numerous social, economic, and cultural factors involved in the reproductive process function differently in the two contexts and that one cannot therefore simply transfer the estimates from one country to the other.

There are other elements regarding the nature of the data in the article in question that should have induced greater caution, since they might cause the estimates to be highly distorted, namely:

■ The data come from a study originally aimed not at estimating the number of sterile couples; indeed, Marchbanks et al. used data coming from research into cancer of the breast, endometrium, and ovaries (Marchbanks et al. 1989, 260); to be precise, the data concerns the control group. It is interesting to note that the original sample decreased by 11.9 percent due to refusals and by a further 4.7 percent because certain respondents could not be traced. There is no mention of the characteristics of the women, but the large numbers involved make it very likely that the estimates could vary considerably on samples effectively observed.

■ Whereas the data concerning the two definitions of infertility that produced the lowest percentages (definitions *c* and *d* in table 7.1) "were based on self-reported answers to direct questionnaire items and were limited to couples specifically trying to conceive," the data regarding the two definitions of infertility that produced the highest percentages (definitions *a* and *b*) are not derived from replies to direct questions but on a reconstruction "based on computations from each respondent's calendar of reproductive and contraceptive events." This reconstruction could clearly give rise to errors, but it is also worth noting that only the data regarding definitions *c* and *d* concern "couples specifically trying to conceive," that is, the only couples about whom it would make sense to pose the problem of infertility, in terms of frustrated desire and therefore a "disease" according to the second definition adopted in medical circles.

Finally, we have to point out an omission that has important consequences for our analysis. Neither of the documents that use Marchbanks et al.'s study to estimate the number of infertile couples in Italy bothers to mention that the American epidemiologists also report in their article the data for conceptions that occur after the couple had been classified as infertile. We discover, for example, that 20 percent of couples considered infertile according to definition "b" ("no conception after two years of unprotected sexual intercourse") conceived within the following six months, and that by twelve months the figure had risen to 32.6 percent. This is the equivalent of saying that the 60,000 couples judged infertile after two years of unprotected intercourse would fall to around 40,000 if the time span were increased to three years—not an unreasonable period of time, especially if the couples are young.

If we consider things from a statistical viewpoint, the impression we get is not that of an epidemic. Granted that the definition of "infertile marriages" used in demographic studies, that is, couples with no offspring born alive in a given period, has nothing to do with their biological ability to reproduce,[9] we find that in Italy after twenty years of marriage only 11 percent of couples are childless. In fact, the number of "infertile marriages" actually fell in the period 1930–60 (Palomba 1992, 121–22). So it is true that if in Italy "the number of men and women who turn to doctors or specialised clinics for problems of infertility . . . has increased greatly, this does not mean that infertility is growing. It only means that people are more sensitive to the problem." And yet the doctors who deal with infertility persist in calling it an "epidemic" (Frontali 1992, 117–18).

The Epidemic in the Media

The use of "data" seems similarly oriented toward supporting the cause of the medical profession while satisfying the media's need for sensationalism. The two texts we will now examine are taken from the national press.

On May 23, 1996, the weekly magazine *L'Espresso* published several feature articles under the general heading "Infertility, Thy Name Is Man" (20–28) The theme was clear right from the headline: "Spermatozoa Halved in the Last Fifty Years." Apart from exploring the other possible causes for this increase in male infertility, such as stress and malformation and dysfunction of the genital apparatus due to pollution, smoking, and excessive use of the car, the article concentrated on the decrease in the concentration of spermatozoa in the seminal fluid.

The first aspect we should look at is the magnitude of this presumed reduction. Although the article starts by suggesting a drop of 50 percent, the data reported in the text is rather different. Thus, the study cited as that of the discoverer of this new phenomenon actually states that the reduction is on the order of 31.5 percent in approximately fifty years. Two other studies, which are briefly summarized, estimate the drop as 25 and 32.5 percent. Not to mention the fact that another study carried out in the United States maintained that, on the contrary, there had been an increase in the sperm count and that an expert in the field of reproduction epidemiology, when interviewed by the journalist, warned of the limited statistical representativeness of many studies on male infertility. In any case, even if we accept the thesis of a decrease, the figure involved is far less than 50 percent. But the fact is that most readers, or rather those who confine themselves to scanning the headlines without going deeper into the content, will fix their attention on that 50 percent.

It is important to stress that the second article contained in the dossier suggests that the "solution" to male infertility is to be found in the techniques of in vitro fertilization (IVF). This suggestion was toned down in an interview with an andrologist reported in the same dossier. According to this specialist, after diagnosis two paths are open to the patient: a surgical operation or pharmacological treatment.

The predominant message is clear, however: Male infertility is growing, and the proof lies in the 50 percent decrease in the sperm count. The solution to the problem of the infertility disease is in any case of medical competence and is to be sought mainly in IVF techniques.

An article that appeared in the national daily newspaper *La Repubblica* on June 29, 1996, takes up the problem again. The article cites an Italian study from which it emerges that the indicator of the increase in male infertility is not the sperm count, which has fallen by only 8 percent in the last twenty years, but the motility of spermatozoa, which in the same period has decreased by between 32 and 50 percent. Predictably, the headline reports the larger figure.

But the point is not so much the media's natural tendency to exaggerate as the fact that a brief item that appeared in the May 1996 issue of *Le Scienze*, the Italian edition of *Scientific American*, questions the credibility of the estimates on which the alarm, fueled by the media, is based. As a researcher from Milan University stated at a conference on infertility organized by the National Health Institute (*Istituto Superiore di Sanità*), "There is no reliable data to prove that male fertility has been reduced by 50 percent in the last thirty years" (27). This is because it is impossible to compare the data on the motility and vitality of spermatozoa gathered with the equipment in use thirty years ago with present-day data based on far more advanced and precise techniques.

Thus, although the scientific basis for the rise in male infertility for organic causes has yet to be proved, this supposed increase is being widely used to justify the equation "infertility = disease" and to legitimize the intervention of the medical profession.

Moreover, in this way the construction of infertility as a disease combines with the definition of infertility as a disease of the couple to allow the medical profession to redefine IVF and AF in general as treatment for male infertility and to further justify medical intervention on women's bodies.[10]

Finally, it is worth noting that, not by chance, both texts—the first indirectly, the second explicitly—promote the idea that the fall in population growth, which is particularly evident and causes much concern in Italy, is due not only to social factors but also to a considerable extent to physiological ones. This is one more reason for calling upon the medical profession to intervene.

THE LACK AND THE NEED FOR REGULATION

"Italy is the Far West of biomedicine." This is how the *New York Times* described our country after the umpteenth case concerning AF had exploded onto the media. The expression had already been used during similar episodes, making the Wild West the most often cited metaphor for the lack of legislation in this delicate area.[11]

This particular case, in April 1995, concerned the initiation of prosecution proceedings against a Neapolitan gynecologist accused of carrying out AF in a fraudulent and unprofessional manner. The special interest in this case lies in the fact that for the first time a doctor was being accused of crimes connected with assisted reproduction and because, in the absence of specific legislation, the examining magistrate was obliged to contend with the crimes of fraud and grievous bodily harm.

Many have called for legislation to regulate the practice of AF. Quite often doctors and researchers themselves are among those who maintain the importance of such legislative action. However, sizable numbers from the same scientific and professional communities seem to be thinking in quite another direction, or rather they express opinions that are highly diversified as to who should regulate and how the task of regulation should be carried out. For example, Renato Dulbecco, the Nobel laureate for medicine and a central figure in the Human Genome Project, when asked about the problems linked to the development of techniques capable of changing human genetics, responded, "Research should be regulated, but not by laws. Loopholes would soon be found for the simple reason that scientific progress poses new and unpredictable problems daily—just think of AF, for instance. What we need are technical and ethical committees who would then judge each case on its merits and grant or deny authorization."[12]

The urgent need to intervene to regulate affairs has been strongly voiced by the Catholic Church since the mid-1980s. In 1987, its position on the matter was made official in the document entitled *Respect for the Unborn and the Dignity of Procreation* by the Holy Congregation for the Doctrine of Faith. On the basis of their traditional doctrine on the subject of contraception and abortion, the ecclesiastical hierarchy expressed its substantial opposition to any form of AF that entails conception outside the womb, even within wedlock, and demanded the introduction of norms that would put an end to this anarchy.[13]

It was probably this legislative vacuum which recently prompted the medical profession to institute self-regulation. On April 2, 1995, their governing body, the National Council of the Orders of Doctors (Federazione Nazionale degli Ordini dei Medici Chirurghi e degli Odontoiatri) approved a resolution that rejected such practices as surrogate motherhood, fertilization of women in non-premature menopause, and postmortem insemination. The general line of this resolution was later confirmed by the new deontological *Code of Medical Practice* approved by the National Council in June 1995. Article 41 reads as follows:

> The principle aim of AF is to provide a remedy for infertility with the legitimate purpose of reproduction. In the interests of the unborn child, the following practices are forbidden:
>
> (a) all forms of surrogate motherhood;

(b) forms of AF in subjects other than stable heterosexual couples;

(c) AF for women in non-premature menopause;

(d) forms of AF after the partner's death.

In addition, all AF practices inspired by racial prejudice are forbidden. No selection of semen is allowed, and all use of gametes, embryos, and embryonic and fetal tissue for commercial, publicity, and industrial purposes is prohibited. Finally, AF performed in medical practices, surgeries, or private health structures not in possession of suitable requisites is forbidden.

This decision, taken by the most authoritative body for the self-regulation of the medical profession, deserves some attention. First of all, we should note that the "normal" family, or rather that which is supposedly best to serve the needs of the unborn child, the defense of whose interests forms a specific reference point, is made to coincide with the stable heterosexual couple. Therefore, the latter is recognized as the legitimate representative of the "demand" for AF. The doctors' definition of the family is broader than that of the Italian Constitution ("the family as a natural association founded on marriage," Article 29) and a similar one upheld by the Catholic Church. The doctors' stand is significant inasmuch as it shows how the problem of AF is intertwined with the broader current discussion on whether it is opportune or necessary to extend the concept of "family" outside marriage.

However, another important question remains unanswered: What do we mean by *stable,* or rather, what are the criteria for assessing stability? Likewise, it is unclear whether, by limiting AF entitlement to heterosexual couples only, the code also excludes heterologous fertilization.

This vagueness of definition is also encountered in connection with *non-premature* menopause and the *suitable* requisites of private centers for AF. In all probability, the National Council did not wish to trespass into the terrain of the legislator in this delicate matter. Curiously, however, it felt no similar compunction when it came to limiting AF entitlement to stable heterosexual couples only.

The second point is that the considerable amount of attention paid by the media to the doctors' stand provoked critical reactions (among which, it should be pointed out, the feminist voice was missing). But it also achieved the effect of consolidating public opinion on the image of the "responsible doctor." Nevertheless, the numerous questions left unanswered by this pronouncement, namely, the admissibility of heterologous fertilization, the stability of the couple, non-premature menopause, and the suitable requisites for AF centers, left doctors ample room for "irresponsible" maneuvers and avoided having to impose on their scientific/professional community a balance that was, and still is, rather uncertain.

The diffusion of the April 2 resolution in the mass media was a timely move that enabled the medical profession to influence—how deliberately we cannot tell—the legislative debate. Between the end of 1994 and the first few months of 1995, there was a noticeable acceleration in the debate in the institutional forum. In June 1994, the National Committee on Bioethics, given the urgency imposed by "the intense discussion which had developed" (1994b, 5), published a brief account and its conclusions on the techniques of AF, many months ahead of the final document, which would be made public only on February 17, 1995. In 1994, a special commission set up by the Ministry of Health was at work. Between July 1994 and March 1995, four bills were submitted in the Chamber of Deputies and the same number in the Senate. In March 1995, first the Chamber of Deputies and then the Senate passed two resolutions on the subject, and on March 29 the Senate Commission on Health and Hygiene began its work, which led to the formulation of a unified bill in September.

The unusual move by the National Council of the Medical Association to divulge the April resolution took place at the end of a period of intense activity in the institutional forum and during the workings of the Senate commission. It would appear to be no coincidence, therefore, that the unified text of the proposition on assisted fertilization approved in September acknowledged the position previously expressed by the medical profession to a very great extent.

THE PRACTICE OF ASSISTED FERTILIZATION

We are still waiting for norms to be introduced, but in the meantime AF continues to be carried out. Little information is available for IVF practice in Italy, and even that is limited to particular local situations. Nevertheless, it is possible to trace an outline of what is going on.

The first "test-tube baby" in Italy was born in 1983. Since then, the number of cases has grown rapidly and spread throughout the country, albeit somewhat unevenly among the regions and between the public and private sectors. The distinction between AF centers within the public health system and private centers is not merely a question of organization (hospital wards rather than surgeries or private clinics). Rather, it marks an important difference between the possibility of access only to homologous AF, on the one hand, and access to both homologous and heterologous forms, on the other. In 1985, a Ministry of Health circular imposed a ban, which is still in force, on heterologous fertilization in structures operating within the public health system. It should be stressed that this was an administrative provision, not a legislative one.

According to data supplied by SIFES (Italian Society for the Study of Fertilization and Sterility), at the beginning of 1988 there were forty-four centers in Italy, of which twenty-one were public and twenty-three were private. A study coordinated by Ventimiglia between 1989 and 1991 revealed that each year approximately 2,100 couples attend the ten centers in Emilia-Romagna alone. This figure should, however, be read in light of the fact that a large number of those attending the centers come from other regions (Ventimiglia 1991).

Since 1994 there has been a National Register for Medically Assisted Reproduction at the Ministry of Health. The data are still incomplete, but the number of centers in Italy may be estimated at approximately two hundred. According to research carried out by ISPES in 1995, the twenty-three centers that used "in vivo" treatment performed 2,481 treatments in 1992–93. The same report also shows that, in the same period, 2,600 couples attended CECOS centers (Centers for the Study and Conservation of Human Sperm) to take part in a program of heterologous AF.

All the data from the various studies, however partial, highlight the absolute predominance of women in taking the initiative of attending a center, even when the application is made on behalf of a couple, something that occurs frequently, since most applicants are either married or cohabiting (ISPES 1995; Ventimiglia 1991; Blangiardo and Rossi 1993). It is therefore the women who represent the "demand" side in the *contingency forum,* not only because they are almost always the subject/object of AF but also because they take it upon themselves to initiate proceedings.

Physicians undoubtedly play a key role in the contingency forum. We examined the attitudes of doctors involved in this forum using data taken from a survey of a sample of 140 physicians in the gynecological sector, 25 percent of whom were not directly involved in using AF (Neresini 1995). Table 7.2 reports the views expressed on those practices closest to what might be called the frontiers of AF.

What is immediately striking is the overwhelming majority in the disagreement area in each of the four items. Over 70 percent of doctors stated they disagreed either partially or totally with the use of all four of these practices. This is even more important if we look at the situation for other procedures, which is very different. For example, table 7.3 shows that the situation is reversed for AF practices that take place within the family in its traditional sense (insemination of a married woman) or in any case within a stable relationship (cryopreservation of the male partner's semen or the female partner's ovocytes). Similarly, the predominance of disagreement is much less marked for practices that go beyond the confines of the traditional family or a consolidated relationship (cryopreservation of the male donor's semen or the female donor's ovocytes, insemination of unmarried women, insemination with donated semen) but that seem to be accepted by a large section of public opinion. In this case,

Table 7.2 To what extent do you agree with the following possible operations concerning assisted fertilization? Distribution of responses (%) among physician respondents (*N* = 140)

	Very Much Agree	Agree to Some Extent	Neither Agree nor Disagree	Disagree to Some Extent	Very Much Disagree	No Reply
Surrogate motherhood	1.4	3.6	10.7	18.6	56.4	9.3
Postmortem insemination	0.0	7.9	12.1	21.4	52.9	5.7
Insemination in menopausal women	2.1	3.6	7.9	17.9	64.3	4.2
Predetermination of sex of unborn child	0.7	2.1	8.6	12.9	71.4	4.3

Source: Neresini 1995.

the high percentage of those who neither agreed nor disagreed, that is, those who were uncertain, produced the greatest degree of balance among the various positions.

Again, with reference to table 7.3, it is clear that the set of practices associated with the manipulation of embryos prompted more cautious attitudes and even rejection by doctors. Nevertheless, even this unequivocal distancing is less decisive than that for the "borderline" practices in table 7.2. Embryo donation was the item that provoked the most disagreement. Here, however, the agreement percentage was 9 percent, higher than for any item in table 7.2.

The general attitude of doctors to these practices may be summed up in the phrase "Not all that is practicable is acceptable." On this point, we should note the almost total unanimity on the possibility of predetermining the sex of the unborn child; this item received the highest score of disagreement (84%) and the lowest agreement (under 3%). In this case, the subject of AF shifts to its farthest extreme and merges into the problem of genetic engineering. Although the two areas should be kept distinct, they often tend to be confused in both the media forum and the institutional forum.

The picture that emerges above is largely confirmed by the findings of Ventimiglia 1991 in the survey of doctors involved in AF in Emilia-Romagna. There are, however, important differences in that this sample of doctors, all directly involved in AF practices, report a lower percentage of disagreement toward embryo donation (55%) and a higher percentage of agreement on fertilization

Table 7.3 To what extent do you agree with the following possible operations concerning assisted fertilization? Distribution of responses (%) among physician respondents (*N* = 140)

	Very Much Agree	Agree to Some Extent	Neither Agree nor Disagree	Disagree to Some Extent	Very Much Disagree	No Reply
Cryopreservation of partner's sperm	29.3	38.6	11.4	9.3	9.3	2.1
Cryopreservation of donor's sperm	18.6	15.7	15.7	23.6	22.9	3.6
Cryopreservation of partner's ovocytes	22.9	34.3	12.1	17.9	10.0	2.9
Cryopreservation of donor's ovocytes	10.7	15.0	13.6	25.7	29.3	5.7
Cryopreservation of pre-embryos	7.1	12.1	9.3	22.9	45.0	3.6
Cryopreservation of embryos	3.6	10.0	10.7	25.0	45.0	5.7
Donation of embryos	2.9	6.4	10.7	21.4	55.0	3.6
Insemination of unmarried women	13.6	16.4	30.0	17.9	17.1	5.0
Insemination of married women	32.9	26.4	21.4	7.9	4.3	7.1
Insemination with donor's semen	12.1	17.1	19.3	19.3	21.4	10.7

Source: Neresini 1995.

of menopausal women (33%) or single women (55%). It is as if direct involvement in AF practices went hand in hand with less restrictive attitudes on the extension such practices.

In conclusion, we were able to establish a connection in our sample of doctors between a "strong" concept of science, that is, recognition of the assumptions of what Mulkay (1979) calls "the standard conception of scientific knowledge," and the tendency to assign to the medico-scientific community a preeminent normative role, independent of the judicial system.[14] In other words, the more the doctors defined science as the depository of objective, universal knowledge, the more they tended to think that legislative intervention to regulate research on human reproduction was a troublesome interference. Consistently with this, regression analysis has shown that there is a link between the position outlined above and the rejection both of laws banning research and experimentation on human embryos and laws that regulate this practice very precisely. At the same time, doctors who share this point of view are more likely to favor "borderline" practices such as the insemination of menopausal women.

Clearly, the opposite tendency also exists: The more doctors are inclined to cast doubt on the certainties of the modern concept of science, the more they feel that laws to regulate research and experimentation are not only legitimate but also necessary. As we have shown earlier, this tendency is the one that accounts for the majority consensus among those doctors interviewed.

This brief survey of doctors' opinions highlights at least three important aspects:

1. There is the attempt to make up for the absence of precise norms with the constraints of professional ethics.
2. Despite this, we note the presence of wide margins of flexibility even with regard to the more borderline practices in AF, especially by doctors directly involved.
3. From the doctors' viewpoint as well, the problem of regulating AF is mixed up with questions concerned with the definition of the "normal" family, the definition of infertility as a disease, and the limits, if any, that should be imposed on research on embryos.

THE WEAKNESS OF THE WOMEN'S VOICE IN THE PUBLIC FORUM

In Italy the conflict between the system of institutionalized religion, the medical system, and feminist culture is perhaps more open and explicit than it is elsewhere. From an empirical viewpoint, the conflict as regards AF chiefly concerns two themes: whether to allow AF also for de facto families (and consequently to single heterosexual and homosexual women) and whether to extend legal protection for the embryo back to the moment of conception. From a symbolic viewpoint, the conflict concerns the institutional and legal configuration of the definitions of the family, sexual intercourse, and women's self-determination. It affects not only gender relations in reproductive choice but also the regulation of abortion. So what is at stake is both the transformation of the patriarchal family model and the amount of legitimacy to be accorded to medical research into AF and its applications.

In the institutional forum, which includes the National Committee on Bioethics, Parliament, and the Medical Association, there is a tendency toward negotiation between the system of institutionalized religion and the medical system. This results in the exclusion of women as social actors, but it does not stop the various bodies from continuing to regulate women's behavior on childbirth. However, the present deadlock in negotiations prompts us to hypothesize that women are not uniformly weak as social actors in all the institutional contexts. That hypothesis will be argued in the rest of this section.

The tendency to exclude women is due in part to the weakness of the feminist movement. It also depends partially on the dynamics of the Italian political scene, where the presence of a noncompetitive democratic model means that left-wing parties have always sought alliance with Catholics especially with regard to family law and women's rights. The limited influence of the women's movement on the institutional forum is the result of a process that began in the 1980s. After a period during the 1970s when the women's movement had a strong influence on politics, there has been a growing disparity between "the considerable diffusion in society of themes, thoughts, and initiatives to do with the condition of women, and the dearth or muteness of collective mobilization" (Melucci 1987, 177).

The women's movement has made a decisive contribution to sociological, philosophical, and political thought on AF (Pizzini 1992, 1994; Bonacchi et al. 1996) also through numerous interventions in public debate. Nevertheless, its ability to produce initiatives and its political impact on the institutional forum has been poor. In particular, it has not had the weight it should have had, given that the regulation of women's behavior is at the very center of the ongoing negotiations.

Toward the end of the 1980s, women's position in the public debate was further weakened for two main reasons. First, the presence of the Green Party in Parliament foregrounded the ecological point of view and the defense of "natural" forms of life in the debate on the limits on research and its application; this might limit—or even call into question—women's self-determination with regard to childbirth. Second, the dissolution of the massive Christian Democrat Party (DC), the only Catholic party, has pushed all political parties—especially the Party of the Democratic Left (DS)[15]—to seek direct negotiation with the Catholic Church to pick up the Catholic vote, which is no longer attached to a single party.

This tendency is at work especially in the debate on two particular documents: the Chamber of Deputies Resolution of June 1993 and the February

1997 DS National Congress memo on the human embryo. These two documents may be considered emblematic, the first for its effort to find some agreement between secular culture and Catholic culture, and the second for the conflict on the woman's right to choose, which emerged even within the left wing.

The *Resolution on questions concerning the subject of bioethics and, in particular, biotechnology and genetic engineering, AF, genic therapy, organ transplants, and the defense of life,* presented by a Green Party MP, after many changes and compromises, got the vote of all parties except the former Fascists (*Alleanza Nazionale*). Its object was to commit the government and Parliament to a definite political line on all the issues in question. In fact, Parliament set itself only two precise tasks for future legislation: the "protection of the human embryo, permitting medical interventions of an exclusively therapeutic nature," and the disposition of "a precise and coherent set of norms on AF" that would aim to guarantee "the rights of the unborn child to an identity, health, and safety and the rights of women to health and safety." As we can see, the resolution left room for negotiation for the medical system and pro-life Catholic culture, but there is not a trace of relevance for women's self-determination.

The second document arose from the fact that in 1996, the Pro-Life Movement presented a bill giving rights to the embryo from the moment of conception and opening the way to a possible review of the abortion law and a limiting of the principle enshrined also by the Constitutional Court that a woman's right to choose should prevail over the partner's or husband's decision and also over medical opinion. At the DS National Congress (February 1997), a motion against this proposal was approved and signed by a group of women politically close to the minister for equal opportunity (a member of the DS). Both the DS leader and the minister for social solidarity (also from the DS) criticized the motion, the former referring to "the individual's freedom of conscience" on this issue, the latter fearing that this document might create difficulties in the political debate on family and welfare policies.

Between 1993 and 1997—the publication dates for the two documents—the Italian political system underwent considerable change. Not only did the former Communist Party come to power for the first time in fifty years (June 1996), but there was also finally a minister for equal opportunity and the post was held by a feminist. From this stem two contradictory and conflicting aspects: on the one hand, the leaders of the DS have stepped up their search for an alliance with Catholic culture; on the other hand, the government is enriched by the presence of an explicitly feminist culture.

Since the early 1990s, the weakness of women's voices in the institutional forum has been partially compensated by two factors: first, the presence of a feminist voice linked to the feminist culture in Parliament, which explicitly supports women's self-determination; and second, the medical system's need to support, at least in part, the ethical pluralism of couples demanding AF, to counteract the strict limits proposed by the Catholic Church. Recent parliamentary bills show the influence of the first factor, while the second has had but a very weak influence on the National Committee on Bioethics.

In the twelfth period of office of the legislature, up to April 1995, seventeen parliamentary bills were proposed on "medically assisted reproduction" (Chamber of Deputies 1995). Three of them, whose first signatories were three left-wing women MPs, recognize adult women as the primary holders of the right to ask for AF. However, the private member's bill, put forward by a woman MP from the Green Party, made the partner's consent obligatory if the woman was part of a couple, whether married or otherwise.

Five bills proposed to forbid paternal disavowal where the child is the result of "heterologous" fertilization and the husband or partner had consented to AF. Four bills limit AF only to married couples, three bills of which propose that the embryo be considered a "human being" and be protected as such from the moment of conception. Three bills proposed that the couple should hold the right to ask for AF.

None of these bills was passed, nor have they fared better in the present Parliament. The very fact that they have not been approved testifies to the difficulty involved in reaching agreement on these issues. At present the DS, which has a majority in the coalition government, is between two fires, both of which form part of the coalition. On the one hand, there are the left-wing Catholics from the Popular Party who support the traditional standpoint of the Catholic Church and wish to reevaluate even the law on abortion. On the other, there are the feminists who are, however, divided on the subject of seeking an alliance with Catholics. The DS is trying to resolve this conflict by means of "the individual's freedom of conscience," thus freeing its MPs from a collective position of the party. Members of the Popular Party agree to this approach, but feminist MPs disagree, since women MPs represent just 8 percent of the total and few male MPs favor of women's self-determination.

DS leaders are also aware that outside Parliament the public opinion of women and gay movements might be very much in favor of the individual's right to choose and women's self-determination, as was amply demonstrated at the time of the referendum on divorce (1974) and that on abortion (1981). Moreover, the influence of Catholic morality is much weaker today than it was in the past. What is more, educated young women and the gay movement form two catchment areas for left-wing votes. So, in the institutional forum, women are politically weak, but the game is by no means over.

A woman's right to choose is taken much less into consideration by the

National Committee on Bioethics as regards both entitlement to AF for unmarried couples and for single heterosexual or homosexual women and the question of whether the defense of the embryo should extend back to the moment of conception.

In the first place, the number of women on the National Committee on Bioethics since 1990 has never exceeded 18 percent of the total, and the few women members have little or no inclination to support women's self-determination, since they almost all belong to the Catholic cultural area. The committee has always been chaired by a Catholic, who, regardless of political ideology, has had little regard for feminism. At the time of writing (1999), feminist culture has, therefore, not yet been represented on the committee. Moreover, the committee has never taken into consideration ethical pluralism on two equally significant counts: feminism and religious minorities. Furthermore, among the moral theologists on the committee who are experts in bioethics, the strictest Catholic position prevails.

The most authoritative researchers in the field of physiopathology and reproduction have sat in turn on the committee. But given the predominance of conservative philosophers, jurists, and moralists, the doctors' stance has been mainly defensive, aimed at gaining at least some degree of freedom for experimentation, research, and application. So the doctors try to adopt a neutral position on social and ethical issues. It is no surprise that in the document *On the Techniques of AF* (National Committee on Bioethics 1994b) there was agreement on not allowing the insemination of single heterosexual or homosexual women, while the Catholic predominance prevented agreement on other ethical priorities, in that the doctors were unwilling to accept the limits that the other members of the committee had proposed. Only one member, a utilitarian philosopher, put the best interests of the woman first over that of the man and the unborn child.

In the document *Identity and Rights of the Human Embryo* (National Committee on Bioethics 1996), the committee, whose composition was even more conservative than before, set out its unanimous opinion recognizing the moral duty to treat the human embryo *as if* it were a person from its conception. It did not reach unanimity, however, on the equivalence of the embryo to the human being. It unanimously held to be illicit the suppressing of the embryo at the stage before implantation in the uterus, as well as all forms of experimentation, except those aimed at safeguarding the health of the embryo that is to undergo the intervention and those "on dead embryos, resulting from miscarriages or abortions, with the parents' consent." As we can see, not only does this open the door to reviewing the legality of abortion, but it also means that the woman's decision alone is not sufficient even in the case of dead fetuses.

Further analysis of the documents produced by the National Committee on Bioethics reveals many interesting instances of sexism that we will now briefly illustrate. In the document on the rights of the embryo, the scientific and philosophical basis for the unanimous decision to treat the embryo *as if* it were a person was the following: "[S]ince each and every one of us has been an embryo . . . we cannot but feel that the embryo is our fellow creature." This reasoning would appear to disavow completely the fact that every human being was "of woman born." It is strange that the legitimation for limiting women's self-determination should be founded solely on the memory of having once been an embryo, as if the embryo could exist without its relationship to the mother's body and will.

Other documents are distinguished by a negation of women's experience and their capacity for moral decision making. In *Coming into the World* (National Committee on Bioethics 1995b) and *Bioethics of Infancy* (National Committee on Bioethics 1994a), women are only regarded as caregivers or as parents to be educated to parenthood. In *Prenatal Diagnoses* (National Committee on Bioethics 1992), the woman is referred to as the "gestant," whose "informed consent" is required by doctors for the development of techniques that embody "the concept of the fetus as patient, the result of modern obstetric assistance and prenatal medicine." There is a singular failure to recognize the problematic nature of the matter in question.

But it is in *Problems of Collecting and Treating Seminal Fluid for Diagnostic Purposes* (National Committee on Bioethics 1991) that we find some genuine expressions of scientific misogyny. In this document there are three significant elements:

1. It is decided to set out some rules for the protection of seminal fluid, since the male germ cell has "the power, by uniting with a female gamete, to give origin to a new human being." But no document awards the female gamete similar ethical dignity.

2. It is declared that every operation on the semen, although carried out "strictly for diagnostic purposes," has ethical importance "when a process of fertilization is started which will not conclude with the complete development of each single element." In the absence of similar motivation for the ethical interest for research on the ovocytes, the reasoning bears a marked similarity to the premodern notion that the ability to start the life cycle was typical of the active principle of men, whereas the female principle was merely receptive and passive.

3. It is declared that "the methods of collecting and taking samples of male germ cells, *unlike those of all other types of cells of the organism,* involve very special moral problems."[16] What emerges from the wording is the anathema

on masturbation and clear sexist prejudice that attributes intrinsic moral qualities only to the male organism (Keller 1995).

The document was approved unanimously. This goes to show that a pragmatic attitude prevails among the medical profession (in order to keep open negotiations for research and its application), rather than one based on principle (as shown by their willingness to subscribe to definitions with very little scientific basis).

The comparative analysis of the presence and absence of women in the institutional forum, politics, and the National Committee on Bioethics reveals that, in Italy at least, women are weaker in the latter area where sexist prejudices that find much less legitimacy in the political arena still persist. The most evident reason for this difference would appear to lie in the predominance of conservative Catholic culture in the National Committee on Bioethics. However, the documents we have considered require further study. Perhaps another factor that weakens the institutional legitimacy of women as social actors stems from the fact that in Italy feminist culture is considered not qualified to enter the technical-political forum as it lacks scientific discourse and technical expertise on the subject of assisted childbirth.

CONCLUSIONS

In the current debate on AF, the stakes would seem to be far higher than those that emerge from other areas of medicine. We are, indeed, witnessing the social construction of a "new natural order of reproduction." The process is by no means over yet, and numerous issues are involved.

In the first place, in the AF debate there is an ongoing conflict of historic importance on whether it is necessary and opportune to redefine the significance of the concept of the family even in its common meaning. Since this conflict is taking place in a period of lack of public debate on the concept of the family in many other contexts, it is not hard to see how important it is for each social actor involved to establish as far as possible the limits and contents of the socially adopted definitions.

Moreover, in Italy especially, the conflict on what constitutes the family for the purposes of AF merges into the broader debate on ethical pluralism. Indeed, doctors who refer to infertility as a disease of the "stable couple" are butting into a semantic field in which the Catholic Church believes it has a special right to intervene and where it negotiates with the various ideologies in the political system. This configuration of the context for the social conflict on the family is to the disadvantage of women's rights to self-determination, because the various feminist cultures are expressly kept in the background and especially because none of the other social actors challenges the central reference to the "stable heterosexual couple."

Another changing situation concerns the definition of the place of the body and sexual intercourse in the social scenario of AF. We are witnessing the birth of a "new natural order of reproduction" in which the presence together of male and female bodies is becoming no longer necessary; neither is the presence together of the body and its reproductive cells (ovocytes and semen). It is a process of desexualization of fertilization and the separation of reproduction and the body,[17] although the latter phenomenon does not yet completely regard the female body, at least not until it is possible to have a pregnancy outside the mother's body. In any case, reproduction no longer seems to be an exclusive aspect of the privacy of the couple, and so the process of reproducing life takes on new social dimensions.

In the third place, negotiations are taking place on the extent to which scientific research and medical practice may legitimately expand their activities. The highest stakes concern the extension and legitimacy of research and experimentation on the embryo. In Italy, the question has not yet been posed explicitly, but it seems to be gaining importance also in the debate within the political system.

Of the various social actors we have examined, the doctors seem to have the lion's share, since they have a predominant role to play in each of the forums under consideration. Nevertheless, in Italy the position of doctors involved in research into the physiopathology of reproduction seems to be rather limited by the standpoint of the Catholic Church, which is very well represented on the National Committee on Bioethics. The position of doctors who apply the various AF techniques appears to be stronger, in that the lack of regulation leaves open the possibility of applications that do not only take into consideration the "stable heterosexual couple." We could say that the contingency forum within which the market for AF techniques is defined is stronger than the biomedical research forum, although the social availability of the applications stems from the relationship between research and medical practice.

The various women's cultures are generally weak in all the forums considered. However, they do seem to enjoy a certain degree of legitimacy in the political forum. In Parliament, more than one single viewpoint on women's decision and choice is represented, often even within the same party. It is not always the case that those who incline toward ethical pluralism also incline toward self-determination for women. We should nevertheless bear in mind that the possible recognition of the rights of the embryo as a human being right from the moment of conception might lead to a limitation on both women's decision and choice and a limitation on research and its application. Thus, the outlook is for a possible new alliance between doctors and women, who, though pursuing sometimes very different goals and despite its not being explicitly negotiated for this reason, could aim to overcome certain constraints that give the *social* order of reproduction its present form.

NOTES

1. By "institutional forum" we refer to all formal regulatory organs, such as the Parliament in all its parts, its various emanations such as the National Committee on Bioethics, the special consultative commission set up by the Ministry of Health and the Senate Commission on Health. The "medical research forum" is the space in which take place the process of social construction of the medical knowledge, represented mainly by the medical scientific reviews, the medical congresses, and the other arenas in which the medical knowledge is presented, discussed, and legitimized. The "social research forum," much like the medical research forum, is the space of social relationships in which the knowledge of social sciences is built up. The mass media forum consists of newspapers and magazines, television, and the Internet; in this forum we find those spaces where public debate on any given issue occurs. The "contingency forum" consists of the network of social actors dealing with the everyday world of (in this case) assisted fertilization practices.

2. See discussion below on heterologous vs. homologous fertilization.

3. Harris (1992) pointed out very clearly that the bioethical debate on genetic engineering concerns the problem of experimentation on the embryo and that this, in turn, is closely linked to the techniques of assisted fertilization.

4. "Homologous fertilization," in the medical language, refers to the assisted fertilization process using semen and ovocytes coming from the couple undergoing treatment; "heterologous fertilization" refers to cases involving donor semen or ovocytes.

5. See National Committee on Bioethics 1995a and Commission on Medically Assisted Procreation 1995.

6. See, e.g., the articles that appeared in *L'Espresso* (October 29, 1995) and in *La Stampa* (January 26, 1995).

7. The data are taken from the 1991 census.

8. National Committee on Bioethics 1995a, 12; Commission on Medically Assisted Procreation 1995, 1.

9. Note that in this way the demographic estimates inevitably tend to inflate the incidence of involuntary childlessness.

10. See van der Ploeg 1995.

11. At the time of writing (August 1998), no law about AF has been passed yet.

12. Taken from an interview that appeared in *La Repubblica,* November 14, 1990.

13. The Vatican's position was reaffirmed in 1995 by the encyclical *Evangelium Vitae.*

14. A regression analysis was carried out applying the stepwise method with a set of independent variables that included structural aspects (gender, age, position in hierarchy, number of infertility cases treated) and attitudes/opinions on science, religion, the function of bioethical committees, the so-called borderline practices, and the problems of the regulation of donation. The four variables selected account for 27 percent of the total variation of the independent variables overall.

15. The Party of the Democratic Left has replaced the Italian Communist Party. At the time of writing, it has been renamed Democratici di Sinistra (DS) and is the leading party in the coalition government.

16. Our emphasis.

17. Note that this process involves considerable violence to the body of the woman because it is necessary to go literally *through* the female body to obtain this separation.

REFERENCES

Arditti, R., R. Duelli Klein, and S. Minden (eds.):
  1984   *Test-Tube Women: What Future for Motherhood?* London: Pandora Press.
Bimbi, F.:
  1989   La riproduzione sociale come costruzione sociale [Artificial reproduction as a social construction]. In A. Di Meo and C. Mancina (eds.), *Bioetica,* 315–30. Bari: Laterza.
Blangiardo, G., and G. Rossi:
  1993   Viaggio tra le contraddizioni del comportamento riproduttivo: Dal rifiuto alla ricerca del figlio "a tutti i costi" [Journey among the contradictions of reproductive behavior: From the refusal to the search for an "at all costs" child]. In P. Donati (ed.), *Terzo rapporto sulla famiglia in Italia.* Cinisello Balsamo: Paoline.
Bonacchi, G., et al.:
  1996   La legge e il corpo [The law and the body]. *Democrazia e Diritto* 36(1): 3–86.
Chamber of Deputies:
  1995   *Procreazione medicalmente assistita* [Medically assisted procreation]. Documentazione e ricerche, XII Legislatura, no. 72.
Cittadini:
  1976   *La sterilità umana* [Human sterility]. Padua: Piccin.
Commission on Medically Assisted Procreation [Commissione di Studio per la Procreazione Medico-Assistita]:
  1995   *Relazione conclusiva* [Final report]. Rome: Ministero della Sanità.
EURISPES:
  1990   Madri ad ogni costo [Mothers at all costs]. In ISPES, *Rapporto Italia '90.* Rome: Vallecchi.
  1995   *Il corpo e la madre: Madri e figli tra norma e scienza* [The body and the mother: Mothers and children between laws and science]. Rome: EURISPES.
Frontali, N.:
  1992   *La cicogna tecnologica* [The technological stork]. Rome: Edizioni Associate.
Guizzardi, G.:
  1996   Le frontiere della bioetica [Frontiers of bioethics]. *Orientamenti,* nos. 6–7: 47–63.
Harris, J.:
  1992   *Wonderwomen and Superman.* Milan: Baldini and Castoldi.
Holy Congregation for the Doctrine of Faith:
  1987   *Il rispetto per la vita umana nascente e la dignità della procreazione* [Respect for the unborn and the dignity of procreation]. Milan: Paoline.
Keller, E. Fox:
  1995   *Refiguring Life.* New York: Columbia University Press.
Kuhse, H.:
  1987   *The Sanctity-of-Life Doctrine in Medicine.* Oxford: Clarendon Press.
Largey, G.:
  1978   Reproductive Technologies: Sex Selection. In T. R. Warren (ed.), *Encyclopedia of Bioethics,* 1439–44. New York: Free Press.

Latour, B.:

1984 *Les Microbes: Guerre et paix* [Microbes: War and peace]. Paris: A. M. Métailié.

Marchbanks, P. A., et al.:

1989 Cancer and Steroid Hormone Study: Research on Infertility: Definition Makes Difference. *American Journal of Epidemiology* 130(2): 259–67.

Melucci, A.:

1987 *Libertà che cambia* [Changing freedom]. Milan: Unicopli.

Mulkay, M.:

1979 *Science and the Sociology of Knowledge.* Boston: Allen and Unwin.

National Committee on Bioethics [Comitato Nazionale per la Bioetica]:

1991 *Problemi della raccolta e trattamento del liquido seminale umano per finalità diagnostiche* [Problems of collecting and treating human seminal fluid for diagnostic purposes]. Rome: Presidenza del Consiglio dei Ministri.

1992 *Diagnosi prenatali* [Prenatal diagnoses]. Rome: Presidenza del Consiglio dei Ministri.

1994a *Bioetica con l'infanzia* [Bioethics of infancy]. Rome: Presidenza del Consiglio dei Ministri.

1994b *Parere sulle tecniche di procreazione assistita: Sintesi e conclusioni* [On the techniques of assisted procreation: Summary and conclusions]. Rome: Presidenza del Consiglio dei Ministri.

1995a *La fecondazione assistita: Documenti* [Documents on assisted fertilization]. Rome: Presidenza del Consiglio dei Ministri.

1995b *Venire al mondo* [Coming into the world]. Rome: Presidenza del Consiglio dei Ministri.

1996 *Identità e statuto dell'embrione umano* [Identity and rights of the human embryo]. Rome: Presidenza del Consiglio dei Ministri.

Neresini, F.:

1995 Bioetica e medicina tra scienza, diritto e società [Bioethics and medicine in science, law, and society]. *Sociologia del Diritto* 2: 95–126

Overall, C.:

1987 *Ethics and Human Reproduction.* Boston: Allen and Unwin.

Palomba:

1992 Il contesto demografico in Italia [The Italian democratic context]. In N. Frontali, *La cicogna tecnologica,* 118–26. Rome: Edizioni Associate.

Pizzini, F.:

1992 *Maternità in laboratorio* [Motherhood in the laboratory]. Turin: Rosenberg and Sellier.

1994 *Madre provetta: Costi, benefici e limiti della procreazione artificiale* [Test-tube mother: Costs, benefits, and limits of assisted procreation]. Milan: Angeli.

Shorter, E.:

1982 *A History of Women's Bodies.* New York: Basic Books.

1985 *Bedside Manners: The Troubled History of Doctors and Patients.* New York: Simon and Schuster.

SIFES [Italian Society for the Study of Fertilization and Sterility]:

1991 *Libro bianco sulla riproduzione assistita* [Report on assisted reproduction]. Palermo: Edizioni SIFES.

Steinberg, L. D.:

1997 A Most Selective Practice: The Eugenic Logics of IVF. *Women's Studies International Forum* 1: 33–48.

van der Ploeg, I.:

1995   Hermaphrodite Patients: In Vitro Fertilization and the Transformation of Male Infertility. *Science, Technology, and Human Values* 20(4): 460–81.

Ventimiglia, C. (ed.):

1988   *La famiglia moltiplicata* [The multiplied family]. Milan: Franco Angeli.

1991   *La procreazione medicalmente assistita in Emilia-Romagna: Indagine sulla domanda e sulla risposta dei servizi* [Medically assisted procreation in Emilia-Romagna: An inquiry into demand and the response of public services]. Rapporto di ricerca. Parma: Università di Parma.

Walters, A. W., and P. Singer (eds.):

1982   *Test-Tube Babies: A Guide to Moral Questions, Present Techniques, and Future Possibilities.* Melbourne: Oxford University Press.

8

Riddled with Secrecy and Unethical Practices: Assisted Reproduction in India

Jyotsna Agnihotri Gupta

Use of assisted reproduction technology has proliferated rapidly in medical practice. Technologies used to assist reproduction including artificial insemination (AI) and in vitro fertilization (IVF) have reached many countries in the developing world, too, including India, even though population controllers generally exhort women in these countries to produce fewer children. For gynecologists in private practice, particularly in the major cities of India, their practice consists largely of infertility treatment. The number of practitioners or clinics offering IVF and related services has grown spectacularly.

Infertility is a serious problem for some couples. Those with less means seek the help of traditional healers and make use of potency-increasing charms, herbs, etc., whereas those who can afford it seek the help of modern medical practitioners and make use of technologies such as AI and IVF. Either way, infertility treatment is big business. However, in the absence of ethical and medical guidelines in this field in India, there is hardly any legislation and little control on practitioners providing these services. There is also a marked secrecy among both providers and users—due to a taboo on discussing sexuality openly—and a lack of good information regarding sexuality and fertility matters. Besides, there is a sense of shame regarding infertility. All this contributes to malpractice among providers—trade in sperm, eggs, and other human material, as well as sex selection in favor of males. Time and again the media have picked up certain events such as the birth of the first Indian "test-tube baby" and drawn attention to some of the malpractices in the trade.

The women's (health) movement in India has had its hands full in dealing with the adverse effects of the government's population control program, the contraceptive technologies introduced within family planning programs, and the use of technologies for sex preselection and sex detection. There has been little consideration of the consequences of the technologies used for assisting reproduction for health, their ethical and legal implications, and the social conditions in which the technologies are applied. Consequently, there has been little public discussion regarding what these technologies mean for women's health and autonomy.

INFERTILITY AND SOME NONMEDICAL SOLUTIONS

A worldwide survey done by the World Health Organization (WHO) on the incidence of infertility reports the incidence of infertile women in India as 3 percent. About 10 percent of couples in India have problems of infertility. "Nearly 16 million couples—or 32 million individuals—in the 18- to 35-year age group, are afflicted by the problem, making infertility one of the most widespread conditions in the country" (Katiyar 1993).

How has infertility traditionally been dealt with before the arrival of artificial insemination and IVF? The problem of infertility has generally been solved at the family level, often behind a curtain of family secrecy. Assuming that it is the woman who is infertile, one of the common solutions is to bring in the wife's sister as a co-wife to ensure heirs for the family. Bigamy was recently outlawed, but since only a small percentage of marriages are registered, there is no way that the offenders will ever be punished.

Many still seek other traditional solutions such as visits to local *vaidyas* (those practicing indigenous medicine), astrologers and *sadhus* (holy men), pilgrimages to famous shrines to ask for the boon of children, fasting, conducting *havans* (fire ritual) and praying, and using an assortment of herbs, charms, etc., either home-made or given by a "holy person" or a charlatan. The psychological trauma of childlessness and the social stigma it carries can often lead to either divorce or desertion of the woman concerned, as it is almost always considered the woman's fault. Infertile women are considered "barren" and inauspicious; they are often driven to desperate measures, including suicide, and men often remarry in the expectation that a new wife will give them the children they hope for. When all traditional methods fail, the desire for a child in some cases is also fulfilled by adoption, particularly intrafamily adoption. Most doctors are now recommending AI and IVF over adoption, as in this way either both or at least one partner is the biological/genetic parent of the child.

TECHNOLOGICALLY ASSISTED REPRODUCTION

Artificial Insemination

There is a tremendous demand in India for artificial insemination (AI), whether the procedure uses the husband's sperm (AIH), donor sperm (AID), or a mixture of both. Between five and six hundred cases of AI are recorded each month. Government hospitals do not provide the facility, so private gynecologists have a booming practice. Most men are reluctant even to go for semen tests. Requests for AID are accompanied by appeals for utmost secrecy: husbands do not want their wives to know that donor sperm is being used for insemination, or wives do not want their husbands to know, or parents do not want their daughter-in-law to learn that their son is sterile. A number of women seem to be concerned that the husband should not be told about his "lack of manhood." Married women come with their mothers without the knowledge of their husbands and in-laws, because if they do not produce a child, they may be deserted. Some doctors, however, do not entertain such requests (Malpani and Malpani 1992). Most doctors have a consent form that needs to be signed by both husband and wife before donor sperm is used.

Sometimes donor sperm is sought by couples who already have children born with genetic disorders, often due to defects in the husband's sperm. In recent years, an even more important reason for seeking artificial insemination by women/couples who have no problem with their reproductive system is to increase the chances of getting a male child by inseminating with sperm which has been separated for its X (female) and Y (male) chromosomes and selected for Y-bearing chromosomes. Also preimplantation diagnosis of the embryo is used for sex selection in favor of males. In this way scientific advances are misused to conform to patriarchal ideologies as well as to the small family norm propagated by the national government and international population controllers. As one provider of these services put it, "To me it is the best way to avoid unwanted pregnancy." They seem to even use the feminist terminology developed in the context of abortion rights, women's right to "choose." In the words of another practitioner, "It helps what I call planned families. A woman has every right to opt for a male or female baby. . . . I think women would not go for abortions if they got babies of their choice."

Sperm Banks

Donor semen is becoming an increasingly accepted option. In spite of an increasing demand for medically assisted reproduction, particularly AI and IVF, India has few sperm banks. WHO guidelines do not support the use of fresh semen, which might transmit diseases, including HIV/AIDS. A major problem is to ensure a regular supply of liquid nitrogen (tanks have to be replaced every three or four days) without which the extremely low temperature at which the semen has to be stored cannot be maintained. Big cities like Bombay and Delhi have sperm banks.

There are three or four semen banks in Delhi, but they supply fresh semen because they do not have storage and preservation facilities. A few years ago, Delhi's first sperm bank for cryogenically frozen sperm, called "Cryo Gene," was established. A quarantine period of 180 days for sperm is mandatory, according to Dr. Bhashini Rao, one of its directors. Usually one ejaculate of sperm is used to inseminate a maximum of three women, a measure taken to minimize the probability of incestuous relationships later on (Rai 1994). There are also a few sperm banks of dubious quality that have sprung up in recent years due to the huge demand.

Apparently there is a shortage of high-quality sperm, in spite of a handsome payment that is made to donors to defray what the Malpanis (1992) call "travel expenses." Donors are generally discouraged by the long battery of laboratory investigations that need to be performed before a donated sample can be declared safe for use. Also, donors are tested for sexually transmitted diseases, hepatitis, blood group, genetic disorders, as well as IQ levels—standards which have been laid down by the American Fertility Association. Donors' height, weight, and complexion are recorded. International standards require that only those who have produced two normal children should be accepted as donors. Yuppie donors are considered rather attractive, as many specialists believe that their genes might confer a certain advantage on the child. Medical students are often used as donors, some even recruited through newspaper advertisements. The identity of donors is not revealed, as specialists want to avoid complications such as paternity suits or blackmail later on.

However, not all medical laboratories work according to such high standards. According to a report by Thakur (1993), some diagnostic laboratories in Delhi are using unsuspecting men as donors for artificial insemination. Those who go to the lab for various tests are made to undergo a semen test as well, or if they go for a semen test they are called back on the pretext that additional tests are needed. When a woman comes with a problem of being unable to conceive, her husband's semen is also taken for examination. If his semen is found to be healthy, his address is noted and whenever there is a demand from a gynecologist for sperm, he is called back for further examination and his fresh semen is collected and used for artificial insemination of other women without his knowledge.

Another report speaks of a similar malpractice in Bombay (Baria 1993). Gynecologists eager to cut costs and effort have found pathology laboratories prepared to supply them with fresh semen, which they would otherwise throw away after the mandatory tests. Gynecologists do not consider setting up sperm banks, where sperm can be frozen for later use, to be cost-effective. Besides, the success rate with fresh sperm is considered higher. Some doctors speak of having "cultivated" their own donors over time. Many doctors use the same donor to inseminate a large number of women and do not match the physical characteristics of the donor with the woman's husband properly.

Drs. Aniruddha and Anjali Malpani (1992) believe that legislation cannot catch up with the extremely lucrative business in infertility; one must rely on self-regulation and upholding of ethics by those in the business.

Women seeking artificial insemination are injected about once a month on the most fertile days of their cycle. Most women have the process repeated every month for about six months, unless they conceive earlier, and are willing to go on as long as it is required. The costs are about Rs. 1,000 (about U.S. $25) per insemination. The success rate varies between 50 and 60 percent. Most doctors are now recommending artificial insemination in place of adoption, as in this way at least one partner is involved in the birth of the child. Also, more men seem open to the idea of their wives being inseminated with donor sperm, as long as this remains a secret. However, some consider it unethical on moral or legal grounds.

Microscopic Tuboplasty

There has been a surge in the use of microscopic tuboplasty, an operation to surgically reverse tubectomy. The success rate of this surgical operation is claimed to be 60–70 percent, higher than that achieved by surgery without use of the special microscope. This operation can be useful in infertility treatment, or a first trial treatment before starting with IVF, but most doctors carry out this procedure only on women who have undergone tubectomy. The emphasis is on the reversibility of tubectomy, as doctors feel that more women will be encouraged to be tubectomized if they are assured about its reversibility.

Therefore, at the policy level, preference is given to women who have undergone tubectomy and then desire to have more children either because they lose a child or because they remarry and want to have children with their new husbands. Women who are infertile because they have some problems with their tubes, due either to some infection or to adhesions, are directed straight to IVF programs (Deval 1990).

IVF in India: A Lucrative "Growth Industry"

Durga Agarwal, born on October 3, 1978, was hailed as the first test-tube baby in India and the second in the world, but her claim to birth through IVF was contested due to a lack of sufficient documentation. This led to the suicide of Dr. Subhas Mukherjee, who claimed credit for the achievement.

Until the mid-1980s, infertility treatment basically consisted of trying to diagnose the cause of infertility, rather than providing a way out. Then came corrective surgery in the form of tuboplasty, lately microscopic tuboplasty. Generally, it ended with the doctor giving up and the couple accepting childlessness or going in for adoption, either within the family or through an adoption agency. However, a whole range of options now exist, from the relatively simple artificial insemination, by husband or donor sperm, to in vitro fertilization in all its variations, such as gamete intrafallopian transfer (GIFT) and zygote intrafallopian transfer (ZIFT). These services are increasingly offered by private clinics, as few government hospitals provide them. In the late 1980s, the All India Institute of Medical Sciences in New Delhi did offer services for the infertile but stopped after about a year for reasons unknown.

The Institute for Research in Reproduction (IRR) in Bombay, in collaboration with King Edward Memorial (KEM) Hospital, has been foremost in research in this field since 1983. Dr. Indira Hinduja was responsible for producing the first documented Indian IVF baby, Harsha Chawda, who was born to a lower-middle-class couple on August 6, 1986. More babies have been born since. Now both IRR and KEM Hospital have stopped offering IVF, reportedly due to pressure from feminist groups who pointed out that most clinics practicing IVF also indulge in sex determination and sex selection. Criticism from the religious orthodoxy also played a role. Now private gynecologists are providing these services. Dr. T. C. Anandkumar, former director of IRR, and Dr. Hinduja of KEM Hospital started a clinic (called Hope) in Bangalore to offer IVF and related services to the infertile.

With the developments in reproductive technology, doctors, especially in the big cities of India, are offering some of the latest and most sophisticated techniques to infertile couples. Dr. R. P. Soonawala (1993), a leading gynecologist from Bombay, confirms that infertility forms 60 percent of most gynecological practice today, whereas a decade ago a gynecologist was consulted mainly for management of pregnancies and deliveries or for family planning thereafter.

Although population control remains India's main objective in the application of human reproduction technologies, IVF is encouraged as a treatment for infertility. The argument given by Dr. Hinduja is that IVF is offered to boost the acceptance of sterilization (a terminal method of contraception preferred by population controllers). She believes more couples will accept sterilization if they know that in case they change their minds afterward they can have a child through IVF (Wichterich 1988). Dr. Anandkumar is reported to have said that even if all women now seeking treatment were to become pregnant, there would be "no undesirable effect on our population" in terms of additional births. He envisaged that IVF techniques would have beneficial effects in medicine as a whole, especially in the treatment of hereditary diseases by gene therapy (Jayaraman 1986). This argument is not really valid, as IVF is too expensive for most Indians to pursue.

Another reason for pursuing research in IVF is to identify and study factors contributing to infertility. In an interview Dr. Anandkumar declared, "An understanding of these factors may provide clues as to how to induce infertility in fertile couples as a means of family planning" (Sheth 1987). A lot of public funds have gone into this research through government grants, while funds for research into common diseases, such as malaria and tuberculosis, which affect a large population, are limited. The Indian government is known to pursue glamorous research into high-tech science in various fields for the nation's prestige. In this case, Anandkumar's argument is likely to have been even more appealing, as it promises to deal with what the government identifies as problem number one—population explosion.

Medical practitioners offering infertility services feel that infertility is a significant problem and if they do not offer the services it is likely to be exploited by quack sexologists. Initially many couples were even keen to go abroad for infertility treatment. In the early years a British hospital appointed an agent in New Delhi to handle inquiries from Indian women seeking treatment. For most people the prohibitive costs (not only of the treatment itself but also of travel) deterred them from seeking help outside the country.

For some time now, young Indian doctors have been training abroad and returning to set up private clinics with state-of-the-art apparatus. Although most of the advanced services for infertility are centered in Bombay, these sophisticated treatments are now becoming available in other cities, too. In 1993 there were more than twenty private IVF clinics, including three in Bangalore and Madras, two each in Delhi and Calcutta, and one each in Jaipur, Manipal, and Coimbatore. In Bombay alone, the number rose from two to twelve within five years (Katiyar 1993).

Assisted reproduction is a "growth industry." Doctors who have invested large sums of money in expensive medical equipment are keen to recover the capital outlay in as short a time as possible. With an increasing number of couples desperate for a child and starting on a roller-coaster of various treatments—the two parties usually find their match. Some of the simpler procedures—such as AI, ovulation cycle study, and semen analysis—are performed by gynecologists themselves, many of whom have acquired the necessary infrastructure. However, couples requiring IVF and more complicated services are referred to special infertility clinics that have the latest equipment from abroad. The economic liberalization policies of the government in the 1990s have made imports easier and could result in an even larger number of clinics offering more sophisticated services in this field. Another aspect is the sale and export of human material (ova, etc.) to developed countries in the North, as there is no regulation and control on the extremely lucrative business in infertility.

Dr. Firuza Parikh, an infertility specialist at Jaslok Hospital in Bombay, says that despite the high cost of treatment and the low success rate, which is between 5 and 22 percent per cycle, the number of patients coming for assisted conception is growing phenomenally. She started offering a new procedure, the micromanipulation of sperm to improve chances of fertilization of eggs. This technique is used only at a few clinics in Singapore, Sydney, Brussels, and in the United States. Another technique that she uses is intracytoplasmic sperm injection (Parikh 1992). With India providing the state-of-the-art techniques, the specialists speak of a flow of foreign couples, from the United Kingdom, the United States, and the countries around the Persian Gulf, to avail themselves of these services. The fees for treatment and accommodation in a nursing home in India are much lower than those charged at clinics abroad (Parikh 1992).

The Malpanis delivered a baby, possibly the first of its kind in the country, using the eggs of one woman, the frozen sperm of a donor, and the womb of another woman. They are extremely excited about their work, which they see as helping childless couples to have children. They started "Infertility Friends," a support group for couples with similar problems (Malpani and Malpani 1992). In North India, IVF is being offered at the Jaipur Fertility Medical Research Centre (JFMRC), a private clinic in Rajasthan, and at the Gangaram Hospital in Delhi. Significantly, most of the children born through IVF at these two centers are males. JFMRC prides itself in producing only male babies in its clinic, while attributing it to sheer chance and denying that they are using any special techniques such as separating sperm and selecting sperm rich in Y (male-producing) chromosomes. Seven male babies in a row cannot be a sheer coincidence, contend most infertility specialists, who at least in principle reject the unethical use of this technology to produce only male babies. Dr. M. Kochchar (1993) of Gangaram Hospital gives a biological explanation for it based on the faster motility of Y-bearing sperm.

IVF treatments are extremely expensive, anything from Rupees 50,000 to 100,000 (currently approximately U.S. $1,500 to $3,000, although cheap by international standards) depending on the number of attempts necessary. As there is no system of health insurance and government hospitals do not provide the facility, people have to pay for it themselves. Although the first IVF baby was born to a lower-middle-class couple, who did not have to pay for the experimental treatment, IVF treatments in India are only for the wealthy. However, some people are desperate enough to raise the money even if it means selling their valuable assets.

Dr. Sadhana Desai, an infertility expert from Bombay with over twenty-five years of experience, says of the latest options available in the field of assisted reproduction that "patients are confused by the alternatives they have, and so are the doctors." Their social and working lives are disrupted, as they come to revolve around doctors, clinics, and hospitals. Sometimes this can take couples through an endless maze of infertility clinics and cause considerable emotional strain in the process. But it seems many couples (read women) seem to be prepared to pay the high price to be rid of what some see as their body letting them down and what others see as the "curse" of infertility, going through up to six cycles of treatment.

IVF and Embryo Transfer (Surrogacy)

In the joint family system, surrogate mothering (social, not biological) is common; widowed family members and older daughters also "mother" children. It is the social role fulfillment that is stressed rather than the biological process of childbirth. The first known case of technological surrogacy in India, reported by Sudha Menon (1993), concerned a childless couple from Bombay who were both infertile and thus opted for surrogacy. Menon asks what the repercussions of renting a womb are likely to be in a society that puts self-sacrificing motherhood on a pedestal.

In July 1997, thirty-year-old Nirmala from Chandigarh caused an uproar when she announced her decision to bear a child for an infertile couple for Rs. 50,000 (Srinivasan 1997). By acting as a surrogate she hoped to raise money to pay her invalid husband's medical bills, which was otherwise beyond her capacity, her monthly income being only Rs. 700. Nirmala expected to conceive through sex with her employer. She openly admitted that she was doing it for the money. According to Dr. Firuza Parikh, the woman was using her resources—in this case, her womb—to earn money for an honorable cause. Nirmala was threatened with action under the Suppression of Immoral Traffic Act. She filed a lawsuit seeking legal sanction for her action.[1]

Surrogacy is still in its infancy in India. Some infertility specialists are hesitant to do commercial surrogacy yet, although they do buy ova (Rs. 5,000 apiece). Dr. Parikh had used IVF on seven surrogate mothers in the period 1990–92. Two children were born as a result. The other couples did not come back for a second attempt. In each case a legal agreement was signed whereby the commissioning couple agreed to look after the surrogate mother during the pregnancy and pay all her medical bills. The latter agreed to look after herself during the pregnancy and not harm the fetus. The surrogate mothers were always related to the couple in some way. According to the doctor, the arrangements were assumed to be altruistic, although money or property may have changed hands (Parikh 1992).

DEBATES ON TECHNOLOGIES USED TO ASSIST REPRODUCTION

At the moment, technologies in the field of assisted reproduction affect a small number of people in India, although they are proliferating at a very rapid pace. The recently constituted Indian Society for Assisted Reproduction lists 186 members. However, there are few public debates on the issue. Newspapers report on these issues from time to time. These technologies have generally received little attention from either policymakers or feminists. Feminists and women's health advocates have taken up the subject for discussion only in a limited way. This reflects the Indian government's population policy, which is geared toward reducing births, and most funds have been channeled into that aspect of family planning. Women's health advocates and feminists have focused mainly on the effects of the government's population control policies on women's bodies and lives and on sex (pre)selection and sex determination followed by abortion of the female fetus. This leaves very little scope for a discussion on other aspects of family planning, which ideally should include measures to deal with infertility, too, and not just contraceptive provision, although not necessarily through high-tech methods such as IVF. In that sense, technologies in the field of assisted reproduction fulfill individual needs.

Some gynecologists who specialize in low-cost and comparatively low-tech methods of assisted reproduction are critical of so much money and effort going into high-tech methods with rather low success rates (Meherji 1993). They contend that simple solutions and conventional infertility treatments are valued less, while IVF is popularized because of the glamour and prestige it brings to the practitioners, the institutions at which they work, and even the nation. Dr. Hrishikesh Pai, better known for his contributions in the field of abortion (he runs Pearl Centre, Asia's largest abortion clinic, in Bombay), is one such critic. He warns against what he calls "rip-offs," and claims to be able to achieve better results using vaginal ultrasound instead of expensive laparoscopy, recycled needles, and leftover nutrient fluids from previous IVF attempts, which he describes as "Third World IVF" (personal communication, 1993). Other infertility specialists providing artificial insemination, especially those working in institutions that also do various forms of IVF, also express their guarded criticism and do not appreciate the importance given to IVF in terms of budget allocations and media coverage as they consider their own work more meaningful and successful. Some are of the opinion that the enormous investments made by IVF specialists in expensive equipment can cloud their medical judgment.

The reporting in the media has been either a glorification of the success stories of conceptive technologies or criticism in terms of their effects in a country with an already large population. Opposition to technologies used in assisted reproduction from a feminist perspective is less known. Women's health groups and feminist organizations are trying to spread information on the issue in a limited way. Lakshmi Lingam, lecturer at the Women's Studies Unit of the Tata Institute of Social Sciences in Bombay, compiled a dossier of articles from magazines and newspapers on new reproductive technologies (NRTs) in India (Lingam 1989). While doing a print media analysis, she argues that it is crucial to view assisted reproduction technologies as links in the same chain [as sex determination technologies] based on uniform ideologies of "abusing, disrespecting, manipulating and exploiting women as 'objects.'" Writing of IVF, she says, "This technology too is anti-woman for it is set within the ideological structure of 'marriage,' 'children within wedlock,' 'the supremacy of biological motherhood' and it reinforces fertility as an important indicator of women's status" (Lingam 1990).

The idea of "biological motherhood" through IVF is being encouraged in preference to adoption, which could be a logical solution for infertile couples. Lingam notes that in patrilineal systems the blood bond is extremely important for rituals and property transfer. Adoption is not favored by infertile couples or their families, as they suspect "that the child may carry the genes of a rapist, for example, making the child tainted in their eyes" (Lingam 1990). Adoption laws in India are different for the different religious communities according to their independent personal laws. Adoption of a child is not alien to Hindus; the Hindu Adoptions and Maintenance Act of 1956 secures equally the interests of parents and child. Adoption under the Wards and Guardianship Act of 1890, which is open to all other religious communities, does not ensure rights of insurance or succession to the child or security of parental status for the adoptive parents. A comprehensive bill on adoption, which could help infertile couples, has been lying in Parliament for more than twenty years. Three separate attempts to pass the Indian Adoption Act failed due to objections from the minority communities on the basis of their personal laws (Nair 1988; Anklesaria 1983). The personal laws of the various communities do not support adoption and give primacy to biological motherhood; therefore, IVF and surrogacy are likely to find support. These same communities, however, reject artificial insemination, as they consider masturbation immoral and adulterous. Lingam (1990) speaks of an interesting deadlock in this situation.

Until very recently, there were no laws on AI or IVF and no body of experts to supervise the ethics of the business or to certify the institutions. A few states have passed laws requiring clinics offering infertility services to register themselves, but there is no body that monitors the quality of the services provided. The Nirmala case (mentioned above) reemphasized the importance of legislation as well as clear-cut ethical guidelines to cover the developments in the field of reproductive technologies. For the first time, attempts were made in early

1998 to formulate guidelines to regulate it. A Statement of Ethical Considerations involved in Biomedical Research on Human Subjects, or the "ICMR Code," was drafted by the Central Ethical Committee on Human Research of the Indian Council for Medical Research (ICMR) under the chairmanship of a former Supreme Court chief justice, M. N. Venkatachalaiah. Revised after seventeen years, the long-overdue ethical guidelines now also encompass the developments in the field of human genetics, organ transplant (including fetal tissue transplant), and assisted reproduction technology. Regarding IVF and in particular surrogacy, the ethical committee experts arrived at the following consensus:

- Surrogate motherhood should be legal only when it is coupled with authorized adoption.
- It should be "rebuttably presumed" that a woman who carries the child and gives birth to it is its mother.
- The intending parents should have a preferential right to adopt the child subject to six weeks' postpartum delay for necessary maternal consent.
- Surrogate motherhood should be legal only on certified medical indication.
- Abortion under the law on medical grounds should be an inviolate right of the surrogate mother, and the adopting parents have no claim over the amounts already paid in the surrogacy contract.

A child born through the use of assisted reproduction technology is presumed to be "the legitimate child of the couple having been born within wedlock, with the consent of both the spouses and with all the attendant rights of parentage, support and inheritance." Further, "sperm or ovum donor should have no parental rights or duties in relation to the child and their anonymity should be protected," according to the committee (Rana 1998).

In January 1994, the Indian Science Congress in Jaipur sponsored a session entitled "New Reproductive Technologies: Boon or Bane?" Most speakers agreed that women were at the receiving end of new developments in reproductive technology. They argued that these technologies (particularly the use of sex determination tests and contraceptives) should be seen against the background of the existing discrimination and violence against women. IVF, according to one of the speakers, is a complicated and expensive procedure that takes a heavy toll on women's lives in terms of their physical and mental health.

The Forum for Women in Bombay is one of the organizations which has taken a stand on NRTs, generally opposing the proliferation of these technologies within a patriarchal ideology. Access to AID and IVF for single women and lesbians, an important rallying point for radical feminists in the West, is not an issue in India, probably because the stigma of having children outside marriage is very strong. Feminists have questioned the nature of science and its antiwoman values and the priorities in science and technology in terms of allocation of scarce funds. Also, women's health advocates have drawn attention to the health hazards of IVF and the fact that more attention needs to be given to the causes of infertility—infectious diseases (such as tuberculosis and malaria), sexually transmitted diseases, environmental factors, etc. The question of the control that NRTs provide over women's bodies is expressed in Lingam's (1990) question, "Is it scientific progress or progressive control?" Many feminists have dismissed the idea of NRTs contributing to expanding women's choice in any way, since women have no choice in other areas of life, subject as they are to patriarchal control and as instruments of population control. Women's role as producers/workers is negated and undermined, and the maternal role is reinforced through these technologies.

CONCLUSION

It is important that feminists and women's health advocates in India take up the discussion of technologies used in assisted reproduction on a national level, just as they have done on other reproductive technologies (contraceptives, amniocentesis), so as to limit the adverse effects of these technologies on women. It is imperative both to demand legislation and control of the practice by private practitioners and enterprises offering services in the field, as well as to provide information to women regarding sexuality, fertility, and infertility, so as to contribute to their health and autonomy.

Supporters of IVF and its critics both use the argument of culture. For IVF supporters, the idea that every woman should be a mother is part of Indian culture. Instances of nontechnological surrogacy in the ancient epic the *Mahābhārata* are cited as examples. IVF and surrogacy are therefore legitimate modern tools for attaining this in case of inability to conceive naturally. For the critics, IVF and allied technologies are considered a threat to the same, and therefore some believe that Indian culture will not allow the practice to become commonplace. "The infertility industry is only one part of an unregulated private health care system which is based on profitability rather than need. . . . As in other situations these health services are capitalising on cultural demands, and on people's poverty," according to Dr. Amar Jesani, coordinator of the Centre for Enquiry into Health and Allied Themes and editor of the journal *Medical Ethics*. It is economic pressures that drive women to rent their wombs or to sell their body parts. For already vulnerable social groups, these pressures are only likely to exacerbate the adverse effects of the economic liberalization policies of the Indian government and the concomitant withdrawal of the state's responsibility in providing basic health services, on the one hand, and the globalization of the growing reproductive technologies market, on the other.

NOTES

This chapter is based on reviews of the literature and interviews conducted during my Ph.D. research. The dissertation was published under the title *New Freedoms, New Dependencies: New Reproductive Technologies, Women's Health, and Autonomy* (Leiden: Leiden University Press, 1996).

1. At the time this book is going into print, I have been unable to track down the final outcome of this case.

REFERENCES

Anklesaria, Shahnaz:
    1983   Storm over Adoption—I: Who Interprets Religious Precepts? *Statesman,* July 26.
Baria, Fara:
    1993   Whose Seed Is It Anyway? *Sunday Observer,* October 17.
Deval, Meena:
    1990   Personal written communication. May 23. (Ms. Deval is a local research assistant for the project.)
Jayaraman, K. S.:
    1986   India Embraces Test-Tube Babies. *Nature* 319 (February 20): 611.
Katiyar, A.:
    1993   Making Babies . . . Special Feature on Infertility. *India Today,* June 15: 54–60, 96–101.
Kochchar, M.:
    1993   Interview. New Delhi, February 22. (Dr. Kochchar is a senior specialist with the Department of Obstetrics and Gynecology, Sir Ganga Ram Hospital and Nursing Home, New Delhi.)
Lingam, Lakshmi:
    1989   *Made in India: A Dossier on the New Reproductive Technologies.* Bombay: Women's Studies Unit, Tata Institute of Social Sciences.
    1990   New Reproductive Technologies in India: A Print Media Analysis. *Issues in Reproductive and Genetic Engineering* 3(1): 13–21.
Malpani, Aniruddha, and Anjali Malpani:
    1992   Interview. Bombay, February 4. (Drs. Malpani are a young husband and wife team who run the Malpani Nursing Home in Colaba, Bombay, in collaboration with Sydney IVF of Australia.)
Meherji, P. K.:
    1993   Interviews. Bombay, January 29 and February 15. (Dr. Meherji is an infertility specialist with the Institute for Research in Reproduction, Bombay.)
Menon, Sudha:
    1993   Who Will Bear Our Baby? *Independent,* December 12.
Nair, Hema:
    1988   The Adoption Option. *The Indian Post, Postscript,* June 19.

Pai, Hrishikesh, and Datta Pai:
   1993   Interview. Bombay, February 10. (Drs. Pai are directors of the Pearl Centre, Bombay.)
Parikh, Firuza:
   1992   Interview. Bombay, February 5. (Dr. Parikh is an obstetrician and head of the Department of Infertility Management and Assisted Reproduction, Jaslok Hospital, Bombay.)
Rai, Usha:
   1994   This Is No Immaculate Conception. *Indian Express,* April 4.
Rana, Pradeep:
   1998   Surrogate Mother Is the Legal Mother: ICMR. *Times of India,* February 9.
Sheth, Parul:
   1987   To Harsha: Best Wishes for a Normal Life. *Times of India,* August 13.
Soonawala, R. P.:
   1993   Interview. Bombay, February 16. (Dr. Soonawala is a gynecologist who owns a private clinic in Bombay.)
Thakur, P.:
   1993   Blind Dates. *Sunday,* May 30: Medical Science sec.
Wichterich, Christa:
   1988   From the Struggle against "Overpopulation" to the Industrialization of Human Production. *Reproductive and Genetic Engineering* 1(1): 21–30.

9

Regulating Reproduction

Naomi Pfeffer

Established and new technologies that involve the manipulation and some-times destruction of the human embryo provoke irreconcilable disputes. Op-ponents of the techniques frequently demand regulation, which, they believe, will shield the human embryo. Paradoxically, regulation is also sought by their adversaries on the grounds it will allow them to continue manipulating and sometimes destroying human embryos. How can regulation serve apparently conflicting ends? Because it has multiple meanings and can be justified in different ways. It can, and does, exploit different tools, each of which can work toward different ends.

This chapter is concerned with what might clumsily be described as legal, or quasi-legal, politically driven approaches to regulation, hereafter called "for-mal regulation." Although there is an assumption of a common meaning of formal regulation, in fact, it is shot through with differing political practices whose origins can be traced to one of several justifications.

The first part of this chapter outlines justifications of formal regulation. The second part examines different formal regulatory mechanisms and gives examples of how they have been used in formal regulatory processes. The chap-ter concludes with a discussion of the politics of formal regulation and a brief consideration of its impact on women. My purpose is twofold: to explain how formal regulation of reproduction works in England, and to develop a frame-work for comparing approaches to the formal regulation of reproduction. Al-though England provides the substantive examples, the critical approach taken here is applicable to thinking about formal regulation of reproduction else-where. Internationally, there is no unanimity on whether and how abortion and in vitro fertilization (IVF) should be regulated or how regulation should be carried out. This lack of consensus has been confirmed repeatedly in surveys (Somerville 1982; Knoppers and LeBris 1991; Morgan and Nielsen 1993; Nielsen 1996). The approach outlined here is intended to facilitate a comparative analysis of regulation that moves beyond the "this procedure is permitted here, but not there" thinking that has tended to dominate the literature, and to encourage instead a political and sociological analysis of the conditions that give rise to what Raymond Williams has called "different formations and distributions of energy and interests" (1985, 12).

WHAT IS FORMAL REGULATION?

Perhaps the central element of the class of behavior that might be termed "regulation" is an interference of some sort in the activity subject to regulation—it is to be governed, altered, controlled, guided, regulated in some way (Mitnick 1980).

This definition, taken from a classic textbook on regulation, is a list of synonyms, a catalog of related meanings like those found in a thesaurus.[1] In making no reference to context or agency, it conflates and confuses the many different activities that might be called regulation. Yet it is only possible to make sense of regulation by locating it in a context and attributing agency. Unfortunately, these are rarely made explicit. For example, in discussions of reproduction, reference is sometimes made to the regulation of menstruation and the regulation of synthetic hormones. Although both types of regulation interfere, they mean radically different things. The former describes a physiological process: the action of synthetic hormones on the menstrual cycle. The latter is shorthand for legal tests of safety and efficacy, perhaps of the same synthetic hormones, by an official body such as the Food and Drug Administration, involving review by research ethics committees, biomedical experiments on animals and people, and interferences aimed at governing access, usage, and costs.

Regulation can also be categorized in terms of formality. Informal regulation is called "social control." Its mechanisms include speech and language, stereotypes, and seemingly innocuous everyday social processes (Smart and Smart 1978). Formal regulation is enshrined in public law—in England, parliamentary legislation and case law—and quasi-legal mechanisms introduced and administered by the state or another corporate body such as a professional association.

Undoubtedly, informal and formal regulatory processes have much in common, often influencing one another. For example, they may target the same people and seek to interfere in the same types of behavior. However, there are crucial, often overlooked differences between them. Theories of informal social control are unlike justifications of formal regulation. Informal social control mechanisms are said to seek to maintain social stability by describing normative attitudes and values and policing deviant behavior. In contrast, formal regulatory mechanisms engage with theoretical weaknesses in the market and are concerned with political, legalistic, economic, and technical matters. As a result of their theoretical differences, the two approaches to regulation invoke different human attributes and behaviors.

The relationship of the moral economy and the political economy is unpredictable. What might be considered morally (or strategically) desirable may not be legislatively possible or on politicians' agendas. Moreover, a moral consequence may not reflect moral intentions. However, social control has been the prism through which most social scientists and medical ethicists have examined the development of the formal regulation of reproduction. In effect, their work has focused on exposing normative values. Edward Yoxen, for example, found in the British public opposition to human embryo research in the 1980s "a return to Victorian values, with its conscious allusion to different modes of self-reliance, respect for traditional authority, patriotism and sexual inequalities." Respect for the sanctity of human embryonic life was one of the issues pursued by the "moral Right," a politically nonaligned lobby that emerged in Britain when Margaret Thatcher's Conservative government held office (Yoxen 1990). For Sarah Franklin, an anthropologist, parliamentary debates on the same topic reveal both hopes and fears about the unfamiliar kinds of kinship entities that may be created by the new reproductive technologies (Franklin 1993).

Normative values undoubtedly influence the introduction of formal regulation, but they cannot adequately account for its various structures or the choice of mechanism. Hence, although *The Embryo Research Debate,* Michael Mulkay's reflexive analysis of the arguments by British lobbies for and against human embryo research during the 1980s, cogently describes how the pro-research lobby mostly got its way, Mulkay cannot explain the structure and workings of the Human Fertilization and Embryology Authority (HFEA), the regulatory body created by the Human Fertilization and Embryology Act of 1990. This is because the legislation was designed by the state, which, as I argue below, was pursuing its own policies. And, as Habermas (1964) warned, although the state might appear to be the executor of public opinion, it does not always listen to it. The state and what Habermas calls the public sphere do not necessarily overlap; indeed, they may confront one another as opponents. In trying to understand the structure and work of formal regulation, what needs to be examined are its justifications and the political context in which it emerges.

JUSTIFICATIONS OF FORMAL REGULATION

The market is the starting point of theoretical justifications for formal regulation.[2] In a perfect market, competition is the regulatory mechanism. The cash nexus enables private, autonomous individuals to choose between goods and services offered by competing providers. In selecting goods and services for private ownership and exchange, individuals regulate standards of safety and quality. Selection is undertaken on rational grounds, based on a cost/benefit analysis. Individuals ask, Is a higher price worthwhile in terms of safety and quality, or is the identical product or service available elsewhere at a cheaper rate? Because the market claims to be impersonal, providers and customers can act unburdened by guilt or social obligation.

Regulation by the market "works" only where there is economic liberty, that is, where private individuals are free to produce, sell, acquire, use, or consume whatever they want. Hence in the marketplace, no one would, should, or could object when a sixty-year-old woman "buys" or contracts for fertility treatment from a gynecologist in order to become a mother, or when a younger fertile woman "sells" her eggs to the older women, using the cash she receives to pay for new clothes for herself. Only cost/benefit analysis—using market considerations as a metaphor not only for cash transactions but also for trade-offs in risk, effort, and benefits in kind (e.g., "free" treatment in exchange for eggs)—can determine which exchanges will take place. If, for reasons of risk assessment, very few women are prepared to sell their eggs, then as scarce commodities the price of human eggs will be relatively high; a high price will deter many women past menopause from pursuing motherhood, and as the number of patients diminish, the practice of gynecologists who offer the treatment will fail, which, in turn, will discourage others from setting up in business. This is one of the ways in which regulation by competition might make it impossible for—not, mark you, prohibit—women past the menopause to become mothers by "buying" fertility treatment. If something untoward takes place, the remedies available to private individuals are found in contract law and tort. In both, the parties to an action face one another as individuals on an equal footing.

In democracies, advocates of formal regulation have to provide electors with reasons for restraining their private individual autonomy. Broadly speaking, four justifications are used. They are discussed below using the regulation in England of abortion and IVF as substantive examples. However, the theories can be applied, albeit in different weight, to other activities, such as buying a computer, driving a car, and living close to a pollution-emitting chemical factory.

1. Individuals have unequal bargaining power Regulation by competition and private law remedies cannot work where a private individual's bargaining power is diminished because of a personal attribute, such as a health problem or an impairment, or because their disadvantaged position in the social structure makes them relatively powerless. Some form of protective method of regulation is required to prevent a "mischief," such as someone acting against their best interests, or being unable to obtain a remedy when harm occurs (Breyer 1982). This justification of formal regulation is used to prohibit certain activities by making them a criminal offense. It is resisted on the grounds that it is paternalistic, denying people the right to opt for riskier alternatives. It is tolerated politically only where a significant social loss may be incurred. For example, the HFEA decided to prohibit surrogacy for social or convenience reasons and to allow it only where it is physically impossible or highly undesirable for medical reasons for the commissioning mother to carry the child. Where surrogacy is not "treatment," according to the HFEA, passing on the risks associated with pregnancy to the surrogate mother is unfair. Where the surrogate mother insists she is prepared to accept the risks, the HFEA falls back on its concerns for the welfare of the unborn child, since surrogacy arrangements are unenforceable in English law, and the carrying mother would be the legal mother unless and until the commissioning mother becomes the child's legal parent through a formal adoption process (Gunning and English 1993).

By stipulating who is the weaker party and who is the potential exploiter, normative values are evident in this justification of formal regulation. In the example given above of how regulation might intervene in the market, which role should be given to the gynecologist, the older woman, and the younger woman? Casting usually reflects social values. Once past menopause, older women seeking motherhood are considered offenders and offensive (unlike older men in whom fatherhood is applauded); their "victims" are the younger women whose bodies they "plunder" for eggs and any children resulting from successful treatment. Saviors of the human embryo extend the victimhood of children backward to the moment of conception. The corollary is also used in support of access to safe, legal abortion: women have to be protected from the demands of an unwelcome fetus.

2. A collective interest in public goods If the first justification of formal regulation focuses on the inability of the market to protect vulnerable individuals, the second rests on a belief in the existence of a collective interest. A collective interest is denied by supporters of the market who understand social welfare as the aggregate of all private individual welfare. A collective interest is more than the sum of private individual interests: it describes a plane where what are called "public goods" are found. Public goods are commodities and services the benefit of which is shared by the collective as a whole. The advantages they bestow cannot be provided for any one person without simultaneously being provided for a substantial number of others. The classic examples of a public good are national defense, clean pavements, and street lighting. Because it is clearly not in the collective interest to allow demand for national defense to be determined through private individual preferences, as reflected in willingness to pay, the state intervenes, raises taxes from its citizens, and equips and maintains armed forces.

Public goods can bestow both material and nonmaterial benefits. Nonmaterial benefits include living in a society in which people generally behave courteously toward one another or everyone lives according to certain personal principles, such as honesty and tolerance. Hence women who would never consider terminating their own pregnancy might support regulation that permits safe, legal abortion and allows other women to decide for themselves (Himmelweit 1987). However, as might be expected, there is little agreement on what is in a collective's interest. Pacifists, for example, would exclude national defense.

During the twentieth century, some campaigners have struggled to have knowledge and technologies associated with fertility control recognized as a public good. Their success requires the redefinition of individual women's reproductive capacity, hitherto considered a private concern, into a public issue. This redefinition has both risks and benefits attached to it. Where reproduction has been exposed in public, women have become subjects of pro-natalist, anti-natalist, and eugenic population policies. The benefits, however, have also been considerable, especially where the public purse pays for appropriate services so that, irrespective of their economic and social status, women are provided with the means of becoming mothers whenever they so choose. While in England, contraception and safe, legal abortion have been recognized, albeit reluctantly, as public goods, circumventing involuntary childlessness has never been defined as such. Medical tests and treatment are available mostly to those who can afford the fees charged in the private medical sector.[3]

The collective interest was evoked in 1986 when data began to emerge on the risks associated with multiple pregnancies conceived as a result of IVF in England. Pediatricians increasingly gave voice to their anxieties about neonatal consequences, especially birth injuries, and social researchers found many parents unable to cope, emotionally and practically, for any length of time with triplets, quads, or more (Botting, Macfarlane, and Price 1990). Most IVF clinicians work in the private, for profit sector, regulated by the market and the HFEA. These clinicians are isolated from the costs and practical realities of delivering and caring for multiple births. It is the taxpayers who wind up paying for many of the medical, social, and financial consequences of multiple births. Many of the babies are delivered and cared for by the National Health

Service (NHS). Hence formal regulation could be justified by invoking the interests of the collective. Clinicians are required to limit to two the number of embryos placed in a woman's uterus, even though this might reduce the chance of pregnancy.

Sometimes the collectivity is enlisted by those pursuing private self-interest. Private self-interest is central to public choice theory, which is said to apply to every individual who stands to gain where what is called the cost of entry is raised and competition is impeded. Crudely speaking, this happens where the powerful convince the collective of their competitors' potential harmfulness. The classic example here is the medical profession, whose system of licensing has subordinated and marginalized other types of health care practitioners. However, many other providers of goods and services stand to benefit from a measure that excludes competitors. Private self-interests are said to motivate politicians with an eye on the next election; they may introduce or support legislation on regulation that may appeal to the electorate.

As the inclusion of politicians suggests, profit is not the only reward sought by private self-interest. Formal regulation can also permit socially undesirable activities. An English example of private self-interests seeking regulation for this purpose, which also raised the cost of entry to the "IVF business," is the Voluntary Licensing Authority (VLA), a system of licensing human embryo manipulation, established by scientists and gynecologists in 1985. In adhering to the rules laid down by the VLA, scientists and doctors could claim they were operating within a regulatory framework that excluded anyone unwilling to accept limits on their work.

3. A belief in allocative fairness Enthusiasts of the market believe it allocates resources efficiently. Moreover, they claim, efficiency is conducive to social welfare. Two incentives for efficiency found in the marketplace are said to maximize social welfare: individual consumer choice forces providers to satisfy social welfare needs effectively and hence efficiently (dissatisfied "customers" are wasteful of resources because they have to seek a further source of satisfaction); cost/benefit analyses may encourage consumers to self-care and obviate their need for welfare. The third justification of formal regulation rejects efficiency in favor of allocative fairness as a means of maximizing social welfare. It speaks of a collective interest in the achievement of a "just" distribution of resources. Contrasting sharply with private self-interests, it is based on a belief in abstract principles, especially altruism: people promote allocative fairness not for themselves but because of what they envisage for the community as a whole.

Two formal regulatory mechanisms are used to promote allocative fairness. The first is sometimes called structural regulation, wherein the types of organizations that are allowed to engage in certain activities are specified (Kay and Vickers 1988). In theory, structural regulation removes incentives for undesirable behavior, such as discrimination, by, for example, creating a statutory monopoly which, because it is embodied with the values of allocative fairness, acts as a "custodian of the public interest." This is what happened in Britain in 1948 with the creation of the NHS when health care services were taken into public ownership. The second mechanism is conduct regulation, in which the incentives for undesirable behavior persist but are discouraged or even prohibited by yardsticks and rewards that discipline behavior, for example, antidiscrimination laws. Prior to 1991, both regulatory mechanisms were used to ensure equity of access and procedural fairness in the NHS (Whitehead 1994).

Because abortion and the treatment of infertility have never been wholly accepted as falling within the collective interest in England, many women have been unable to secure free treatment within the NHS. If they can afford it, some have paid for it in the private sector; others have gone without. As a result, the private sector provides more abortions and infertility treatments than any other elective medical procedure (Williams and Nicholl 1994), which means structural regulation applies partially. Moreover, although strict conduct regulations govern abortion, IVF, and other infertility treatments that involve the manipulation of human gametes and embryos, they are concerned mostly with safeguarding the human gametes and embryos and not with the women undergoing treatment.

Allocative fairness is the most susceptible of the four justifications to political ideology and is discussed in greater detail in the final section of this chapter.

4. Structural problems in relation to information   In a perfect market, buyers have sufficient information to evaluate competing products and services. They can identify the range of alternatives and understand the characteristics of the choices they confront. The buyer, faced with alternative suppliers, spends time, effort, and money in her search. The seller spends money on research, labeling, and advertising to make the product's or service's qualities known and attractive.

Not every potential "buyer" or "seller" has access to relevant information, or, if it is available, they may be unable to evaluate it. Research suggests some patients overestimate the technical effectiveness of IVF (Johnston, Shaw, and Bird 1987); others underestimate the burden—physical, emotional, and social—of a higher order multiple pregnancy, probably because the prospect of triplets or more is too remote to be imaginable (Price 1993).

There are several ways of overcoming structural problems of information. The first considered here is prior approval: products and services are required to meet certain specified standards before being released to consumers as happens with licensing of medical practitioners, drugs, and, increasingly, new medical technologies. The second method, describing minimum standards of safety and quality that must be met, is less costly and allows greater freedom of consumer choice; people can decide for themselves how high (or low) a standard is acceptable to them. However, difficulties arise where the quality of the product or service can only be verified through consumption, as happens with medical care and IVF. What happens when the product turns out to be poor or even harmful? Patients cannot return an unsuccessful cycle of IVF to the clinic in the same way they can return an unsatisfactory product. Sometimes "implication" counseling is offered to help people think through the possible consequences of their treatment. However, "implication" counseling does not solve the issue of redress when something untoward happens. In the private medical sector, redress is available only through the courts.

A third approach is to regulate the information itself. In England, clinics licensed by the HFEA to carry out IVF and artificial insemination are required by law to provide data on "outcomes" of different licensed procedures. These data are published by the HFEA in its annual report and in its *Patients' Guide to DI and IVF Clinics*. However, data on medical procedures are often difficult to interpret; they are based on aggregates when what patients want to know is whether it will work for them. Moreover, making sense of them often demands considerable technical expertise that few patients possess. Using recently developed computer-intensive statistical techniques, statisticians analyzed published data of live birth rates of IVF clinics in the United Kingdom, and concluded that few firm inferences could be drawn from them without additional statistical analysis (Marshall and Spiegelhalter 1998).

If experts on medical statistics cannot make sense of the HFEA data, what hope is there for would-be purchasers of IVF? The problem is that many clinicians are reluctant to divulge potentially discrediting data to the HFEA. Sometimes, in this sort of situation, a second agency acts as a proxy for consumers, or a well-informed patient pressure group may provide useful information. Unfortunately, neither of these solutions has arisen as yet in England in relation to IVF. For these reasons, improving information is considered a weak method of formal regulation.

CHOOSING A REGULATORY MECHANISM

Although they are justified in terms of deficiencies of the market, regulatory mechanisms are not simply "tools for a job," if such things can ever be said to exist (Clarke and Fujimura 1992). The reason why a regulatory mechanism is seen as the right one can only be understood as part of a situation: "rightness" varies across time and space and according to the requirements of participants in the formal regulatory process. For example, different legal cultures and traditions promote some regulatory mechanisms and reject others. David Vogel, a U.S. political scientist, distinguished three distinctive styles of formal regulation: the British, the continental, and the American (Vogel 1986). In France, for example, people can seek redress in courts devoted to review of government administration, whereas in Britain, it is the ordinary courts that review the activities of public authorities. The U.S. system is distinctive in handing over the power to enforce compliance to an independent regulatory agency and in allotting to consumers a share of regulatory power; hearings are conducted in public, and interested groups have participation rights denied consumers in other countries. Another factor that influences the choice of regulatory mechanism is the system of health care. In England, where health care has enjoyed structural regulation for over fifty years, preference has been given to informal mechanisms of redress. In contrast, in the United States, where private health care is dominant, damages in tort are mostly sought.

Sometimes mechanisms are deliberately selected for their capacity to hit or miss targets. Rules, for example, can vary in clarity. The rules of the Unborn Children (Protection) Bill were precise, befitting its unambiguous intention of affording human embryos almost complete protection from researchers. The bill was put before Parliament in 1985 by a controversial member, Enoch Powell. As its title suggests, the bill sought to prohibit human IVF except for treatment purposes and, by so doing, prohibit human embryo research. Moreover, the fertilization of a human ovum in vitro was to be allowed only with the authority of the secretary of state for health, a government minister. Possession of a human embryo produced in vitro for purposes other than treatment would be a criminal offense. Powell's bill found some support in Parliament but was not endorsed by the government and so, for reasons discussed below, failed to become law.

Worried by the threat to research and practice posed by Powell's bill and its supporters, and conscious of developments elsewhere (for example, in the United States, where a moratorium on federally funded research involving human embryos had been in place since 1975), in 1985 the government-funded Medical Research Council (MRC) and the Royal College of Obstetricians and Gynecologists (RCOG) established what was initially called the Voluntary Licensing Authority (VLA) (Gunning and English 1993, 33–46). As a system of self-regulation, the VLA licensed research and medical procedures using human embryos, claiming both were public goods: the potential benefits to humankind in circumventing involuntary childlessness and eradicating congenital disabilities made it worthwhile (the ends justifying the means, where the means had been given prior approval). Moreover, before it was fourteen days old, the human embryo, or pre-embryo as the VLA insisted on calling it, could not count as human.

The VLA's rules were vague. For example, Guideline 13d states that "laboratory conditions must be of a high standard (e.g., good culture facilities, facilities for microscopic examination, appropriate incubators and training in "non-touch" techniques)" (VLA 1986, 32). Readers are not told what is meant by "high standard," "good," and "appropriate." Vague rules encourage what lawyers call "creative compliance," that is, they allow flexibility in interpretation by both regulators and those being regulated. As the VLA explained, "The intention was not to draw up restrictive and rigid guidelines which might have been unworkable in practice, nor to constrain further progress in areas in which research was considered essential for medical advance" (VLA 1986, 8).

Although rules regulating clear-cut moral issues are easy to draw up (you shall not do this or you must do that), their legal force is often weak because they deal mostly with private behavior, which is extremely difficult to police. Moreover, in the British parliamentary system, attempts at introducing legislation on a single moral issue rarely succeed because they are usually introduced by an individual MP, without the support of government. Called a private member's bill, they stand little chance of success unless an overwhelming majority of MPs support them. Indeed, no private members bill has succeeded since 1959 if it was opposed by even a single MP or it was not given time by the government to proceed through all the required stages. Hence Powell's bill failed (Marsh, Gowin, and Read 1986).

A bill addressing several different albeit related concerns has a greater chance of becoming law because of what public choice theorists call "logrolling": deliberately complex legislation encourages "trading" of votes by various sectional private interests, sometimes ensuring that neither side of a struggle emerges as outright winner or loser, which is often a politically satisfactory outcome (Ogus 1994, 60–62). The Human Fertilization and Embryology Act of 1990 provided ample opportunities for "logrolling." In introducing the bill to the House of Commons, the then secretary of state for health, Kenneth Clarke, described it as "complex" (Clarke 1990). It consisted of forty-nine sections, dealing with surrogacy, abortion, definitions of a human embryo, human embryo research, kinship, clinic licensing arrangements, and the remit of the HFEA, among other things. Although it was sponsored by the Conservative government, the policies it contained did not follow a party line. MPs were allowed to consider and vote on each clause in turn in accordance with their personal dictates. Both sides of the human embryo debate can claim some successes and some failures. For example, the act permitted licensed human embryo research up until the embryo was fourteen days old, but it also reduced the upper limit on termination of pregnancy from the twenty-eighth week of pregnancy to the twenty-fourth.

Formal regulatory mechanisms can serve different purposes. Prior approval, one of the most interventionist mechanisms, can prohibit an activity under one set of conditions and facilitate it under others. According to the Unborn Children (Protection) Bill, introduced expressly to ban human embryo research, prior approval would have had to be sought for each attempt at fertilizing a human ovum in vitro for subsequent implantation in a specific woman, and it would be considered only for clinical purposes. It was a case-by-case approach: Each woman's "suitability" for motherhood would have been assessed by a government minister who would have delegated the task to civil servants. If rules were flouted, the police would have been called upon to seek out offenders, and the judiciary would have been asked to prosecute them.

Prior approval was used by the VLA in order to permit the manipulation of human embryos for both treatment and research purposes. It gave blanket approval to medical practitioners of suitable credentials who agreed to abide by its guidelines and who worked in premises it had inspected and approved. The VLA's annual reports list centers offering a licensed clinical service and the name of the license holder. The selection of suitable patients was left to clinicians, although one of the conditions of its license was that clinics had to have access to an ethics committee to provide supervision and advice on "difficult" cases.

Proposals for research on human embryos were considered by the VLA on a case-by-case basis. It claimed to be scrutinizing research in the public's interest, describing itself as "particularly anxious, given the public's concern, that only soundly based research with clearly defined aims and methods should be accepted" (VLA 1986, 9). In submitting to the VLA's rules and scrutiny, researchers working with human embryos could claim to be showing them respect. However, it is also possible to argue that the VLA favored private self-interest. In granting licenses and reviewing research protocols, the VLA staved off threats to outlaw human embryo research, thereby enabling scientists and clinicians to continue manipulating and sometimes destroying human embryos. Between 1985 and 1991, when it was replaced by the HFEA, ninety-three research projects using human embryos were approved by the VLA (Gunning and English 1993, 114). In 1990, it was estimated that five thousand human embryos were being used for research purposes each year in the United Kingdom (McNair-Wilson 1990).

The efficiency and effectiveness of a formal regulatory mechanism is determined by the power of its operator. The VLA was a system of professional self-regulation in that its members were appointed in an individual capacity, and up to half were lay people; it was established by the Medical Research Council

(MRC), which represents the interests of the research community, and the Royal College of Obstetricians and Gynecologists (RCOG), which represents the interests of gynecologists (Price 1989). Professional self-regulation rests on a mixture of the justifications of formal regulation described above. According to its enthusiasts, only those practicing expert work know which standards should be set and attained and only they can identify where they have not been met. Moreover, because nonprofessionals do not possess the relevant knowledge, it is in the collective's interest for professionals to regulate themselves and determine their own standards of practice (Allsop and Mulcahy 1998, 74).

The VLA Guidelines were derived from the recommendations of the influential report of the government-sponsored investigation into the ethics of human fertilization and embryology (Warnock 1985) and guidelines issued by a committee of the MRC (1982) and an RCOG ethics committee (RCOG 1983). However, as a voluntary self-regulating professional body, the VLA found compliance difficult to achieve; it had only informal penalties such as "naming and shaming" with which to discipline recalcitrants. When a leading infertility specialist refused to comply with the rule of replacing a maximum of three embryos in a woman's uterus (introduced because of the problems associated with higher order multiple pregnancies), the VLA withdrew its approval of the clinic. However, it could not prevent the doctor concerned from practicing. Instead, a combination of peer pressure and the commercial interests of the private hospital in which the clinic was located appear to have made him conform. The private hospital was probably unwilling to have its position in any possible action for negligence jeopardized by its failure to conform to a recommended code of practice (Gunning and English 1993, 56).

THE POLITICS OF REGULATION

The willingness of a government to support formal regulation and the type of regulatory mechanism it decides to introduce are determined by its ideological position in relation to the role of the state and the market.

The postwar British welfare state had been organized around a belief in allocative fairness, using both structural and conduct regulation to achieve this end. Central government served as both planner and direct owner of the means of production of goods and services, taxing citizens and spending on their behalf. However, in 1979, a Conservative government under the leadership of Margaret Thatcher came into power determined to replace regulation for allocative fairness with policies promoting allocative efficiency. It began to dismantle structural and conduct regulations and introduce mechanisms that placed responsibility for regulation on consumers (Majone 1997). The impact on reproduction of these radically different approaches to regulation can be gathered by comparing the Abortion Act of 1967 and the Human Fertilization and Embryology Act of 1990.

The Abortion Act of 1967

In English law, the legal grounds for terminating a pregnancy gradually widened during the twentieth century. By the late 1930s, it was possible to have a pregnancy terminated legally if a doctor said a woman's physical and mental well-being were at risk if the pregnancy continued to term. After World War II, politicians repeatedly attempted to introduce legislation that would further widen the conditions under which an abortion could be performed legally (Lovenduski 1986). The 1967 bill, the sixth put before Parliament in fifteen years, was passed with a firm majority a year after the then left-wing Labour Party had won the general election. In addition to medical grounds for terminating a pregnancy, the act introduced a new social reason: a doctor would escape prosecution for terminating a pregnancy if it was held that "the pregnant woman's capacity as a mother will be severely overstrained by the care of a child, or another child as the case may be." The act extended the number of categories of women for whom abortion should be made available. Before 1967, approximately 27,500 abortions were performed legally each year (Simms 1974). An unknown number were carried out illegally.[4] In 1969, the first full year of the act, which also introduced statutory notification of the operation, 49,829 abortions were carried out; by 1995, the number had risen to 153,135 (Office of Population Censuses and Surveys 1996).

Parliamentarians were specifically concerned not to legislate abortion on demand; instead, the act enlarged the conditions under which doctors performing an abortion could escape prosecution under the Offenses Against the Person Act of 1861. Outside of the act, abortion is still a criminal offense. Doctors are not compelled, but consent to perform the operation. Two doctors are required to certify that indications for abortion exist. In effect, the act confirmed and extended doctors' control over women. A woman seeking an abortion within the NHS has to convince two doctors that her circumstances fall within the provisions of the act. In 1971, as a result of differing interpretations of the act by medical practitioners, the abortion rate varied twofold to threefold in different parts of England and Wales (Potts, Diggory, and Peel 1977, 305).

The act specified that the operation itself was to be performed within an NHS hospital or some other place officially approved. As Richard Crossman, the government minister then responsible for the act, put it, "The Minister's job is not to tell the doctor how to do his job, but to see that the job is done in adequate physical conditions" (Crossman 1969, 948). However, the only physical conditions examined were those of "approved places": private nursing homes run either for profit or by a nonprofit charity set up to provide low-cost abortions in parts of the country where women were poorly served by the NHS. Covered by structural regulations, NHS premises and facilities escaped inspection and prior approval. As a civil servant put it, "The difference between the independent sector and the NHS is that the NHS has a whole range of checks and balances with respect to management and there is the ultimate responsibility to the Secretary of State. That is not shared, except only in part, as far as the independent sector is concerned. It is those checks and balances which make it unnecessary to apply the same sort of strictures to the public sector."[5]

Conduct regulations encourage allocative fairness. The act requires any practitioner who terminates a pregnancy to notify the chief medical officer within seven days of performing the operation. Moreover, notification includes submission of the following information about the woman on whom the operation was performed (published data exclude some of the information collected that might identify individual women):

Date of birth of woman
Occupation of woman
Usual place of residence of woman
Citizenship of woman
Marital status of woman
Previous pregnancies
Number of existing children
Gestation of pregnancy
Grounds for pregnancy termination
Category of premises where abortion is performed
Geographical location of premises
Type of operation performed
Medical sequelae of operation

The data published by the Office of Population, Censuses, and Statistics, a government department, speak of a political commitment to allocative fairness. Because doctors state the type of premises in which the operation was performed, it is possible to gauge the extent to which the NHS is fulfilling its commitment to equity of access, to whom, and in which parts of the country. These data were used by pressure groups campaigning to widen women's access to NHS facilities that are free at the point of delivery.

Approved places run by charities were considered second best to the NHS. They were a necessary evil, filling in gaps in abortion services created by unsympathetic NHS doctors. Clinics run for profit were abhorred. The climate of opinion was against profiting from medical care. Indeed, between 1974 and 1976, the Labour government was locked in a crusade against private for-profit medical practice within the NHS on the grounds that it was "a flaw in the pure crystal of the NHS's underlying conception: the idea that the treatment of patients should be determined exclusively by criteria of need, as distinct from the ability to pay" (Klein 1989, 118). Newspapers regularly featured stories of private nursing homes financially exploiting women seeking abortions, through grossly overcharged fees, and "fee-splitting," where the clinic and referring doctor shared the fee. The profits of some private abortion clinics were reputed to be enormous. As one doctor put it, as a result of the 1967 act, private abortionists "were driven from the back-streets not into obscurity, but in a Rolls-Royce to more fashionable accommodation in the High Street or on Ascension Square" (Hordern 1971, 106).

The act was interpreted and administered by civil servants, using powers delegated to them by the minister of health. They inspected "approved places" and published guidelines in departmental circulars. After numerous stories in the press about the "abortion racket," further conditions were imposed on private clinics relating to the scale of fees charged, and special investigators with police experience were employed so that factual checks as to the management and administration of approved places could be made (Lane Committee 1974, 131). Considerable discretion was delegated to civil servants because it was said to be impossible for Parliament to draw up a set of rules that would be appropriate in all possible cases. However, the working of the Abortion Act was monitored by Parliament in other ways. Between 1974 and 1980, the act was reviewed by six parliamentary committees, set up in response to newspaper stories of profiteering or to pressure from the anti-abortion lobby.

The Human Fertilization and Embryology Act of 1990

In 1978, Louise Brown, the first baby conceived in vitro, was born in Oldham General Hospital. Because of its concerns about the ethics and safety of IVF (but not the legality, as the procedure was not then covered by law), in 1971 the MRC had denied financial support of the research of gynecologist Patrick Steptoe, embryologist Robert Edwards, and other members of the team who successfully pioneered the technology. Nonetheless, working in what might be described as a provincial backwater, outside of elite gynecological circles, they were able to experiment on patients. Steptoe exercised considerable influence over several local NHS committees, including a research ethics committee he had set up and chaired at Oldham General Hospital, and the Oldham Area Health Authority, an administrative tier of the NHS, which agreed to accommodate Edwards's team and equipment at the NHS Kershaw Cottage Hospital. Edwards's work on human embryology at Cambridge University was supported by the U.S. Ford Foundation; donations from private individuals covered the team's research expenses (Steptoe and Edwards 1981, 67). Patients paid for what was experimental treatment.

Some people heralded the birth of Louise Brown as a triumph of British medicine; others saw it as a sinister development, threatening the moral fabric of society. The government responded to these concerns by convening an official committee chaired by a moral philosopher, Mary Warnock. It published its report in 1984. In claiming protection of the public as the primary objective of regulation of human embryo research and manipulation, the committee was citing the second justification of formal regulation. It recommended regulation by prior approval through the creation of a statutory licensing authority independent of government, health authorities, and research institutions. Independence was desirable to persuade the public that decisions had not been unduly influenced by sectional interests (Warnock 1985, 75–76). Coincidentally, independence of government was also demanded of regulatory bodies, albeit for different reasons, by the Conservative government, led by Margaret Thatcher.

Thatcher's government was committed to making the machinery of government smaller. Before she became prime minister in 1979, she had pledged she would reform the civil service and professions, both perceived by her as pursuing private interests, holding back progress, and making efficiency impossible. Civil servants were one of her first targets; their number was reduced by 102,000 to 630,000 people by 1984, and by 1986, 151,689 jobs had been eliminated (Davies and Willman 1991, 8). Moreover, the idea that ministers could be genuinely responsible for day-to-day regulatory tasks delegated to civil servants was deemed a "fiction"; not only were ministers overloaded with work but they were mostly unsuited to management. The solution was to separate policy making from regulatory practice. The task of formal regulation was delegated to agencies, often called "quangos," that is, judicial or quasi-judicial, autonomous bodies. Quangos emulate commercial organizations. Their employees are responsible to boards of unelected directors, who, in turn, are accountable upward to ministers but never downward to the electorate (Cole 1998).

In 1990, the Human Fertilization and Embryology Act was passed by Parliament and, the following year, the HFEA began work. The HFEA is an independent statutory body funded partly by the fees charged by licensed IVF centers and partly by the taxpayer. Its primary aim is to "safeguard [although because it does not say from what, it allows itself a roving brief] all relevant interests: patients; children; the wider public; and future generations." Its objectives are "to ensure that both treatment and research are undertaken with the utmost respect and responsibility." Its principal task is "to regulate, by means of a licensing system, any research or treatment which involves the creation, keeping and using of human embryos outside the body, or the storage or donation of human eggs and sperm" (HFEA 1993, 1).

HFEA personnel are responsible to a committee of twenty-one members, appointed by the secretary of state for health, a politician. The chair and at least half of the committee's members are neither doctors nor scientists involved in research or practice. Their work is laid down in a code of practice, which has twenty-nine sections. Members determine the HFEA's policies and scrutinize treatment and research licenses. Clinics seeking a license or renewal of an existing one complete an application form and are visited by HFEA members and by clinical, scientific, and "social and ethical" inspectors. Like the Abortion Act, the HFEA requires clinicians to submit data on their practice, which it publishes in an annual report. The data, which include

Total number of patients receiving IVF, DI, etc.
Number of different types of procedures
Number of treatment cycles
Size of center
Source of gametes
Number of clinical pregnancies
Number of miscarriages
Number of terminations
Number of ectopic pregnancies
Number of live births
Number of stillbirths and neonatal deaths
Single or multiple pregnancy
Developmental defects and syndromes in children born as a result of IVF,
    DI, or micromanipulation of sperm

measure the efficiency of the technology: it is possible to gauge from them whether, for example, conception is more likely to result from IVF using women's own eggs or donated ones, or if donor insemination (DI) is more effective where women take fertility drugs. With the exceptions of age and cause of infertility (tubal disease, endometriosis, unexplained, and other), the data exclude any information about the women undergoing IVF or DI. Women are invisible. Moreover, although clinics are categorized according to their size (large or small), nothing is said about ownership, although for complex reasons, knowing who owns the premises is no longer a guide to who paid for treatment.[6]

Unlike its Labour predecessors, the Conservative government was not interested in collecting or publishing data on allocative fairness. Moreover, it believed private medicine offers patients choice, and resisted proposals to single it out for special regulatory attention. In its report, the Warnock Committee had also recommended treating both NHS and private clinics in the same way, but it probably did so for another reason: neither structural nor conduct regulation had prevented Steptoe from plowing his own controversial furrow within the NHS. However, in urging the NHS to remedy deficiencies in services for infertile women and men, members of the committee were evidently exercised by the lack of concern for allocative fairness in the treatment of infertility. They expressed surprise at the lack of data on both the prevalence of infertility and on treatment services, and they pressed NHS policymakers and planners to fund the collection of statistics on both, perhaps similar to those on abortion. Moreover, in recommending the establishment at national level of a working group that would draw up guidance on the organization of services, it demonstrated an increasingly unfashionable belief in centralized planning by government.

The Conservative government failed to act on the Warnock Committee's recommendations in relation to statistics. Instead, rough and ready data on NHS provision of infertility treatment were collected by campaigners concerned that access to IVF was determined by ability to pay, not by need. In 1986, Frank Dobson, a Labour MP, then shadow minister of health, sponsored a survey of NHS provision. The report, which claimed to give "a much clearer picture of the services available, or to be more accurate the services not available," concluded with the following: "This Government frequently proclaim their commitment to family values and to the health service. Their utter indifference to the problem of the infertile gives the lie to both these claims" (Mathieson 1986, 28). In 1988, the Greater London Association of Community Health Councils, a voluntary organization examining and commenting on the capital's health services, recommended the Department of Health and Social Security issue clear guidance on development and funding of specialist services for infertility (Pfeffer and Quick 1988, 5). When Dobson's survey was updated in 1990 by Harriet Harman, a Labour MP, then shadow minister of health, she found geographical disparities in provision had worsened (Harman 1990).

Set up in 1991 by a Conservative government convinced of the virtues of the market and competition and individual private choice as regulatory mechanisms, it is not surprising that, instead of data on allocative fairness, the HFEA publishes *The Patients' Guide to DI and IVF Clinics*. Its purpose is "to help people who are considering DI or IVF to understand the services offered by licensed clinics and decide which would be the best clinic for them" (HFEA n.d., 4). The Guide places responsibility for obtaining appropriate treatment squarely on patients. A typical piece of advice is, "You should feel quite free to decide against a clinic" (HFEA n.d., 5). While this advice speaks in favor of regulation by competition, it can be heeded only by women with information and resources necessary to "shop around."

In the early 1990s, organizations representing patients began to collect data on NHS funding of licensed infertility treatments. According to the *Report of the Third National Survey of NHS Funding of Infertility Services,* published in July 1995, at the most, 2,990 IVF cycles had been purchased in the previous year by the NHS (Wiles and Patel 1995). According to the HFEA, in the fifteen months between 1 January 1995 and 31 March 1996, 36,994 IVF treatment cycles were carried out, which, roughly speaking, means that nine out of every ten cycles are paid for by the patient (HFEA 1995, 29). Women have to find the money themselves; private insurance schemes do not cover IVF.

One possibly unintended beneficiary of the system of regulation established by the Human Fertilization and Embryology Act is the government. In delegating rule making and by handing over the power of prior approval and its enforcement to the HFEA, the issue of human embryo research that had consumed so much of its attention was effectively depoliticized. Since 1990, controversies relating to human embryos or provoked by new developments in reproductive technologies have been dealt with by members of the HFEA, not by British politicians. Parliamentary debate and the deliberations of official committees have been replaced by a "continuing dialogue with all those involved in, or concerned about, the area of assisted reproduction," which is conducted at an HFEA annual conference attended by staff of licensed clinics and HFEA members and staff, and by formal and informal consultations with professional bodies and organizations.

CONCLUSION

When both the Abortion Act and the Human Fertilization and Embryology Act were introduced, public and parliamentary debate focused mostly on the human embryo. Nonetheless, both acts have had a considerable impact on women's lives. I want to conclude by highlighting how the different approaches to formal regulation of reproduction represent women.

When the Abortion Act was passed in 1967, welfare politics were still in the ascendancy. Doctors who profited from abortion were vilified. Women forced to pay for the operation were seen as recipients of exploitation and their numbers sullied the reputation of the NHS. In practice, the Abortion Act of 1967 saw women as citizens, with entitlements to free treatment. Emerging in a political climate that applauded regulation by the market, it is not surprising the HFEA treats women as consumers, with no rights as citizens and many responsibilities as consumers. Moreover, in this ideological context, inability to pay for private treatment discredits women. This is evident in the many newspaper stories about women unable to find the money necessary for a licensed infertility treatment. For example, in April 1995, the front page of the *Daily Mail* was emblazoned with the headline "Shame of the Test Tube Mother." The article described how a twenty-seven-year-old accountant had stolen £20,000 from her employers in order to pay for infertility treatment. It had "worked." However, days after she had found out that she was expecting triplets, the police had arrested her. As Zygmunt Bauman has argued, where individual choice is exalted, those excluded from making choices are the "new poor," disenfranchised and oppressed.[7]

NOTES

1. I am grateful to Doris Zallen for drawing my attention to the circularity of many definitions of regulation.

2. This section draws heavily on Ogus (1994).

3. See Pfeffer 1993. For an excellent analysis of the situation in the United States, see King and Meyer (1997).

4. Before the 1967 act, there was no statutory requirement of notification of abortion, hence precise figures are unavailable. Many abortion were disguised as D&C (dilation and curettage). It was known that abortion formed a substantial part of gynecologists' workload, up to one in five admissions to hospitals (Lane Committee 1974, 12).

5. *Special Reports and Minutes of Evidence of the Select Committee on the Abortion (Amendment) Bill Together with the Proceedings of the Committee, Session 1974–75* (London: HMSO, 1976), 64.

6. In the 1980s, the distinction between NHS and private clinics was blurred by clinicians offering IVF when they introduced private practice and charitable schemes into NHS hospitals (see Pfeffer 1992). The internal market introduced into the NHS in 1991 has confused the situation even further.

7. Quoted in Gabriel and Lang (1995), 38.

REFERENCES

Allsop, Judith, and Linda Mulcahy:
  1998   *Regulating Medical Work: Formal and Informal Controls.* Buckingham: Open University Press.
Botting, Beverley J., Alison J. Macfarlane, and Frances V. Price (eds.):
  1990   *Three, Four, and More: A Study of Triplet and Higher Order Births.* London: HMSO.
Breyer, Stephen:
  1982   *Regulation and Its Reform.* Cambridge: Harvard University Press.
Clarke, Adele E., and Joan Fujimura:
  1992   What Tools? Which Jobs? Why Right? In Adele E. Clarke and Joan Fujimura (eds.), *The Right Tools for the Job: At Work in Twentieth-Century Life Sciences,* 3–44. Princeton: Princeton University Press.

Clarke, Kenneth:
  1990 *House of Commons, Official Report,* 2 April, col. 915.
Cole, Michael:
  1998 Quasi-Government in Britain: The Origins, Persistence, and Implications of the Term "Quango." *Public Policy and Administration* 13: 65–78.
Crossman, Richard:
  1969 *Hansard Parliamentary Debates,* vol. 782 (1968–69), col. 948.
Davies, Anne, and John Willman:
  1991 *What Next? Agencies, Departments, and the Civil Service.* London: Institute for Public Policy Research.
Franklin, Sarah:
  1993 Making Representations: Parliamentary Debate of the Human Fertilization and Embryology Act. In J. Edwards, et al. (eds.), *Technologies of Procreation: Kinship in the Age of Assisted Conception,* 96–131. Manchester: Manchester University Press.
Gabriel, Yiannis, and Tim Lang:
  1995 *The Unmanageable Consumer.* London: Sage.
Gunning, Jennifer, and Veronica English:
  1993 *Human In Vitro Fertilization: A Case Study in the Regulation of Medical Innovation.* Aldershot: Dartmouth.
Habermas, Jürgen:
  1964 The Public Sphere. *New German Critique* 1(3): 49–55.
Harman, H.:
  1990 *Trying for a Baby.* London: House of Commons.
Himmelweit, Susan:
  1987 Abortion: Individual Choice and Social Control. In *Feminist Review* (eds.), *Sexuality: A Reader,* 98–102. London: Virago.
Hordern, Anthony:
  1971 *Legal Abortion: The English Experience.* Oxford: Pergamon Press.
Human Fertilization and Embryology Authority (HFEA):
  n.d. *The Patients' Guide to DI and IVF Clinics.* London: HFEA.
  1993 *Code of Practice.* London: HFEA.
  1995 *Fourth Annual Report 1995.* London: HFEA.
Johnston, Marie, Robert Shaw, and David Bird:
  1987 "Test-Tube Baby" Procedures: Stress and Judgements under Certainty. *Psychology and Health* 1: 25–38.
Kay, John, and John Vickers:
  1988 Regulatory Reform in Britain. *Economic Policy,* October, 285–351.
King, Leslie, and Madonna Harrington Meyer:
  1997 The Politics of Reproductive Benefits: U.S. Coverage of Contraceptive and Infertility Treatments. *Gender and Society* 11: 8–30.
Klein, Rudolf:
  1989 *The Politics of the National Health Service.* London: Longmans.
Knoppers, Bartha M., and Sonia LeBris:
  1991 Recent Advances in Medically Assisted Conception: Legal, Ethical, and Social Issues. *American Journal of Law and Medicine* 17: 329–61.
Lane Committee:
  1974 *Report of the Committee on the Working of the Abortion Act.* Vol. 1. London: HMSO.

Lovenduski, J.:

1986   Parliament, Pressure Groups, Networks, and the Women's Movement: The Politics of Abortion Law Reform in Britain (1967–83). In J. Lovenduski and J. Outshoorn (eds.), *The New Politics of Abortion,* 49–66. London: Sage.

McNair-Wilson, Michael:

1990   *House of Commons, Official Report,* 20 June, col. 964.

Majone, Giandomenico:

1997   From the Positive to the Regulatory State: Causes and Consequences of Changes in the Mode of Governance. *Journal of Public Policy* 17: 139–67.

Marsh, Dave, Peter Gowin, and Melvyn Read:

1986   Private Members Bills and the Video Recordings Bill (1984). *Parliamentary Affairs* 39: 179–96.

Marshall, E. Clare, and David J. Spiegelhalter:

1998   Reliability of League Tables of In Vitro Fertilization Clinics: Retrospective Analysis of Live Birth Rates. *British Medical Journal* 316: 1701–4.

Mathieson, David:

1986   *Infertility Services in the NHS: What's Going On? A Report Prepared for Frank Dobson MP, Shadow Health Minister.* London: House of Commons.

Medical Research Council (MRC):

1982   Statement on Research Related to Human Fertilization and Embryology. *British Medical Journal* 285: 1480.

Mitnick, Barry M.:

1980   *The Political Economy of Regulation: Creating, Designing, and Removing Regulatory Forms.* New York: Columbia University Press.

Morgan, Derek, and Linda Nielsen:

1993   Prisoners of Progress or Hostages to Fortune? *Journal of Law, Medicine, and Ethics* 21: 30–42.

Mulkay, Michael:

1997   *The Embryo Research Debate: Science and the Politics of Reproduction.* Cambridge: Cambridge University Press.

Nielsen, Linda:

1996   Legal Consensus and Divergence in Europe in the Area of Assisted Conception— Room for Harmonisation? In D. Evans (ed.), *Creating the Child,* 305–24. The Hague: Martinus Nijhoff.

Office of Population Censuses and Surveys (OPCS):

1996   *Abortion Statistics: England and Wales.* London: OPCS.

Ogus, Anthony I.:

1994   *Regulation: Legal Form and Economic Theory.* Oxford: Clarendon Press.

Pfeffer, Naomi:

1992   From Private Patients to Privatisation. In Meg Stacey (ed.), *Changing Human Reproduction: Social Science Perspectives,* 48–74. London, Sage.

1993   *The Stork and the Syringe: A Political History of Reproductive Medicine.* Cambridge: Polity Press.

Pfeffer, Naomi, and A. Quick:

1988   *Infertility Services: A Desperate Case.* London: GLACH.

Potts, Malcolm, Peter Diggory, and John Peel:

1977   *Abortion.* Cambridge: Cambridge University Press.

Price, Frances:

1989   Establishing Guidelines: Regulation and the Clinical Management of Infertility. In Robert Lee and Derek Morgan (eds.), *Birthrights: Law and Ethics at the Beginning of Life,* 37–54. London: Routledge.

1993   Beyond Expectation: Clinical Practices and Clinical Concerns. In Jeanette Edwards, et al. (eds.), *Technologies of Procreation: Kinship in the Age of Assisted Conception,* 20–41. Manchester: Manchester University Press.

Royal College of Obstetricians and Gynecologists (RCOG):

1983   *Report of the RCOG Ethics Committee on In Vitro Fertilization and Embryo Replacement or Transfer.* London: RCOG.

Simms, Madeleine:

1974   Gynaecologist, Contraception, and Abortion—from Birkett to Lane. *World Medicine,* 23 October, 49–60.

Smart, Carol, and Barry Smart:

1978   Introduction. In Carol Smart and Barry Smart (eds.), *Women, Sexuality, and Social Control,* 1–7. London: Routledge and Kegan Paul.

Somerville, Margaret A.:

1982   Birth Technology, Parenting, and "Deviance." *International Journal of Law and Psychiatry* 5: 123–53.

Steptoe, P., and R. Edwards:

1981   *A Matter of Life.* London: Sphere.

Vogel, David:

1986   *National Styles of Regulation.* Ithaca: Cornell University Press.

Voluntary Licensing Authority (VLA):

1986   *The First Report of the Voluntary Licensing Authority for Human In Vitro Fertilization and Embryology 1986.* London: Medical Research Council.

Warnock, Mary:

1985   *A Question of Life: The Warnock Report on Human Fertilization and Embryology.* Oxford: Blackwell.

Whitehead, Margaret:

1994   Who Cares about Equity in the NHS? *British Medical Journal* 308: 1284–87.

Wiles, Richard, and Hament Patel:

1995   *Report of the Third National Survey of NHS Funding of Infertility Services.* London: College of Health/National Infertility Awareness Campaign.

Williams, Brian T., and Jonathan P. Nicholl:

1994   Patient Characteristics and Clinical Caseload of Short Stay Independent Hospitals in England and Wales, 1992–93. *British Medical Journal* 308: 1699–1701.

Williams, Raymond:

1985   *Keywords.* London: Flamingo.

Yoxen, Edward:

1990   Conflicting Concerns: The Political Context of Recent Embryo Research Policy in Britain. In Maureen McNeil, Ian Varcoe, and Steven Yearley (eds.), *The New Reproductive Technologies,* 173–99. Basingstoke: Macmillan Press.

10

Gender-Based Management of New Reproductive Technologies: A Comparison between In Vitro Fertilization and Intracytoplasmic Sperm Injection

Françoise Laborie

In vitro fertilization (IVF) and intracytoplasmic sperm injection (ICSI) are two reproductive techniques. ICSI, which appeared ten years after IVF, both complements and reinforces IVF. The difference comes from the fact that in IVF, oocytes and spermatozoa are simply placed together in the hope that the spermatozoa will penetrate the oocytes on their own. With ICSI, a spermatozoon is forcefully introduced into the oocyte. Thus we see that the invention of ICSI is addressed to men with male sterility, while IVF was invented to fight against sterility of tubal origin in women.

Although on biological and medical levels, these two techniques carry both uncertainty and risks, numerous differences exist in the arguments made by doctors and correlatively in the ways of developing these techniques. In the case of IVF, it is especially, and almost exclusively, feminists who speak of the risks; more often than not, practitioners withhold comment. In the case of ICSI, it is biologists, geneticists, doctors, and those who practice IVF who, worried, call out loudly and with justification for further experimentation on animals and a slowing down of the progression to human trials. Their fears concern risks for the descendants, surgical risks for the patients, insufficient experimentation on animals, and a lack of knowledge with regard to the fundamental processes. However, it is important to notice that these criticisms are exactly the same as those that the feminists have directed toward IVF—more often than not without any echo.

How can we explain such a difference in the standpoints of some specialists? Furthermore, how can we explain the persistence of this difference now that (as of 1996) approximately nine hundred children have been born as a result of ICSI, and experts' fears have not been confirmed that the mechanical and violent penetration of the oocyte would endanger offspring? One of the possible explanations of the difference lies in the gender-based dimension of both techniques and of their risks. Having investigated the theoretical and practical conditions of ICSI production, I will point out how gender plays a role in the economy of its development.

THE STORY OF THE RESEARCH

For a decade (1984–93) I tried to analyze various social stakes that underlie and organize the development of NRTs (new reproductive technologies) and their legal and ethical regulations in France and Europe. More particularly, having analyzed the scientific literature, I emphasized the very strong sexual differentiation of these technologies: the severity of the interventions and the health risks concerning essentially women. I also analyzed data about the number of risks of abnormality in the children who were born. I had pleaded publicly for an objective, independent, and long-term evaluation to be carried out on these technologies, an evaluation that in fact still does not exist (Laborie 1985 to 1996).

I abandoned all this in 1993, having a feeling of monotony and failure regarding the social usefulness of such research work. I thought I had roughly "understood" which interests were at stake and located different forces in balance. The critical analyses produced by different actors, including feminists,[1] scarcely had any effect on the course of things. If the worries expressed should one day become justified, this would perhaps be on the occasion of the discovery of very harmful consequences for women, their children, and possibly even to society as a whole. Obviously, no one wishes such consequences on a world that has already met asbestos scandals, mad cow disease, and contaminated blood.

From 1994 until May 1996, I turned my professional activities largely to other fields, but I continued to read in the press all that concerned the development of NRTs. I could therefore measure to which point my decision was not inevitably judicious as I read the announcement—heralded by trumpets, as usual—of a new revolutionary technique of micromanipulation of the gametes, named ICSI. Started in 1992 by a Belgian team in Brussels, two years later this new technology was proclaimed a "veritable technological revolution" because it had led to such a large number of births in cases once considered hopeless. Of course, the usual triumphant tone of the media announcing a discovery or a great "first" was there as usual. But speaking of ICSI, certain articles, spectacularly entitled "rape of the ovary," for example, expressed different fears or warnings (Jean-Yves Nau in *Le Monde*).

In France, 1994 was the year of the vote on the laws regulating the NRTs and the year in which two opinions were published: one from the Conseil de l'Ordre des Médecins, and the other from the National Ethics Committee for health and human sciences (in French: CCNE, Comité Consulatif National d'Ethique). Both strongly criticized NRTs in general and ICSI in particular: they addressed several unusual warnings to practitioners for caution in the indications because there were different risks for the health of women, and they recommended long-term objective evaluations of those technologies.

Various techniques of micromanipulation of gametes were already described by the early 1990s, all of which aimed to "help" faulty sperm penetrate the oocyte. After some experimentation on animals, one had tested chemical zona drilling and then partial zona dissection (PZD) of the zona pellucida (ZP) of human oocytes.[2] In a technique called subzonal insemination, practitioners also attempted to introduce (by use of a microsyringe) several sperm *under* the zona pellucida, expecting that the ensuing membrane would take care of selecting only one. These attempts generally failed. Therefore, there was a tendency toward a more and more violent enforcement to oblige/assist the sperm to penetrate as closely as possible to the center of the oocyte. In every case, the success rates were lower than the already slim results of classic IVF, which in good teams does not obtain more than twelve to fifteen evolutive pregnancies (and still fewer deliveries) for one hundred punctures of many oocytes.

The announced "technical revolution" introduces a higher degree of invasion. With ICSI, one injects *into* the cytoplasm—that is, deeper and closer to the nucleus of an oocyte—one single sperm by using a micropipette.[3] This technique was made to allow men who, up to that point, had been considered hypofertile or sterile to father a child without having to resort to using donor sperm—as was frequently the alternative in these cases. The children would therefore carry the genes of their legal or social fathers.

The social consequences were immediately visible: disinterest in sperm banks and a renewal of the long lists of people waiting to enter the IVF centers that practice ICSI, just like ten to twelve years earlier when the first births after IVF began to fuel the flames of hope in numerous sterile couples and lead a lot of people, often without any real need, rapidly toward the IVF centers. The time and the money involved in this new technical procedure are added to the usual costs related to the IVF operations that still remain necessary.

In May 1996, I returned to one of my familiar fields: the annual scientific symposium of French NRT professionals, which I had attended since it began in 1985. The usual symposium's title—"Annual meeting of periconceptology"—had been changed and seemed to indicate the entrance into a new era. So I assisted in the "First meeting of the French Federation of Reproductive Studies," which included, for the first time, the urological and andrological societies. This was an act that symbolically and visibly confirmed the ever-increasing importance that the indication of male sterility has in the development of IVF—a technique intended for women suffering from tubal sterility. ICSI was clearly not there for nothing.

At the very beginning of the symposium, a controversy erupted that, for me as a sociologist of science, was a wonder to behold. On the one hand were those (NRT practitioners and researchers) who pleaded for the absolute necessity of using animals to carry out research on ICSI before developing it any further on a human trial level. On the other hand were those who considered themselves more strongly linked to the world of the clinicians, trying to demonstrate that "experiments on animals add nothing to the research or to the trials done on people." One of them (whom I shall name later on) declared that he could not evaluate a risk that was only speculative. So I found myself back in the fray, studying the sociology of NRT development again.

MATURATION OF THE PROBLEM

The arguments presented through this controversy looked like those developed by some sociologists (Marcus-Steiff 1990, 1991), feminists, and a very few doctors (including Marsden Wagner of the World Health Organization) criticizing many forms of IVF development. These criticisms emphasized the lack of objective evaluation with regard to low success rates and the silence of the practitioners on the risks and the application of improper indications. Some were pleading to put a stop to using women essentially as guinea pigs. Some (Vandelac 1989) expressed their fears concerning the catastrophic developments risked for future generations.

However, at the time of my return to the IVF practitioners, the novelty came from the fact that this time the plea for experimentation on animals before progressing to human trials was made in the setting of a symposium of professionals and was led by Bernard Jegou, director of a research unit at French National Institute of Health and Medicine Research (INSERM). Jegou began by refuting various arguments:[4]

> Just because several stages of classic IVF have been done without experiments on animals doesn't mean that it has to continue! To continue is an argument of Russian roulette with accumulation of risk taking! It is not enough to say that one has not proved that it is dangerous![5] Nor that experiments on animals take too long! Nor that all medical acts involve taking risks! Here, it's not a question of medical adventure but of medical adventurism! The history of ICSI shows that there is a mad acceleration and absence of visible connection to research! Now, we need animal models. We need experiments on animals to be verified and to precede with treatment on humans! We need research independent from the pharmaceutical industries! Some people

have talked about "PMA vigilance," animal models having to be one of the cornerstones of that! There is no lack of questions to be examined: The epididymis—how is it useful?[6] What relationship is there between the morphology of sperm and integrity of its DNA? What are the relationships between different degrees of alteration of the spermatogenesis and the genotype of the sperm? One must analyze the problems of transmission of genetic illnesses—human testing has been badly done!

But there were more surprises in store for me. Among those opposed to animal models was Jacques Testart. Like Jegou, he was director of a unit at INSERM and therefore an independent researcher. He and René Frydman were responsible for the birth of the first French "test-tube baby" in 1982. Then he was one of those refusing to carry out some research on the embryos, notably on pre-implantation diagnosis of the embryos (PID), which he believed risked inducing a rapid demand for "made-to-order babies," that is, responding to wishes for eugenic orders. Moreover, he never had evaded controversy with some clinicians.

He also criticized the practices—in his view, eugenic practices—of the federated network of sperm banks, called Centers for Studies and Conservation of Eggs and Sperm, because they choose the sperm donor assigned to a couple according to the morphological characteristics of the social father. That may be why Testart is sufficiently opposed to resorting to sperm donation to prefer ICSI. Moreover, several years earlier, he took up and publicly developed (Testart 1990) one of the theses of the critical feminists, according to which women had been used as free, intelligent, talking guinea pigs providing the indispensable raw material used for IVF research—namely, their oocytes.

Testart now reversed his alliances, putting himself in opposition to those who, criticizing the development of ICSI, plead for prudence and for experiments to be carried out on animals first. In order to refute the necessity of resorting to animal subjects, he declared during this symposium:

I am even more linked to the world of the clinicians who are putting on the pressure so that we go more quickly. . . . There is no animal model which is comparable to the human model. . . . I have criticized the Belgians who have not carried out research on the mechanical risks of ICSI on animal models. . . . The hormonal stimulations of the ovaries have been done on women without having carried out experiments on animals and without first having understood everything. Why do we ask ourselves questions on male genetics and not on female genetics, which can also constitute a cause of sterility in women?

Far from advocating the caution that had largely contributed to his public reputation, he is reportedly one of those who, working on ICSI, takes the most risks. It appears that in injecting not a spermatozoid but a spermatid (that is, an immature sperm that is only in the primary stages of spermatogenesis),[7] he takes two kinds of extra risks—not to mention the already numerous problems involved in ICSI. First, there is the risk of damaging the oocyte more severely because the size of the spermatid is greater and requires a syringe of a larger diameter. Second, there is the risk of introducing even more disturbance on a genetic level.

Oh, what a surprising change of scenery after such a long absence! My landmarks were so strongly blurred that I was formulating three remarks simultaneously in my mind:

1. In such a context, one could expect some mention of problems concerning the health of babies. Now, as the symposium continued, the results were revealed concerning almost nine hundred children born by ICSI in Belgium. It appears that in these children, the incidence of major malformations (23/900) does not exceed that of children born by IVF, that is to say, that of the population in general (Bonduelle 1994, 1995). Prenatal mortality is, however, 19 out of 1,000, double that which is given for the Belgian population in general (Wisanto et al. 1995). In other words, in the hands of the team from Brussels (and undoubtedly of those who are sufficiently experienced), ICSI gave rather reassuring results, at least in the short term (Liebaers et al. 1995; Martin du Pan, Campana et al. 1995).

2. Furthermore, all of the arguments put forward by Jegou could have been made about classical IVF (as Testart had pointed out, giving one or two examples; now there are a lot of examples that confirm Testart's criticism, and I am going to detail them further on), but that has not been the case: the development of IVF has not been the object of major criticism by most practitioners.

3. Finally, it seemed to me that experiments on animals had already been carried out for ICSI, in all likelihood no more or less than with classic IVF (a point which I intend to verify accurately). But in all likelihood, the progression to human trials had been very fast and carried out *before* the solid results of a consistent evaluation had been established.

POSITION OF THE PROBLEM: CERTAINTIES, COMMENTS, AND QUESTIONS

Having read a great number of scientific publications on ICSI, I am able to present a few certainties and ask some questions. First level of certainty: With regard to ICSI, animal research has been carried out before, during, and after undertaking clinical human trials. Therefore, it is not an absence but an insufficiency of experiments on animals that is emphasized by the specialists.

Second certainty: The plea for the need of further experimentation on animals is not limited to France. Reading the papers in international scientific journals was enough to convince me of that. The arguments put forward are varied and interesting; I shall summarize and present them later on. To avoid all misinterpretation, I must specify that I put forward the latter point without aiming to conclude that there has been sufficient animal research carried out for ICSI. I only suggest that when some practitioners of human reproduction technologies deplore, in the case of ICSI, an absence of consistent research on animal models, they are treating the cases of ICSI and IVF differently. This, more than likely, testifies to greater worry over, and more marked concern for avoiding, certain risks when ICSI is on the agenda.

Of course, with ICSI there is no lack of reasons for worrying a lot, and all the more reason to worry in that indications for using ICSI are increasing very rapidly,[8] like in the history of the development of IVF. However, having examined the reasons given to justify the necessity of developing and deepening research on animals and of slowing down the progression to human clinical trials, I would like to show, confirming my first impression, that many of these concerns could just as easily have been addressed previously to classic IVF. Now, that has not been the case.

Thus, several questions arise: Where does this change in the treatment of the problems come from? What kinds of stakes are revealed by the controversy? Are they cognitive stakes? Or are they ethical stakes? Is it a manifestation of concern for public health? Are the unknown elements surrounding ICSI potentially so much more serious than those which one has ignored concerning IVF? Who risks suffering the possibly damaging consequences? With surgical puncture of sperm, would men become, in their turn, objects of possibly painful and risky experiments? Are the risks of transmission of genetic abnormalities with ICSI entailed by all potential offspring or only by certain categories of offspring? Are some risks entailed specifically by male descendants? Facing these new "concerns," how do we read the previous insufficiency regarding classic IVF? One sees the questions that I ask myself as vast and not devoid of considerations in terms of gender.

RESEARCH ON ANIMALS/CLINICAL RESEARCH

Establishing the precise chronology of the knowledge acquired and the results obtained thanks to research on animals on the one hand, human experimentation on the other hand, would probably be a very fruitful research program.

It is more or less what has been done for ICSI by a team of Australian practitioners (Catt et al. 1995) who presented their work in October 1994 during an international meeting held in Australia.[9] Their article emphasizes to what extent, in the case of ICSI, practical and theoretical knowledge acquired from experimental attempts carried out on human subjects has allowed an improvement of the attempts on other mammals. The authors pointed out that ICSI has been practiced since 1962 in echinoderms and since 1974 in amphibians. They underlined that with mammals, the application of this technique is more delicate and gives variable results. First successful in 1976 in the hamster, where it proved to be easiest, ICSI later allowed the birth of rabbits in 1988, cows in 1990, humans in 1992, and, finally, mice in 1994. According to the authors,

> All the reports showed that injection of sperm into oocytes can cause terminal damage. . . . *This report re-investigates some of the basic parameters of sperm injection in domestic species using knowledge gained from human oocyte injection.* [Emphasis is mine]. The ability to use human oocytes for research is severely limited and so the development of an animal model for the human would rapidly increase our understanding of the mechanisms underlying successful sperm injection. Given the relative ease with which large numbers of oocytes suitable for injection can be obtained, domestic species ICSI would also serve as a training tool for human ICSI.

As with conventional IVF, one sees that the first research and successes have been carried out on amphibians in the last twenty or thirty years. The progression to mammals is much later: at the same time, it both precedes and follows the first births of human babies which, in the case of ICSI, were obtained in 1992 (i.e., after the births of rabbits and cattle, but before the births of mice). But more than that, it is the research carried out on humans (and therefore from the oocytes punctured with some risks to women) which allow the understanding and conquering of certain difficulties encountered in animals. It was explicitly the same case with classic IVF, where births in humans preceded, and made it possible to achieve, those of cattle and pigs—a point which further reinforces the similarity in the ways of development of both techniques.

ANALYZING THE ARGUMENTS OF PROFESSIONALS PLEADING FOR EXPERIMENTS ON ANIMALS

How might we understand the differences outlined above in the debates regarding IVF and ICSI? To examine this problem, I have studied the arguments being forwarded by professionals pleading for further animal experimentation. My sources are the articles published in scientific journals; minutes of symposia, sometimes followed by discussions among various practitioners of ICSI; some letters to the editors that appeared in the "debates" section. During the last three months of 1995, some scientific journals opened their pages to rich debates on the safety or the dangers of ICSI. In October 1995, *Human Reproduction* published five articles in its "debates" section under the global title "Rewards and Risks in ICSI" (C. de Jonge and J. Pierce 1995; S. C. Ng et al. 1995; P. Patrizio 1995; A. Van Steirteghem, H. Tournaye, et al. 1995; R. Yanagimachi 1995). Furthermore, after publishing a very alarming article in September 1995 (In't Veld, H. Brandenbourg et al. 1995), pointing out that a very high incidence of chromosome abnormalities was observed in a fairly weak series of fetuses produced by ICSI, the *Lancet* published in October 1995 five letters to the editor responding to or commenting on the previous article. Among the five letters, there is an article written by the Brussels team of Van Steirteghem, who had obtained the first and the most numerous births by ICSI.[10]

Analyzing and summarizing these publications, I shall present the following synthesis of the principal arguments, which some practitioners used to plead for caution with regard to the development of ICSI in humans and achieving more experiments on animals.

I have singled out six patterns of arguments: the first three emphasize that, until now, we do not know, we do not understand, the fundamental mechanisms of human reproduction nor the disturbances that are inevitably introduced by ICSI. There will be perturbation in the complex processes of maturation, selection, and preparation of the sperm to be able to achieve fertilization. Neither do we know what happens in the very early stages of fertilization. Thus, there is the forced mechanical introduction of deficient, abnormal, even immature spermatozoan, which leads us to examine the possible links between aberrant morphology and genetic defects of the sperm. On the other hand, this injection risks allowing the involuntary entrance of virus or foreign substances, even foreign genes into the oocyte.

The fourth type of argument raises the question of risks linked to surgical interventions carried out on men in order to extract their sperm. Starting with these previous considerations, the fifth focuses on the necessity of carrying out more experimentation, thus disposing of a very large number of oocytes and, consequently, resorting to female animals as possible providers of oocytes. Finally, in the sixth type or argument, ethical considerations are developed that are correlated with the use of procedures that, like ICSI, are still experimental.

Let us now present and comment on the different types of arguments.

Argument 1. Fundamental mechanisms have to be understood

It is first argued that one must understand the fundamental mechanisms which explain that, with ICSI, "it works"—even with a sperm that has the most "abnormal" morphology, provided that it is still living. That ICSI "works" has been shown first by the results of the Belgian team, then later confirmed by others. Thus, the Australian authors previously quoted (Catt et al. 1995) wrote: "The basis of how and why ICSI works is poorly understood and virtually nothing is known about what happens to the spermatozoon and oocyte in the few hours following sperm injection. Research with human material is of necessity limited, so the use of domestic species should promote research into the fundamental mechanisms of ICSI."

So, in order to improve understanding, what to do? According to many authors, there are two main programs:

a. One must get to know better the complexity and the chronology of the biological and morphological processes which, in normal fertilization, delicately regulate the very early stages of maturation of the gametes, preparation for their conjunction, their fusion and the fertilization, and the early cleavage of embryos. This is the mandatory prerequisite to correctly evaluate any disturbances introduced by ICSI and their possible consequences.

R. G. Edwards, who first obtained the birth of a baby by means of IVF (and thus cannot be suspected of being critical or wary of innovative technologies in the field of NRT) shows to what degree the complex molecular processes of fertilization can be disturbed by ICSI. Nevertheless, his position seems ambivalent with regard to ICSI: despite his remarks he does not plead for animal research, while at the same time writing (Edwards 1995):

> A high percentage of two-pronuclear eggs form after ICSI, which is surprising since it apparently bypasses the closely-knit interactions which normally occur during fertilization, including sperm-egg fusion, membrane hyperpolarization, calcium discharges and activation of the egg. *However, success with ICSI may have been a narrow victory, since many oocytes display a disordered activation.* . . . The successive stages of fertilization after ICSI seem to proceed at the same rate as, or more quickly than, normal fertilization. Nevertheless, pronuclei form asynchronously in 25% of human oocytes after ICSI; approximately 7% of the eggs have three pronuclei after ICSI; the frequency of asynchrony seems to be greater than after IVF. . . . ICSI clearly disturbs the normal course of events. . . . Piercing the *oolemma* with the injection pipette might induce calcium discharges and activate the egg. . . . Many eggs with two or more pronuclei have apparently passed through a near-normal activation process and are fully capable of growth to full term fetuses. *We will not know which activating systems are involved until we have acquired more data on the nature of hyperpolarization and the ultrastructural events which occur in human oocytes after ICSI.* . . . *The injection of spermatids or spermatozoa might*

disturb the fine architecture of the oocyte. . . . Chromosomal segregation would be disturbed, leading to the formation of complex monosomic or trisomic embryos. Evidence from IVF shows that an imbalance of these factors in the oocyte and in the sperm nucleus may cause various disturbances at fertilization. Such disorders could occur with increasing frequency after the injection of spermatozoa or spermatids into oocytes. . . . Chromosome movements could be disturbed during ICSI. [Emphases are mine]

Reading Edwards, one understands that ICSI obviously disturbs, not only mechanically because of the violent intrusion of a syringe but also through the delicate molecular processes that organize the subtle and well-timed ballet of conjunction of the gametes.

Well, of course! But one question springs immediately to mind. How is it possible that Edwards never addressed this kind of remark to in vitro fertilization, when one knows (and that knowledge would obviously be shared by Edwards, who invented this technique) the detail of the stressful operations to which not only women but also their oocytes are subjected before the step of in vitro fertilization? What about the delicate procedures described by Edwards when carrying out classic IVF: one uses a large number of oocytes (sometimes several dozen) that have been collected simultaneously during the same cycle after having been forced by huge doses of various hormones and which consequently present an often insufficient maturation? What about the delicate processes when we remember that oocytes are sometimes harmed by the acts—also violent—of surgical punctures? If, in case of IVF, the biologist can generally eliminate the nonfertilized oocytes, why would this same procedure of elimination, of selection of nonfertilized gametes, not be sufficient in the case of ICSI? Are not Edwards's remarks concerning ICSI pertinent and applicable in the case of conventional IVF? Once again, why are the discourses so radically different in situations where they could well be the same, or at least similar, differing only in the degree to which ICSI introduces new risks relative to those already present in IVF, and thus introducing a gradation in warning against it?

b. Returning to the arguments of the professionals pleading for further animal experimentation on ICSI, we have discussed their demands for a better understanding of the general mechanisms of maturation and fertilization. On the other hand, they demand a specific understanding and evaluation of the importance of the role of the epididymis in the maturation of sperm. There seem to be some differing points of view here. Two English authors (Tsirigotis and Craft 1995) even write: "The old concept that spermatozoa need to go through the full length of the genital tract before they are able to achieve fertilization is no longer valid." This is also the opinion of André Van Steirteghem and his colleagues (Nazy et al. 1995).

Many authors, however, do not seem to agree with this remark, nor are they ready to conclude the innocuousness of the suppression of biological barriers in selecting sperm. Among them, Axel Kahn, geneticist and member of the National Ethics Committee, declared in March 1994, during an interview that appeared in the daily French newspaper *Libération:* "With ICSI, one short-circuits all competition between spermatozoids. However, one ignores the biological function of this competition: if such sperm succeeds in penetrating the oocyte, is that by chance or thanks to a natural selection? In the cases for which ICSI is used, sperms are deficient: is there not then a risk of favoring the transmission of an unsuspected genetic abnormality linked to this failure?" (Bensimon and Dufau 1994).

So Axel Kahn deplores the fact that ICSI suppresses the biological barriers which, surrounding the oocyte, select sperms that are competing to achieve fertilization. Let us comment on his position:

Here again, one can only make the parallel with the methodology of IVF. With ICSI, many practitioners wonder about the possible risks resulting from two processes: on the one hand, the mechanical forcing of the biological barriers of the oocyte, on the other hand, the possible nonmaturation of sperm when they have been aspirated before having circulated in the genital tract (epididymis). With IVF, two very similar processes have not given rise to such critics. The retrieval of many oocytes during the same cycle after hormonal stimulation renders most of them immature. On the other hand, puncturing the oocytes on the ovaries suppresses the step in which oocytes move along the fallopian tubes, a step in which they usually achieve their maturation. Then one must be allowed to ask the question: Are the first two processes (mentioned in case of ICSI) disturbing the sperm maturation riskier than the two latter (used during attempts of both IVF and ICSI), which disturb the maturation of oocytes?

In addition, inspired by the remarks of Axel Kahn, one could ask if the ovulatory dysfunctions of women may not sometimes come from genetic defects. Will it not also be a matter of concern with regard to IVF progeny? In other words, could little girls whose mothers suffer from ovulatory deficiency have inherited their mother's ovulatory problems? Why has this not, to my knowledge, ever been brought up?

Argument 2. Long-term risks for children, males in particular

It is necessary to clarify a problem linked to the preceding question—whether or not there are any links between aberrant morphology and genetic defects in sperm. If the answer is positive, one would therefore have to ask whether ICSI induces any long-term dangers to children, males in particular. If these links exist, knowing that with ICSI one injects sperm whose morphology is abnormal (their movement is very slow, even nonexistent, or they are immature), there is a risk of transferring one or several genetic defects to descendants. One must therefore test, even in the long term—that is, in the pubescent offspring—the risks linked to the type of injected sperm and the links between some types of male sterility and genetic abnormalities of the sperm.

If the links exist, two kinds of consequences are possible: either the genetic defects discovered are carried by the Y chromosome and will therefore be transmitted exclusively to male descendants who, at the very least, also risk being sterile, or the genetic defects or mutations are potentially transmittable to all of the children. Thus it was discovered in 1993 that the absence of vas deferens (a major cause of male sterility) often results from a genetic mutation linked to the serious illness called cystic fibrosis. This father's mutation may be transmitted to descendants, and if the same mutation also exists in the mother, performing ICSI in such conditions may even lead to the cystic fibrosis of the child.

a. In one version of this argument, Patrizio (1995) writes:

> Potential concerns relating to the use of ICSI may be divided into at least two categories: firstly, ICSI-independent problems; secondly, ICSI-dependent problems (i.e., related to the technique itself). In the first category are all the conditions in which ICSI is used without understanding the true reasons for its indication. We are now starting to understand that some forms of incomplete maturational arrest presenting as *azoospermia* and some cases of extremely severe *oligoasthenozoospermia* are due to deletions present on the long arm of the Y-chromosome. What will be the result of ICSI in this instance? Would we be passing on a mutation to a male offspring that will render him infertile? Do the parents accept the risk? How many more cases of genetically associated infertility, either in males or females, may only appear at puberty or later in life?

And he concludes on a question concerning the possible future of children born by means of ICSI: "Should our colleagues, pediatricians, obstetricians, and general practitioners be prepared to ask the means by which reproduction was attained when facing an unusual clinical scenario?"

His interrogative conclusion could as well have been one of those signed by the critical analysts of IVF, notably the feminists (Pappert 1988; Laborie 1988c, 1994a, 1994b; Holmes 1988; Vandelac 1989) who have added to this worry for the children that of the health of the women. In fact, these feminists have very often predicted and denounced a scenario all the more likely in that it actually happened some years ago. Some oncologists or other specialists, faced with different pathologies and even cancers, would not think to correlate the sickness observed in women with the long-term effects of the treatments to which their mothers (or they themselves) were submitted ten or twenty years previously during IVF attempts.

b. In another version of the argument concerning the health of children, C. de Jonge and J. Pierce base their warning on biological and ethical considerations.

> It has been demonstrated that the zona pellucida and oolemma act to select
> normal sperm. These findings raise the question of what the implications
> might be when these selective barriers are bypassed using ICSI. The selection
> of spermatozoa for ICSI from a male factor infertility patient based solely on
> a cursory overview of morphology may unwittingly result in the transmission
> of chromosomal abnormalities. Reports of ICSI success using sperm aspi-
> rated from individuals with congenital bilateral absence of the vas deferens
> are emerging. For some individuals this anatomical defect is expressed as a
> result of a mutation related to cystic fibrosis (CF). Although recent data tend
> to offset those concerns, the evidence presented above stimulates questions of
> whether the passage of genetic defects from spermatozoa to offspring will be
> facilitated by ICSI. *The reproductive ability of these individuals is not able to be
> determined at the present time.* [Emphasis is mine]

c. Finally let us note that the Brussels team members of Van Steirteghem say they address a warning to the future parents about ICSI's risks of transmission of sterility in male children. In order to avoid the birth of children possibly bearing the cystic fibrosis illness, the team states furthermore that there is an imperative necessity to control parental genomes, and those of the embryos, before their transfer in utero: "Although ICSI has been applied in many centres around the world we still feel very strongly about the correct and careful counseling of the patients. The couples should be informed about the unknown aspects of the procedures. It may well be that certain forms of male infertility may be genetic in origin. *The parents should be informed that their male offspring may have similar problems to their father* [emphasis is mine]."

Argument 3. Risks induced by the procedure of injection itself

a. Additional risks exist due to the sperm injection process. There are possible concomitant introductions of contaminant products of chemical and/or biological origin that can carry foreign DNA possibly capable of mixing with the sperm's DNA.

Patrizio (1995) writes:

> ICSI-dependent problems are the concerns that stem from the use of ICSI without complete understanding of the potential "long-term effects" of the technique itself. Exogenous, heterologous DNA can be carried into the oocyte at the time of ICSI by the spermatozoa; and so other potential foreign material contained in the sperm suspension may be inserted into the eggs. *Without the use of ICSI, it was shown that homologous and heterologous macromolecules may be incorporated in mouse epididymal spermatozoa, transferred into the eggs and produce transgenic offspring at a frequency of 30%.*

Emphasis is still mine as I discover—thanks to this quotation about ICSI—some other major risks concerning conventional IVF "without the use of ICSI" that I had never heard about. As far as I know, these risks had until now been hidden and never been brought up. Anyway, one can easily understand that invading the heart of an oocyte by using a syringe increases the risks of introducing chemical, biological toxic substances and, in the worst cases, the risk of injection of bacterial or viral DNA or DNA from some animal species.

b. There is also a risk of damaging the genetic material of the oocyte and perhaps even its fine architectural structure (see Edwards above).

Argument 4. Risks linked to surgical interventions on men in order to extract spermatozoids

The risks linked to the withdrawal of sperm in men are usually invoked not as a reason for demanding more experimentation on animals but as an appeal for caution with regard to ICSI. Surgical aspirations of sperm are done either from the epididymis (the technique called MESA: Micro-Epididymal-Sperm-Aspiration) or from the testicular tissue (the technique called TESE: TEsticular Sperm Extraction). These interventions seem to be carried out with increasing frequency, possibly as the indications for use of ICSI have increased. Such extractions are carried out particularly in cases of obstruction due to infections, accidents, vasectomies, or in case of deficient erections or ejaculations (absence of vas deferens or testicular disorders). Tsirigotis and Craft (1995) wrote: "The MESA technique involves acquired microsurgical skills, and a certain amount of trauma and post-operative morbidity may occur, e.g., potential pain, hematoma formation and infection. In addition, any further surgery may be more complex because of post-operative fibrosis. The cost of the technique is also high and post-operative recovery may be protracted if complications do occur."

In fact, in some cases of azoospermia, or lack of ejaculation, obtaining sperm is done by an aspiration of the contents of the epididymis, or indeed by a surgical extraction from the testicular tissue. In other words, men seeking to be fathers feel obliged to submit themselves to surgical procedures that are possibly traumatic and painful. As for men, this is a whole new attitude, an unseen scenario, an unprecedented way of participating in making babies.

Thus, what a change in men's feelings about the—technological—way of making babies! A considerable social change from a gender-based standpoint!

However, in order for IVF to be carried out—and also obviously in the case of ICSI—many women (some of whom are not sterile at all) have to undergo surgical punctures, under local anesthetic, of dozens of oocytes on their ovaries, without anyone, except the feminists, worrying about it.

One needs to know that this surgical puncture operation has almost always been preceded by a hormonal blockage of the ovaries—putting the women in a state of temporary menopause, in order to avoid their "savage" spontaneous ovulation and more easily control the induction and the occurrence of their next ovulation. Thus, the ovaries are very strongly stimulated by means of various hormones, in stronger and stronger doses year after year.[11]

When it works, very often the pregnancies are, according to a new concept, "highly multiple" (which means that four, five, or even more fetuses are growing in the uterus). This leads practitioners to urge that women and couples accept an "embryonic reduction," in other words, a selective abortion, in order to keep and to allow only two, or at the very most three, fetuses to develop in utero. One should also know that this latter intervention is not without risk of provoking, in about 10 percent of cases, a total abortion. This obviously constitutes a veritable catastrophe, since these couples have already undergone numerous physical and psychological ordeals and have seen success beginning to take shape.[12] One can see that concerning women, their bodies, and their health, things are far from being harmless: "light" or "moderate" hyperstimulations are the everyday procedures of IVF (and, of course, also of ICSI) trials, and surgical punctures of oocytes are considered inevitable.

Let us mention another supplementary reversal of the conventional circumstances required to achieve procreation. By sexual intercourse, millions of sperm are ejaculated in order that one of them might fertilize a single oocyte produced by spontaneous ovulation. On the contrary, with IVF, practitioners want to utilize several oocytes and only a few sperm, and even fewer in the case of ICSI.

Some people will see in these new techniques the manifestation of an equality of treatments of men and women that would be beneficial to the relationship between the sexes. I note an obvious dissymmetry: When it is a question of male gametes, one immediately emphasizes the traumatic and possibly dangerous character of the surgical puncturing procedures, whereas, when dealing with the puncturing of oocytes, one does not stop emphasizing to which point the procedures are easy, well mastered, and perfectly innocuous.

Argument 5. As a consequence of the preceding reasons, one must carry out even more experiments and, therefore, have at one's disposal a great number of oocytes

To Catt et al. (1995), it is the number of oocytes necessary for new research that justifies resorting to animal models. One may ask whether pleading for animal research on ICSI does not correspond, for the authors, even more to a utilitarian or practical argument (one needs an enormous amount of oocytes, more than the women are able to provide) than to an ethical argument (not to use women as guinea pigs) or health concerns (there are unknown risks). This seemed to me to be confirmed by the principal points that Catt et al. gathered in conclusion:

> Given that ICSI in domestic species works, then the following uses of the technique must be considered. (1) Availability of material: The only constraint on the number of oocytes is the amount of time, expertise and money available. Since abattoir-sourced ovaries are essentially waste material, the oocytes are economical and it is ethically sound to use them. (2) Training: Most IVF units have found that technical competency with ICSI takes time and experience. ICSI with domestic species is technically similar to human and thus, is suitable as a training tool. Given the constraints in some units, states or countries on the use of human material for either training or producing zygotes not for transfer, then the alternative of using material from domestic species is attractive.

Once more, it is clear that these remarks could have been made with regard to the great number of experimental research projects that are carried out in "classic IVF," thanks to the oocytes of women.[13]

Argument 6. Ethical considerations

Finally, some authors (de Jonge and Pierce 1995; Hervé and Moutel 1995) plead for experiments on animal subjects in the name of what they say are ethical considerations.

a. De Jonge and Pierce write:

Before ICSI can be condoned as an acceptable clinical procedure, several ethical concerns exist that require careful consideration and discussion. The first set of issues results when a new technique or drug makes the transition from an experimental clinical procedure to a routinely applied clinical procedure. The second set involves "procreative rights" and the conflicts that can result when individual rights are exercised and the potential harm to others. The biological mechanisms of ICSI are not well understood. In addition, animal research data are lacking that could support the current, albeit limited, genetic data on children born as a result of ICSI. Thus, given these two significant issues, perhaps ICSI should still be considered an experimental clinical procedure.

These considerations could be addressed to conventional IVF, and one wishes that they had been written to describe the problems posed by the various forms of IVF development. IVF still involves a great number of experimental protocols and is a largely unsuccessful procedure. Even when successful, it leads to the birth of babies whose frequent and serious prematurity causes difficulties for a good number of them. At birth they must be transferred to intensive care units, which does not always avoid certain handicaps or difficulties, which in turn may lead to social problems. Those institutions are obviously very expensive for the society.

Furthermore, the attempts of evaluation made by many feminists have shown that the various protocols routinely tested on women are anything but benign with regard to the consequences for their physical and mental health (Corea et al. 1985; Dhavernas 1986, 1987; Holmes 1988; Pappert 1988; Spallone and Steinberg 1987; Stanworth 1987; Vandelac 1989). Several women—their exact number is not known—have died during or after these treatments. Aside from these extreme cases, the usual treatments lead to side effects presenting various degrees of severity and duration (Laborie 1994b). A controversy still exists on the question of whether the treatments with very high doses of hormones lead to a significant increase of ovarian cancers; it might be an "epidemic," to use the word of a French practitioner. However, I have never heard that this problem induces, on the part of the practitioners, the demand for testing the possible risks of the procedures more thoroughly on animals—and I deplore that.

b. Returning to the ethical reservations expressed regarding ICSI above: Hervé and Moutel (1995), after they too have mentioned most of the risks presented above, express their ethical position by writing:

A review of published work shows that ICSI constitutes human experimentation not preceded by adequate work in animals; it has been done without any ethics committee approval. Thus ICSI is offered to couples without the usual ethical safeguards in clinical research; and its implementation has not been accompanied by any national evaluation protocol to follow the biological risks and societal effects, nor by any epidemiological surveys. These facts explain that 2 years after the institution of ICSI we are proposing discussion of the observance of the following ethical criteria: (1) evaluation of all centers practicing ICSI, with a uniformly consistent methodology and complete openness with respect to practice; (2) the teams practicing ICSI and those carrying out the evaluation should be independent of each other and continuing information gathering, not only about scientific personnel but also about patients and society, on the status of evaluation work. The public would not understand if no rigorous evaluation had been done, at the same time that ICSI is the object of much attention by the media.

These proposals totally converge with the kind of demands previously formulated by different authors (Wagner and Saint-Clair 1989 and Marcus-Steiff 1990, 1991, among others) about IVF. These authors have pleaded for an independent investigation and evaluation of the ways by which the success rates have been measured and calculated at all centers and how the accidents of varying degrees of severity have been hidden. For example, in France there is no question about these accidents in the inquiries carried out for the publication of the national IVF register, called FIVNAT, which, of course, does not even mention their existence. In brief, as Marsden Wagner, director of the European section of "Women and Children's Health" of the World Health Organization, wrote as early as 1989:

> No new technique should become standard until after rigorous evaluation. Until then, it must remain experimental. Evaluation involves assessment of efficacy, safety and costs, including indirect expenditures on treatment of side effects. IVFET and related assisted reproduction technologies have not been scrutinised in this way. . . . There is a lack of randomised trials to ascertain the efficacy of IVFET compared with more established treatments for specific classes of infertility, which seriously hampers evaluation.

CONCLUSION

Unlike with the conditions of IVF development, concerning the appreciation of the risks of ICSI, this time the professionals are divided. The births of a lot of babies, apparently in good health, does not seem to be enough to convince them of the perfect innocuousness of the technique. Some professionals urge caution and plead for the development of sufficiently conclusive research on animals before extending ICSI to a greater number of couples in a greater number of centers. The various examples provided support the hypothesis that I put forward initially regarding the differences between ICSI and IVF discourses.

I think that at least one part of the explanation is due to the fact that with IVF the risks are principally incurred by women and children, the latter regardless of their gender, whereas with ICSI, the same risks for women and children exist plus additional risks for children of both sexes (cystic fibrosis) and for male children in particular (sterility). Furthermore, with ICSI some risks are highly likely for the health of men from whom one will have collected sperm by surgical means (and no longer by masturbation, as with IVF). Finally, considering that one of the forms of masculine sterility—which is an indication for ICSI—may be linked to a serious illness (cystic fibrosis), risks exist for some children (of both genders) to get this illness (bearing in mind that this last risk may be eliminated by means of a preliminary genetic analysis carried out on both parents, or by a pre-implantation diagnosis carried out on the embryos.)

If with IVF there is a gender-based differentiation in the risks to the detriment of women, then ICSI adds various risks applying specifically to men and to male offspring. One sees, therefore, the ways of developing the two techniques as being very different and that the professionals open an ethical reflection based on the health risks induced by the technique. In other words, the differences in the ways of developing the two techniques and of the scientific discussions about them may result from a worry about the gender-based differentiation of the risks: the male sex and the fertility of the male descendant may be specifically at risk with ICSI, but not with IVF. This way of reasoning reproduces ancestral attitudes with regard to the gender-based consideration of the inherent risks of procreation: isn't it normal for women, but aberrant for men, to suffer and to take risks in order to have children?

Even in the case of hypersophisticated technologies, those for which the technical dimensions themselves (precision of the tools, complexity of the process, the competence and skill of the technicians) are strongly determinant, gender is still active and even at work on the processes of the production of scientific knowledge, on the organization of scientific and ethical debates, and consequently on the forms of technological development.

The comparative example here analyzed allows making clearly apparent the existence of a joint construction process of (reproductive) techniques and of gender. Let us consider how practitioners have convinced (and still convince) so many women to take many risks with the procedures engaged in IVF and some other NRTs, including ICSI. Let us face the generalized absence of ethical concern in this regard to the position—at first sight, very much correct—

which prevails about ICSI. One can see that the asymmetry is—at least in part—grounded on an unequal gendered treatment of women and men seeking to have children by means of technology. Obviously this asymmetry reproduces and reinforces the inequality of treatment of both sexes. In other words, it reproduces gender relationships.

However, one may finally wonder whether the criticisms and warnings that some people address to ICSI are not equally the result of previous criticisms addressed to IVF or indeed the consequence of the recent climate of suspicion and distrust about a number of major topics, such as contaminated blood, asbestos, and mad cow disease. These topics have all shown in different ways to which point the logic of profit, so prevalent in the new technological developments, can induce pathologies to the detriment of public health considerations.

NOTES

An earlier version of this article appeared under the title "Construction conjointe des techniques procréatives et du genre: Comparaison entre FIV et ICSI," in *La recherce féministe dans la francophonie: Etat de la situation et pistes de collaboration* (Montreal: Ed. du Remue-ménage, 1999).

1. It is impossible to name them all. I have mentioned in the bibliography some publications of members of the Feminist International Network of Resistance to Reproductive and Genetic Engineering (FINRRAGE) (G. Corea, H. B. Holmes, R. Duelli Klein, F. Laborie, R. Rowland, L. Vandelac) and some collective books written in French that include feminist analysis.

2. Zona pellucida is a kind of external shell surrounding the oocyte—and the very early embryo. It forms a barrier that the sperm must penetrate in order to achieve fertilization and that it must perforate in order for the embryos to implant and develop.

3. According to Diana Payne (1995), "The manufacture and use of precision glass instruments is critical for success with ICSI." She explains that the glass injection pipettes must be precisely beveled and sharp, and they should have a diameter at the tip of 6–8 μm—neither narrower nor wider. Until 1994, the injection and the holding pipettes were handmade on a microforge from glass capillaries adequately cleaned and dried. Then the pipettes have to be polished, beveled, and drawn sharply to produce a sharp point, and then sterilized at 150°C for two hours before use. Payne writes that, "with the increasing of ICSI procedures, several companies now offer high quality pipettes for sale." She gives a precise description of the procedures: first, the spermatozoa has to be immobilized by cutting its tail with the sharp injection pipette, then it is aspirated into the pipette, tail first. The oocyte is held flat against the holding pipette using gentle suction. The injection pipette is positioned so that the oocyte plasma membrane and the tip of the injection pipette are both in sharp focus—this ensures injection through the middle of the oocyte. The polar body is oriented at 12 o'clock and the bevel of the pipette faces 6 o'clock. Practitioners have found that on some occasions the injected sperm become involved in the chromosomes of the oocyte. So they always orient the injection pipette with the bevel facing 6 o'clock in an attempt to reduce the incidence of this abnormal outcome. The spermatozoon is positioned near the pipette opening. The injection is then pushed steadily against the zona pellucida (ZP) until it pierces ZP. To ensure that the oolemma does rupture, the oocyte cytoplasm is aspirated back into the injection pipette until there is a sudden increase in the speed of cytoplasm movement in the pipette, which indicates that the membrane has ruptured. All these procedures are made with the use of micro manipulator set-ups: a microscope equipped with environmental chamber maintained at 37°C in a constant, humidified atmosphere of 5% CO_2 in air.

4. The minutes of this symposium have not been published. Here, I am giving some extracts from my own notes.

5. Do not succumb to panic and refuse all criticism as long as one has not proved the danger—this is an argument one has also heard in relation to mad cow disease, where some people thought they could not take any measures whatsoever as long as it was not clear that the illness could be transmitted to human beings by the consumption of meat.

6. The epididymis is an organ responsible for urinary and genital functions.

7. Spermatogenesis is the process by which the spermatogonia develop into spermatocytes, then spermatids, and finally spermatozoa in the strictest sense. According to the biologists, it is only by these stages of development that a spermatozoon is capable (as long as it is mobile and normal) of penetrating the zona pellucida. Its nucleus then fuses with the (female) nucleus of the oocyte and, if everything is normal, achieves fertilization.

8. To the hypofertile patients are added those whose sperm have abnormal heads (teratospermia), those whose faulty spermatogenesis only allows gathering of immature sperm from the ejaculation, and those whose azoospermia results in the congenital absence of deferential channels—which we know, since 1993, to be a variant of mucoviscidosis. Mucoviscidosis is a disabling illness of genetic origin on a respiratory level that, more often than not, leads to early death.

9. The minutes of this symposium appeared in *Reproduction, Fertility, and Development* 7, no. 2 (1995). Apart from the texts of the articles, there were also extracts of discussions among practitioners—which are always extremely interesting and full of information—for example, on the doubts, questions, and analyses of failures, such as those which one can listen to when one attends professional symposia but which normally are not published.

10. In October 1995 the *Lancet* published four letters to the editor (by Stanton et al., Govaerts et al., Tesarik, and Hervé and Moutel) that were highly critical of ICSI and one letter from the Brussels team (Liebaers et al. 1995) supporting it. These letters were in response to an alarming article by Int' Veld, Brandenbourg et al., published in September 1995, which mentioned having detected, by means of prenatal diagnosis (PND), an incidence of 30 percent (*sic*) of chromosome abnormalities (four out of twelve fetuses) resulting from ICSI. The Brussels team replied by giving them the results from 585 PNDs: it reported 6 chromosome abnormalities (1 percent). They add that, at the time of publication, 877 children had been born after ICSI, 23 of whom (2.6 percent) had major malformations. A Swiss team gives comparable results in a study of 339 babies, which shows that there is 2.9 percent of congenital abnormalities (Martin du Pan, Campana, et al. 1995).

11. These stimulations may, in a good number of cases, lead to hyperstimulations of varying degrees of seriousness which, in the most violent stages, may lead the women to be admitted to intensive care units, where it happens that some of them die. Why is this? Practitioners say they need large numbers of oocytes in order to increase the number of embryos obtained and the chances of realizing a pregnancy (if not always a birth). Transferring many embryos into the uterus (three, four, five, and even more in some instances), they observe an increase in the implantation rate of the embryos and therefore in the number of pregnancies. Once the transfer of some embryos has been carried out, some remain. The spare embryos will be cryopreserved. Once they have been thawed, those that are not damaged by this operation will be transferred, if the first attempt did not succeed or if a second pregnancy is wanted. If more embryos still remain, they are given to a couple, donated to research, or destroyed. It is important to know that even before the start of the procedure, the couples are asked to state in writing what they would like to see happen to their spare embryos. Yet another unseen social problem that is very difficult to think about!

12. However, even in the cases of successful embryonic reduction—in other words, where there has only been a partial abortion and some fetuses remain to develop in utero— that does not mean that there are not severe psychological problems to overcome. In fact, let us imagine the couples, passionately wanting a child for a long time, and having carried out numerous procedures for a number of years without success, who expect to achieve a successful pregnancy as promised and who feel obliged to agree to abort some of their fetuses. As a woman who has pleaded for a woman's right to abortion, I cannot be suspected of being among those who oppose abortion. I think, nevertheless, that this technological correction of a technological error truly constitutes a strong trauma, an almost unthinkable contradiction. It is, however, a solution to which one must—reasonably—quickly agree, but without really having measured it up, in the absence of time with which to think it through.

13. On account of the innumerable protocols, tested experimentally on women and used in IVF, we mention the variability of the pharmaceutical molecules and the doses used for the intense hormonal stimulations that cause the ovaries to develop, in the course of the same cycle, dozens of oocytes; the variability of the techniques and surgical procedures of puncturing the oocytes; of transferring the gametes into the tubes; the ways of embryonic culturing; the techniques for transferring the embryos in utero or in the tubes; the techniques for maturation or congelation of the oocytes, of the embryos, etc.

REFERENCES

Bensimon, C., and S. Dufau:
  1994   Questions sur une fécondation musclée [Questions regarding a forceful pregnancy]. *Libération,* March 30.

Bonduelle, M., et al.:
  1994   Prospective Follow-up Study of 55 Children Born after SUZI and ICSI. *Human Reproduction* 9(9): 1765–67.
  1995   Comparative Follow-up Study of 130 Children Born after ICSI and 130 Children Born after FIV. *Human Reproduction* 10(12): 3327–31.

Catt, J. W., et al.:
  1995   Comparative ICSI in Human and Domestic Species. *Reproduction, Fertility, and Development* 7(2): 161–66.

Corea, G.:
  1985   *The Mother Machine.* New York: Harper and Row.

Corea, G., R. Duelli Klein, et al.:
  1985   *Man-Made Women: How New Reproductive Technologies Affect Women.* London: Hutchinson.

de Jonge, C., and J. Pierce:
  1995   Intracytoplasmic Sperm Injection: What Kind of Reproduction Is Being Assisted? *Human Reproduction* 10(10): 2518–20.

Dhavernas, M.-J.:

1986 Les nouveaux modes de procréation: L'enfer et le paradis [The new means of procreation: Hell and heaven]. *Les Temps Modernes* 42(482): 2–30.

1987 Comme les carabiniers, les enjeux politiques des NTR [Like the carabinieri, the political efforts of new reproductive technologies]. *Les Cahiers du GRIF* 36 (De la pensée à l'eugénisme [Special issue: On thinking about eugenics]): 71–85.

Edwards, R. G.:

1995 Cell Cycle Factors in the Human Oocyte and the Intracytoplasmic Injection of Spermatozoa. *Reproduction, Fertility, and Development* 7: 143–53.

Hervé, C., and G. Moutel:

1995 Sex Chromosome Abnormalities after Intracytoplasmic Sperm Injection. Letter/ comment, *Lancet* 346(8982): 1096–97.

Holmes, H. B.:

1988 In Vitro Fertilization: Reflections on the State of the Art. *Birth* 15(3): 134–45.

In't Veld, P., H. Brandenbourg et al.:

1995 Sex Chromosomal Abnormalities and Intracytoplasmic Sperm Injection. *Lancet* 346: 773–74.

Laborie, Françoise:

1985 Ceci est une éthique [This is an ethics]. *Les Temps Modernes* 462: 1214–55; 463: 1518–43.

1986 La reproduction, les femmes et la science: Des scientifiques en mal de maternité? [Reproduction, women, and science: Science in the disinterests of maternity?] In *Maternité en mouvement,* 181–86. Montreal: Presses Universitaires de Grenoble et St Martin de Montreal.

1988a La radicalité des mères-porteuses [The radicalization of expecting mothers]. In *Sortir la maternité du laboratoire: Actes du Forum International sur les nouvelles technologies de la reproduction organisé par le Conseil du statut de la femme,* 205–14. Montreal: Government of Quebec.

1988b Texte pour la Conférence de clôture [Text for the Consensus Conference]. In *Sortir la maternité du laboratoire: Actes du Forum International sur les nouvelles technologies de la reproduction organisé par le Conseil du statut de la femme,* 365–68. Montreal: Government of Quebec.

1988c Procréation artificielle: Libération ou oppression des femmes? [Artificial procreation: Liberation or oppression of women?] In *Le Féminisme et ses enjeux: 27 femmes parlent,* 287–311. Paris: Edilig.

1989 De quelques faces cachées des nouvelles technologies de la reproduction humaine [On certain hidden aspects of the new human reproductive technologies]. In *L'ovaire-dose: Les nouvelles méthodes de procréation,* 89–114. Paris: Syros-Alternatives.

1992a Des fantasmes à la mise en actes: Offre et refus de la science [Illusions of enactment: Offering and refusing science]. In *Les enfants des femmes,* 93–100. Brussels: Complexe.

1992b Femmes embryons et hommes de science [Embryonic women and men of science]. *Autrement,* no. 6, issue entitled *Le sexe des sciences: Les femmes en plus.*

1992c Incidences des technologies de la reproduction humaine sur la vie quotidienne [Incidents of human reproductive technologies in daily life]. In Alain Gras, Bernard Jorges, and Victor Scardigli (eds.), *Sociologie des techniques de la vie quotidienne.* Paris: L'Harmattan.

1993   Social Alternatives to Infertility. In Patricia Stephenson and Marsden Wagner (eds.), *Tough Choices: In Vitro Fertilization and the Reproductive Technologies,* 37–50. Philadelphia: Temple University Press.

1994a   D'une banalisation sans évaluation et de ce qui peut s'ensuivre [On routinization without evaluation and the consequences thereof]. In Jacques Testart (ed.), *Le magasin des enfants,* 83–106. Paris: François Bourin; paperback, Gallimard, 1994.

1994b   Procréation artificielle: Santé des femmes et des enfants [Artificial procreation: The health of women and children]. In Godelieve Masuy-Strobant, Catherine Gourbin, et al. (eds.), *Santé et mortalité des enfants en Europe: Inégalités sociales d'hier et d'aujourd'hui,* 477–500. Chaire Quetelet, Louvain la Neuve: Bruylant-Academia; Paris: L'Harmattan.

1996   Parents et médecins face à l'embryon: Relations de pouvoir et décisions [Parents and doctors confront the embryo: Relations of power and decisions]. In Brigite Feuillet Le Mintier (ed.), *L'embryon humain approche multidisciplinaire,* 193–202. Paris: Economica.

Laborie, Françoise, Joachim Marcus-Steiff, and Josyane Moutet:

1985   Procréations et filiations: Logiques des conceptions et des nominations [Procreation and parentage: The logics of conceptions and attributions]. *L'Homme 95* 25(3): 5–38.

Liebaers, I., M. Bonduelle, E. Van Assche, P. Devroey, and A. Van Steirteghem:

1995   Sex Chromosome Abnormalities after Intracytoplasmic Sperm Injection. Letter/comment, *Lancet* 346(8982): 1095.

Marcus-Steiff, J.:

1990   Les taux de "succès" de la FIV: Fausses transparences et vrais mensonges [The costs of "success" in IVF: Transparent falsifications and true lies]. *La Recherche* 21(225): 1300–1312.

1991   La controverse sur les taux de succès de la FIV [Controversy over the costs of success in IVF]. *La Recherche* 22(231): 527–29.

Martin du Pan, R. C., L. Campana, et al.:

1995   Traitement de la stérilité masculine par injection intracytoplasmique: Evaluation critique [Treatment of male sterility with ICSI: A critical evaluation]. *Schweizerische medizinische Wochenschrift* 125(31–32): 1483–88.

Nazy, Z. P., P. Devroey P, A. C. Van Steirteghem, et al.:

1995   The Result of ICSI Is Not Related to Any of the Three Basic Sperm Parameters. *Human Reproduction* 10(5): 1123–29.

Ng, S. C., S. L. Liow, A. Ahmadi, E. L. Yong, A. Bongso, and S. S. Ratman:

1995   Intracytoplasmic Sperm Injection—Is There a Need for an Animal Model, Especially in Assessing the Genetic Risks Involved? *Human Reproduction* 10(10): 2523–25.

Pappert, A.:

1988   In Vitro in Trouble, Critics Say. Critics Worry Women Not Told of Fertilization Program Risks. *Globe and Mail,* Toronto, February 8.

Patrizio P.:

1995   Intracytoplasmic Sperm Injection (ICSI): Potential Genetics Concerns. *Human Reproduction* 10(10): 2520–23.

Payne, D., et al.:

1995   Local Experience with Zona Drilling, Zona Cutting and Sperm Microinjection. *Reproduction, Fertility and Development* 7(2): 45–50.

Spallone, P., and D. L. Steinberg (eds.):

1987   *Made to Order: The Myth of Reproductive and Genetic Progress.* Oxford: Pergamon Press.

Stanworth, M. (ed.):

1987   *Reproductive Technologies: Gender, Motherhood, and Medicine.* Minneapolis: University of Minnesota Press.

Testart, J.:

1990   A la recherche du cobaye idéal [In search of the perfect guinea pig]. *Le Monde Diplomatique,* July.

Tsirigotis, M., and I. Craft:

1995   Sperm Retrieval Methods and ICSI for Obstructive Azoospermia. *Human Reproduction* 10(4): 758–60.

Vandelac, L.:

1989   La face cachée de la procréation artificielle [The hidden face of artificial procreation]. *La Recherche* 20(123): 1112–24.

Van Steirteghem, A., H. Tournaye, et al.:

1995   Intracytoplasmic Sperm Injection Three Years after the Birth of the First ICSI Child. *Human Reproduction* 10(10): 2527–28.

Wagner, M. G., and P. A. Saint-Clair:

1989   Are In-vitro Fertilization and Embryo Transfer of Benefit to All? *Lancet* 2(8670): 1027–30.

Wisanto, A., M. Bonduelle, A. C. Van Steirteghem, et al.:

1995   Obstetric Outcome of 424 Pregnancies after Intracytoplasmic Sperm Injection. *Human Reproduction* 10(10): 2713–18.

Yanagimachi, R.:

1995   Is an Animal Model Needed for Intracytoplasmic Sperm Injection (ICSI) and Other Assisted Reproduction Technologies? *Human Reproduction* 10(10): 2525–26.

■ PART THREE

CLINICAL ENCOUNTERS: Users and the Cultural Appropriation of Fetal Diagnostics

Ann Rudinow Saetnan

We have organized our anthology according to two normative chronologies: a chronology of fertility and a chronology of technological innovation. Each chronology is normative in the sense that a certain order of events is expected, even sanctioned as morally preferable, but may not necessarily be enacted in given case histories. In the chronology of fertility, it is expected that one will seek to avoid pregnancy until one's life circumstances are favorable for child rearing (although precisely what circumstances are seen as favorable certainly varies with cultural location and time), that one will then seek to achieve pregnancy (childbearing being almost universally valued), and be protective of the health of mother- and (especially) child-to-be during pregnancy. We have followed this chronology in our order of technologies—the book's first section being directed at contraception, the next at conception, and this third section at fetal diagnostics—and have seen how each technology to some extent serves to reinforce these chronological norms.

According to the normative chronology of medical technology innovation, new medical technologies should first undergo a period of development and testing. During this period, it is expected that they will be applied to clinical usage, but only fairly late in the testing phase and only under careful controls for scientific evaluation purposes. After sufficient testing, and before being released for general clinical usage, it is expected that medical technologies will be subjected to debates resulting in standardized usage policies, in other words, that they will be regulated. Only after these two phases should we (according to these norms) expect to encounter a given technology in routine clinical applications. As we have seen, however, experimental technologies such as IVF may well be offered as routine clinical options while remaining both untested and unregulated. Or regulations may be debated and passed into law without benefit of clinical trial results.

Among the many actor groups linking these two chronologies, we have focused on the technologies' end users—primarily women, but also male partners and offspring. On the one hand, we have examined how they are represented in different discourses at various points where the innovation chronology takes place. Who speaks for them, and how are they portrayed in research proposals? in the laboratory? in field studies? in debates on technology regulation issues? and finally, particularly in this section, in clinical encounters? On the other hand, we have examined how the outcomes of negotiations at those points interact with gendered social structures, norms, and identities—not least as reflected in normative chronologies of fertility. For instance, who is delegated responsibility for fertility control? Under what circumstances are women (and/or men) allowed, encouraged, expected, pressured, forced to use various technologies to limit fertility? Under what circumstances are they allowed, encouraged, etc., to conceive? How are these norms expressed, and to what extent are they incorporated into women's (and men's) identities and behaviors?

When we now turn to fetal diagnostics, we focus on technologies that—tested or not, formally regulated or not—are situated in routine clinical practices. The users we meet, although also imagined and interpreted by various spokespersons, are at the same time live, flesh-and-blood, reflecting, and acting women. Each of these women is confronted with a set of diagnostic services being offered her. Each, more or less independently, threads her own way through the service infrastructure available to her. Individual choices, seen one at a time, may not have much impact on the overall pattern of services or on their meanings in terms of gender, but the sum of many repetitions of similar choices creates a tapestry of meanings and behaviors that may be quite different from the behaviors and meanings anticipated or encouraged by, for instance, service providers. This section focuses, in other words, on actual end users engaged in negotiations-as-navigation.

A number of concerns have been raised, especially in feminist literature, as to how much leeway women have to "navigate" with respect to these technologies and as to what outcomes are emerging from those navigations or from the constraints that restrict them. For instance, there has been concern that as the fetus gains visibility, the pregnant woman loses visibility and/or autonomy—that her own health, knowledge, interests, etc., will be increasingly ignored and her behavior increasingly controlled. There has also been concern that women themselves would lose confidence in their own bodies and their knowledge of their bodies, deferring to physicians to tell them such things as when they got pregnant and how they are faring. And there has been concern that the existence of certain technical "options" such as the possibility of diagnosing and aborting fetuses carrying serious defects might be experienced as a form of coercion, in effect telling women that since the choice is theirs to make, then the responsibility for caring for such a child will also be theirs alone to take. In short, there have been numerous and varied concerns for the effects that implementation of these technologies might have on women's health, autonomy, and integrity.

The chapters in this section address such concerns. In the first chapter, Lise Kvande shows how a Norwegian media discourse on ultrasound has changed over the past two decades—moving from a focus on statistical evidence, to a focus on physician and technology heroics in which women as users were invisible, to a focus on individual users facing dramatic decisions.

Potential end users of the technology are confronted with these messages, as well as with messages their health service providers deem relevant (often messages claiming the safety and reliability of the technology). But end users are not merely passive recipients of "information." In the second chapter, I present results from interviews with Norwegian women who have chosen to use or not to use ultrasound in their pregnancies. The interviews show that these women maintain substantial faith in their own knowledge of their bodies and their life situations, even in the face of counterclaims based on ultrasound.

The next three chapters highlight the cultural variability of meanings attributed to fetal diagnostics. The essay by Lynn Morgan cautions our readers against a possible pitfall in reading these chapters: One should avoid the assumption that modern, western, technoscience-based knowledge is correct, whereas alternative viewpoints from other cultures are merely "ethnoscientific," implying that they are somehow more primitive and less accurate. Morgan shows that the technoscientific view of conception as creating an individual, observable during pregnancy by means of ultrasound, is just as much a cultural construct as is the Ecuadoran concept of the fetus as a liminal figure, not yet fully human, not yet sure of life. This liminality accounts for the possibility of pregnancy loss and infant death in ways that western knowledge must discount in order to perceive an ultrasound image as representing a "baby," an individual with a social and legal existence independent of its mother. This acknowledgment of uncertainty also affects the ways ultrasound is offered to Ecuadoran women and the ways they experience it.

C. H. Browner and H. Mabel Preloran present another example of cultural differences in women's interpretations of fetal diagnostics. Again, this relates to differences in the women's acceptance of technoscience as representing authoritative knowledge. While Euro-American women and acculturated Mexican American women tend to accept health service providers' invitations to follow up an alarming find from an alpha-fetoprotein test with further diagnostics, more recent Mexican American immigrants often choose not to do so. They maintain their faith in the signals from their own bodies and from their own and their sisters' and mothers' previous pregnancy experiences.

Comparing Canadian and Greek women's ways of interpreting and dealing with ultrasound in pregnancy, Lisa Mitchell and Eugenia Georges find that in both cultures, ultrasound represents a striving for modernity—a modernity that is more taken for granted in Canada than in Greece. Another facet of the technology showing both similarity and difference between the two countries concerns the meanings attributed to sonogram images. In the Canadian context, these images are taken as evidence of fetal personhood, as for instance when personality traits are attributed to the fetus on the basis of how it looks and moves on the screen. In the Greek context, personhood is understood as something that emerges more gradually, and personality traits are not attributed to fetuses during sonogram observation.

In the final chapter, Deborah Blizzard presents fetoscopy—a technology that has for some time been sidelined by less intrusive alternatives but that is now reemerging as a new diagnostic and therapeutic alternative. For the time being, this is a technology that only the most resourceful of end users manage to find out about and gain access to. Examining the rhetorical comparisons through which providers and end users seek to make cultural sense of the technology, Blizzard asks how we might apply comparisons at an early stage of technological development to achieve culturally sensitive services in the event the technology becomes routine. In other words, how might we draw on our experiences and analyses of other technologies and apply them to new technologies now emerging? We do not envisage a single universal answer to this question, but we do think that seeking ways for women and other lay end users to find their own voices in these matters and make their voices heard should be part of any answers developed.

11

Screening through the Media: The Public Presentation of Science and Technology in the Ultrasound Diagnostics Controversies

Lise Kvande

Ultrasound technology was introduced into Norwegian maternity care in the late 1970s, which is late compared with other Nordic and western countries. By the mid-1980s, however, ultrasound had come to be offered, de facto, as a matter of routine prenatal care (i.e., offered to all pregnant women even in the absence of symptoms of pathology). This practice of routine diagnostics in the absence of symptoms is known as *screening*. Most hospital districts offered one such ultrasound scan per pregnancy, some two. A single-digit percentage of hospitals did not officially offer screening, but the majority of their patients received a scan nonetheless at the request of their primary care physicians. Capitulating to this fait accompli, it became official national policy as of 1986 to offer a single, nonmandatory ultrasound at around the eighteenth week of each pregnancy (Backe and Buhaug 1986). Both the practice and policy of ultrasound screening in pregnancy have remained stable since the mid-1980s, but they have also remained controversial throughout that time. These controversies have been presented for the public through the mass media. But, as we know, the media seldom tell "the truth, the whole truth, and nothing but the truth." The way the media presents these controversies to the general public thus constitutes a "window" for investigation through which we may catch some of the political and cultural assessments regarding use of ultrasound in pregnancy. The subject of this chapter is the role of the mass media (mainly the newspapers) in the controversies surrounding the use of ultrasound diagnostics in pregnancy in Norway.

The mass media have several aims and roles. One role they lay claim to is that of "watch dog" over authorities and societal development. Taking this claim at face value, one might expect that changes in maternity care would be an important issue in the news. As viewed through a larger spectrum of media, including medical journals and feminist writings, the controversies surrounding use of ultrasound have been diverse and the subject focuses attention on medical-technological development, the care of expectant mothers, and the status of the fetus in our society—just to mention a few of many themes.

Whether we like it or not, our perceptions of these themes are based to a great extent on the presentations we are given through mass media, of what this "really is about." In this perspective the media presentations are important—both as sources of information and as an arena for bringing scientific, professional, and laymen's opinions together in the public debate. Thus the media are not only passive *channels* (literally "media") in this controversy but also active agents.

I will address several questions in this chapter: *Who* appears in the media, and *what themes* are discussed there? *How* do the media present the actors and the subject, political, and cultural values? The perspective here is not whether mass media have given a *true presentation* of the ultrasound field. I am attempting to look at the media material as artifacts of a technological, political, and cultural debate from the 1980s and 1990s, when the journalists and their newspapers appeared to be important storytellers. Taking this approach, we must relate the media presentations not to some "truth about ultrasound" as a form of reality "out there" but to the complex of debates that the presentations sometimes instigated, sometimes reflected, and sometimes ignored.

Since the mid-1980s, both the technological equipment and the medical practice have changed. A main approach has been to analyze whether the media presentations have changed. Concentrating on the last ten to fifteen years, the analysis shows three distinct phases of media discourse concerning ultrasound screening in pregnancy. These are characterized by different themes, different modalities, and to some extent different participants. These phases will be presented shortly.

THE MEDIA MATERIAL

The material for this analysis has been gathered from some of the main newspapers and the national broadcasting channel in Norway, in an attempt to find out in what way the mass media deal and have dealt with questions concerning the use of ultrasound diagnostics in pregnancy since 1982.

The Norwegian newspaper market is characterized by diversity. For a population of only 4 million, there are about 150 newspapers, and Norwegian households take an average of 1.8 newspapers (Allern 1992; Norske Avisers

Landsforbund 1991). Most of the newspapers are local or regional, based on subscriptions and to some extent governmental financial support. This means that even though they are dependent on advertisers, they have a rather high degree of editorial freedom (at least in theory). The newspapers analyzed here are from the three largest cities in Norway: Oslo (*Aftenposten*), Bergen (*Tidende*), and Trondheim (*Adresseavisen*). The *Aftenposten* and the *Adresseavisen* are conservative and share many of the same political views. The *Bergens Tidende* does not differ much from these, although it is based on a liberal tradition. I have analyzed more than five hundred articles, mainly from these newspapers, and nine television programs.

This chapter does not go deeply into the question of media power, economics, ownership, editorial functions, and journalists' framework. The perspective has been the readers': What has actually been written, or not written, in the news? How have the newspapers presented the technology and the scientists? What attention has been drawn to the various aspects of ultrasound diagnostics? Whose voice has the mass media made room for? And what kind of news has gotten the biggest photos and the front-page paragraphs? These have been the main questions here, in order to analyze what information and impression pregnant women are likely to have got from media when they themselves have to consider whether to be examined or not. The purpose has been to find out the information value of the news and to some extent to analyze the discourse(s) on ultrasound technology, as presented in the media.

Recent media research emphasizes that there is no one-way influence from media reports to people's consciousness and opinions (see, e.g., Høyer 1989). What the public actually knows or believes, what pregnant women feel about being examined with ultrasound, may be quite different from what the media have presented.[1] For example, in the case of ultrasound diagnostics, there is reason to believe that women's talk about pregnancy and maternity clinic checkups play an important role in women's interpretations of what this is all about. Everyone who has been pregnant, or who has been near a pregnant woman over time, can tell about how a big abdomen always leads to informal discussions on care for the unborn and other "pregnancy talk." On the one hand, the mass media thus is only one of several sources for collecting information and assessing issues on maternity care, including ultrasound examinations.

On the other hand, the public is nonetheless confronted with the "reality" as the journalists present it. In one sense the readers have to watch the subject through the journalists' eyes, even though they are free to analyze the news as they want and have qualifications for.

News is much more than reflected fragments of "reality." And news is much more than words. The current study is not a linguistic one but an approach of semiotics. This means that nonverbal signs have been considered important—be they photos, headlines, or how and where the news has been placed. In order to analyze both the information and the cultural values of the news, special attention has been paid to modalities in the way of presenting the ultrasound field.

The term *modalities* points to the various signals a text carries that indicate whether the matters referred to in the text should be taken as fact (positive modalities) or treated with some skeptical distance (negative modalities). A positive modality is, for instance, articles where the news is presented as the journalist's own statements of fact, as in the following excerpt: "For the doctors, it is very important to be able to establish the fetus's exact gestational age, and here ultrasound gives particularly accurate information if the examination is performed early in pregnancy. With ultrasound, one can track the pattern of development, and the doctors can to a large extent see how the baby will manage after delivery. This enables them to instigate therapeutic efforts in a timely fashion when necessary" (*Aftenposten,* January 20, 1984). Such articles usually seem more positive and certain than articles just referring to the participants' statements as claims. More positive effects can also be achieved by the use of photos and headlines. For instance, the excerpt above is from the inner-page continuation of a front-page article headlined "Examinations with Ultrasound Save Newborns' Lives." Headlines and illustrations affect degrees of attention, and thus, though indirectly, give signals of what should be seen as most important in the controversy.

A negative modality is, for instance, articles just referring to the actors' claims and work, without trying to present a view of "how things really are."[2] For example, the journalist in the following excerpt points out that it is a select committee who claim that ultrasound should not become routine in prenatal care. Thus the journalist does not necessarily endorse that claim: "Ultrasound technology, the committee claims, should not yet be implemented as a routine examination for all pregnancies, but should be used only according to clinical indications" (*Adresseavisen,* June 20, 1984). Also, statements questioning opinions that have already been regarded "closed" and definite by the participants may be seen as in negative modality.

This kind of analysis makes it possible to assess mass media as a producer and bearer of cultural meaning. There is no doubt that our perceptions of fetal diagnosis in general, and ultrasound diagnosis in particular, have been changing over the last fifteen years. This may be due to technological development, but this is hardly enough to explain why the ultrasound controversies have become so much of a public debate in the 1990s. By examining the mass media, some new perspectives on the connection between society, culture, and technology may become visible.

MAIN TENDENCIES IN THE MEDIA'S PRESENTATION OF
ULTRASOUND TECHNOLOGY AND PRACTICE

The Battle of Statistics, 1982–1986

The controversies surrounding use of ultrasound diagnostics have changed over time. Beginning in the late 1970s, more and more maternity units got ultrasound equipment, but there were differences both geographically and in practical use. The introduction of obstetrical ultrasound doesn't seem to have led to public discussions itself. The first years, the main question was whether all pregnancies should be examined this way, or only high-risk pregnancies.[3] Larssen et al. (1982) stressed that the death rate among newborn children in Norway was higher than in other Nordic countries, for instance, 50 percent higher than in Sweden, and they concluded that one-third of all perinatal deaths could be avoided by better organization within hospitals and maternity care.[4] However, the researchers did not conclude that screening of pregnancies with ultrasound was what was needed to address the problem. Soon a governmental report about maternity care was presented (NOU 1984). The conclusion was that different aspects of the health care system could and should be improved by, among other efforts, a stronger degree of centralization. An ultrasound screening program was also discussed but not recommended: Medical gains had not been documented, and the costs were too high.

Some interesting articles then appeared in the newspapers, which illustrates one of the main controversies from these first years. The researchers (among them epidemiologists) stressed the point of negative cost-benefit assessment, and got some publicity on this. Rather boring articles, in some ways: informative about the research work, but hardly suitable to engage the general readership.[5] Two days later, the same newspapers presented a hospital medical team who had reduced the death rates for infants by 50 percent—thanks, they claimed, to ultrasound diagnostics and some other efforts.[6] These articles represent the start of a rivalry for public attention and legitimacy through the mass media. On the one hand, epidemiologists presented public health statistics, demonstrating that ultrasound diagnostics for every pregnancy is expensive but does not provide any known medical benefits. On the other hand, obstetricians presented their own figures to show that they saved babies' lives. Figures 11.1 and 11.2 give a visual impression of articles typical for this period.

In this first period, pregnant women, midwives, and female/feminist medical professionals are all absent from the media's presentation. It is strange to see how mass media dealt with this important issue for maternity care without taking pregnant women into account. Instead, the clinical professional men were in a sense presented as speaking on behalf of the women.

In this introductory phase for ultrasound diagnostics, the activities were

313

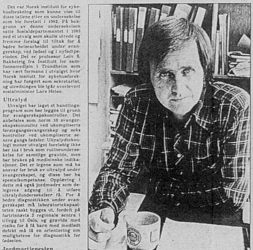

Figure 11.1 A "talking head" (epidemiologist Leiv S. Bakketeig) is used to present statistics on perinatal mortality, *Adresseavisen*, June 20, 1984. The headline reads, "Many deaths avoidable. Perinatal care should be improved, says committee." In the article, the perinatal mortality study group is quoted (i.e., negative modality) as stating that ultrasound technology "should not yet be implemented as a routine examination for all pregnancies."

not a dominant subject in the mass media. Discussions among professionals emerged from time to time, but always on a very general level. In part this may be because the practice was rather unestablished, and there were still no sensations to talk about. The reports were also characterized by journalistic distance (negative modality), in the sense that they mostly referred to what the actors said.

It became clear, however, that there was a need for some regulations in this area. A survey of differences between hospitals in use of ultrasound examinations showed, for instance, that one of the regional hospitals offered six (!) ultrasound examinations to each pregnant woman.[7] By the mid-1980s, between

Figure 11.2 Arguments for ultrasound screening were also offered in the "battle of statistics," here from *Aftenposten,* Oct. 22, 1985. The headline says, "Norwegian research project shows: Profitable to give all pregnant women an ultrasound examination." In a mix of positive and negative modalities, the lead paragraph reads, "Let all pregnant women have access to ultrasound examination. It pays! . . . 'In human terms, medically, and economically, screening with ultrasound has given mainly positive results. Ultrasound has made the fetus a patient in its own right,' says [Dr. Sturla H.] Eik-Nes." The illustration shows Dr. Eik-Nes examining an anonymous pregnant woman with ultrasound.

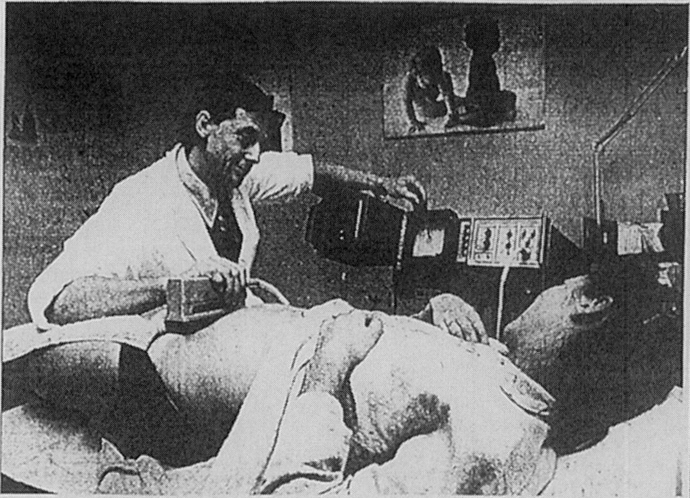

85 and 95 percent of the pregnant women in Norway were offered ultrasound examinations (Backe and Buhaug 1986). Without any special public engagement in this early phase, the clinicians could define their own practice, deciding who and how many to examine within each hospital.

In 1986, the first Norwegian consensus conference was held. The subject was the use of ultrasound diagnostics in pregnancy, particularly the question of whether "to screen or not to screen" all pregnancies this way. The conference went for screening, which later became formalized policy. Since 1986, all pregnant women have had the opportunity to get an ultrasound examination, but they are free to refuse it.[8] A focal point in this decision was the underlining of a need for information to the women before the examination. The principle of "informed consent" should secure women's right to say no and to give them a basis for assessing the risk for finding malformations.

This consensus decision was a strange outcome of the controversy on screening. Although the consensus panel concluded that screening had no known medical gains, they nevertheless went for screening with *one* ultrasound examination per pregnancy—and one of the reasons was a wish to *reduce* the number of such examinations per woman. Research had shown that without legislation, the hospitals had come to be too liberal with the use of this technology.

The consensus conference did not result in closure of the statistical debate but rather in its confirmation. For the mass media, however, the ultrasound issue lost interest as long as it remained a question about statistical benefit analysis. When the question later reappeared on the agenda, it was as a question about ethics—an issue that was largely ignored by the media in this first phase.

Ethical aspects connected to ultrasound diagnostics were largely neglected by Norwegian journalists throughout the 1980s. The media focused on ethical problems concerning IVF (in vitro fertilization) and to some extent amniocentesis, while ultrasound diagnostics were mainly treated as an economic issue. For the clinical experts this was not the case. They examined fetuses, they sometimes found malformations, and they had to deal with the problems of selective abortions. Dr. Sturla Eik-Nes, at that time already the most central man in obstetric ultrasound in Norway, argued for discussing the ethical issues at the first consensus conference, on the basis that findings of malformations would be the central issue confronting ultrasound diagnostics in the following years. During the three-day conference, the professor was allowed only ten minutes to present that theme! The organizers did not want to stress these aspects at the time.[9]

Nevertheless, one might imagine that the media would take ethical approaches into account, but they were silent. Prenatal diagnostics were discussed in general, but the focus was implied to be amniocentesis. The main subject in these discussions became the possibility to choose what kind of babies we want. Actors in these discussions were men: experts within medicine, genetics, or philosophy and laymen—the latter particularly from Christian organizations. But the subject of ultrasound technology was seldom mentioned in these discussions, nor were the clinical experts who worked with ultrasound active. And the mass media let them remain silent, although it was known, of course, that ultrasound diagnostics deals with the same ethical issues as amniocentesis when it comes to diseases.

Other issues were also largely ignored by the media. During this introductory phase, there were a lot of decisions to be made about the organization of ultrasound activities. The media didn't give much attention to this, although some aspects did come up. The expensive technology was mainly obtained by the regional hospitals, while most general practitioners neither had competence to operate it nor money to acquire it. In a small country like Norway, this seemed to be the most rational way to do ultrasound screening. This centralization of health service seems to have been subject to only limited protests from general practitioners.[10] This doesn't have to mean that consensus was achieved, but the media were not concerned about this.

Another issue was which profession(s) would perform the ultrasound examinations. From the beginning it seems to have been gynecologists, some of whom had studied abroad and brought the technology and competence into Norwegian hospitals. When ultrasonography became routine, however, the question about professional competence came up. In 1986, when 85–95 percent of all pregnancies were examined by ultrasound, the Norwegian Association of Midwives laid claim to this work as a part of routine prenatal care and thereby of midwifery.[11] This claim led to some professional controversies until a national educational certification for midwives' use of ultrasound was formalized around 1989.[12] This controversy was quite important to the midwives, who during some years had experienced a decrease in functions and power within the health care system. This issue was nevertheless barely mentioned in the press.[13]

These aspects of the organization of ultrasound services—their geographical distribution, the division of labor, training requirements—have all been subjects of some controversy within and among the professions. Debate can to some extent be found in the professional journals, but it has not been opened up to the general public through the mass media.

The Age of Heroics, 1986–1990

Statistical battles aside, the late 1980s was a time of "good news and great technological improvements" in obstetric ultrasound. In 1985, Dr. Eik-Nes established an ultrasound laboratory at the regional hospital in Trondheim, seeking to make a national competence center in prenatal diagnostics and fetal medicine. There were already established connections to the Norwegian Institute of Technology, and an interdisciplinary team worked with clinical and technological improvements. In 1986, the technicians, in collaboration with cardiologists, developed a new Doppler blood flow instrument that became successful on the international market. Primarily this instrument was developed within cardiology, but it soon became clear that it would be important also for the gynecologists and obstetricians.

Beginning in 1986, the public presentation of ultrasound diagnostics changed. Now we could see the professor and his staff with babies in their arms, babies who (it was claimed) would have died if their mothers had not received a routine ultrasound examination. Of course, this was *good news* in two senses of the phrase—good to hear, and newsworthy. These stories contained all the makings of a front-page article: a newborn child, saved from death; happy parents, humanity, technological "revolution," and clinical masterstrokes.[14] For an example of this type of article, see figure 11.3.

This kind of article was often written as the journalists' own statements, and the journalists didn't conceal that they were great admirers of the ultrasound laboratory staff. The positive aspects of these activities were presented without questions. In this way, the writings were characterized by technological optimism and technological imperative, and they were emphasized by positive modalities.

It is often stated that Norwegians have a great deal of patriotism. This has also been a part of the presentation of successful prenatal therapy. The ultrasound technology has been developed and partly produced in Norway, and the scientific and clinical competence has brought attention abroad. Thus these rescues of diseased fetuses in Trondheim have been reported in several regional and national newspapers, with a tendency to emphasize the aspects of fantastic technology and clever medical professionals.

The perspective of the "marvelous new technology" in the late 1980s gave a lot of attention to Dr. Eik-Nes and his staff in Trondheim. Of course, because of their competence, but also helped by the mass media, they became authorities within this field, an authority they have kept and carried with them into the ethical discussions that will be analyzed below. The public presentation of their activities has also given weight to the arguments for routine screening of all pregnancies, because many of the malformations found would not have been discovered otherwise. At least, this argument has been raised in the articles about rescued babies. Such stories contributed heavily to political discussions about screening. No statistical materials about health care economics can get the same level of media attention. This kind of presentation of the new technology favors the clinical professionals over the critics of ultrasound screening.

This perspective dominated so clearly in this period that one could hardly find any criticism of the ultrasound experiences.[15] But a new problem turned up in the media, which indirectly was a result of the increased ultrasound control. This was also a kind of professional rivalry.

Parallel to the positive talk about technology and competence, some of the hospital neonatal departments experienced a resource crisis because of an increased number of premature births. The worst conditions seem to have occurred in Trondheim, where the National Center for Prenatal Therapy is located.[16] It is rare that physicians criticize one another in public. Furthermore, one group of physicians in this conflict (if indeed it can be called that) had already received considerable positive media attention. And too, resource battles have their own informal codes of behavior, reinforced by the knowledge that breaking them will more likely lead to resentment and defeat than to resource gains. Therefore, one would not expect to find any blame against the

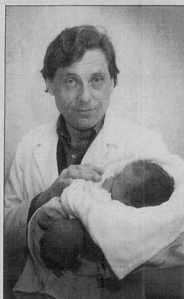

Figure 11.3 A typical presentation of Dr. Eik-Nes in the "Age of Heroics" (*Aftenposten*, July 16, 1987). Eik-Nes is shown as the "proud father-figure" holding a baby saved by early ultrasound diagnostics.

prenatal diagnostics. Nevertheless, some of the media talk was clear: politicians and doctors at the premature department asked, more or less discreetly, whether it could be justifiable to put so much money into ultrasound diagnostics and fetal therapy when the premature department hardly could keep the resulting small babies alive.[17] This was not professional rivalry as such, but a struggle for resources. It is a borderline situation between one group using another for leverage and criticizing resource distributions that favor the other group. Over several years there has been some dissatisfaction among doctors at the regional hospital in Trondheim because the ultrasound team has status as a national research and clinical center, which gives them extra money. Usually this controversy is handled very carefully, or not at all, in the media. Thus, throughout the period covered by this study, this particular debate has not been so much a criticism of the ultrasound team and their activities as it has been a struggle with the politicians where the ultrasound (and the IVF) team have become the allies of the neonatal department. The positive presentations of the ultrasound activities represented in this case an extra possibility for the neonatal department to apply public pressure for more money.

In this period as well, certain themes discussed elsewhere and at other times during the discourse are more or less ignored by the media. For instance, as in the previous period, pregnant women were not given serious attention in the newspapers—apart, that is, from the articles of successful therapy. In these articles, women appeared (if they appeared at all) as relieved mothers, photographed beside the doctors, stating that they were well taken care of. In many cases, they simply did not appear. These exceptions could not present the views of the "normal" pregnant woman, submitting to a "normal" routine examination, and finding the fetus okay—as in most cases. The question about what is going on when the pregnant women are offered ultrasound examinations has therefore not been taken into account in the public presentation of ultrasound diagnostics. In other forums, for instance, in medical journal articles and in feminist literature, it has been claimed that ultrasound screening has several effects on individuals, couples, and society as a whole, for example, changes in the relationship between parents during pregnancy and changes in our cultural perception of pregnancy and unborn babies. These circumstances, however, have not received status as "news," perhaps because they have been considered too "soft" and abstract to have anything to do in the newspapers. One exception from this is a theme emerging in the 1990s concerning to what extent we want only "perfect babies" as the aftermath of technological development.

As mentioned, the conclusions from the first consensus conference state that information to the pregnant women, prior to their consent to an ultrasound exam, must be taken seriously; they should have a real opportunity to refuse ultrasound diagnostics on the basis of information. At the second consensus conference about ultrasound in pregnancy, in 1995, research was presented which showed that many pregnant women believed the ultrasound examination to be mandatory. During the ten years such an examination has been officially offered, the proportion of eligible women examined has always been 98–99 percent. If the women believe they have no choice, then health personnel haven't fulfilled their duty to inform. But it also illustrates that these questions haven't been emphasized by the press. The media have not made a point of the individual approach to be or not to be examined with ultrasound. It seems to have been taken for granted that all women want such an examination—with whatever effects this may have had on the presentations. One reason may be that normal pregnancies and women are not attractive to journalists as themes. The normal and general is not *news*. It's nothing to talk about . . .

The same fate has met the doctors who disagree with the use of ultrasound technology in normal pregnancies. There has always been some opposition, for instance, from the epidemiologists mentioned above and from a group of feminist doctors and midwives calling for greater caution with new technologies and for greater autonomy for women vis-à-vis medical specialists. These groups have had no "news" of interest for journalists. Thus they have had few opportunities to present their views through media, except in the form of letters to the editor or articles submitted on a freelance basis. In this way the practice of ultrasound screening could become "normal" and heavily established without public debate or criticism worth mentioning. Instead, the theme of progress, of technological and scientific development got virtual hegemony for some years.

The Age of Humility, 1990–1995

In the 1990s, however, the ultrasound screening practice became something to talk about, in a sense that interested the journalists as well as other groups in society. The background was a select committee report on the subject of humans and biotechnology (NOU 1991). The committee consisted of doctors (among them Dr. Eik-Nes) and representatives from several organizations, for example, various associations for the disabled, and was called "the committee on ethics" (*etikkutvalet*). Their report dealt with new technologies within medicine and ethical challenges these raised. Ultrasound diagnostics was one of many technologies treated in the report, but did not receive more attention in the report than many other issues within gene and biotechnology. For example, amniocentesis, hereditary diseases, and ethical issues in IVF and the use of frozen embryos were also treated in the report.

The public discussion lasted (off and on) for three years, until the parliamentary debate on the report.[18] Ultrasound diagnostics came to be one of the focal points in the public debate over these years and got much more attention than many other themes in the same report.

Now the media discourse changed a bit—again. Suddenly a dark side to the marvelous technology appeared. Media began to describe what happens when malformations are found, malformations which cannot be repaired.[19] The "therapy" in many of these cases is abortion, unless the parents choose to bear a handicapped child. It was already well known and accepted that the unborn who couldn't survive, or who were very seriously diseased, could be aborted. But the question of what qualified as a "very serious" disease wasn't a subject for public presentation or discussion until the 1990s (aside, that is, from some earlier discussions on amniocentesis).

Since the subject emerged, the most discussed disease has been Down's syndrome. This diagnosis has given the right to abortion, although it isn't in itself lethal. The prognosis for people having this handicap is quite open: some grow up and act almost "normal," while others have great problems with physical and/or mental functions. In 1990, after the presentation of the public report, this diagnosis of anomaly was given special attention in the mass media. It was then connected to ultrasound screening, which in many cases is the technology and the occasion through which the diagnosis is made.

The ethical dilemmas due to prenatal diagnostics should be well known and will not be repeated here. The mass media have to some extent treated these issues as they did with the articles about "the fantastic technology" in the late 1980s: by presenting individual stories, mostly in cases where parents against all odds chose to carry a diseased child to term. In some ways most of these are "sunshine stories," with families who are doing well. The most famous of these is the grandson of two former prime ministers in Norway. He's got Down's syndrome, and this was not discovered during the pregnancy. His mother has been quoted often as saying she's glad she never got the opportunity to choose abortion (see fig. 11.4).[20]

It would seem that such individuals are easier for journalists to find than those who choose abortion or those who regret the birth of a handicapped child and might want to speak of that regret. There are no statistics available as to the number of parents offered an abortion following fetal diagnostics or on the number choosing to abort or to continue the pregnancy.[21] Thus we cannot know how representative the media presentations are. It may be that parents who choose to continue such a pregnancy are more willing to speak out in public. Perhaps it is easier to speak out when you perceive yourself to be on the moral high ground than if you fear being perceived as weak and egoistic. Or perhaps journalists find these families' stories more (news)worthy, either because they are rare or because they represent some sort of moral high ground. In recent years, however, journalists have succeeded in finding a few sad stories, too, so they can "keep the balance," so to speak. From time to time, though

Figure 11.4 A front page from the "Age of Humility" (*Verdens Gang,* Jan. 24, 1996) shows "Phillip Willoch Syse's Mamma: Glad she missed the Abortion-choice." Phillip is the grandson of Kåre Willoch and Jan P. Syse, both former prime ministers.

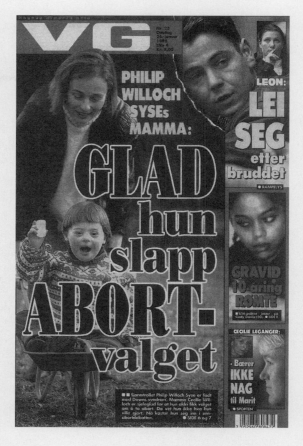

infrequently, such individual stories get big headlines, in particular in the newspapers dependent on sale of single copies. And yet there is another aspect of the personified presentations when connected to ethical problems.

When the media in the late 1980s (and later) talked about the positive results from ultrasound diagnostics and fetal therapy, the "hero" was the doctor. When it came to ethical approaches in the 1990s, the subject wasn't that easy to connect to one or more individual doctors. In other words, media presentations of the early 1990s did not turn the "heroes" of the 1980s into "villains," even though they were defending the practice of doing late abortions.[22] The responsibility now seemed to be much more pulverized, with both the medical profession and the politicians as authorities.

As mentioned, many women even now believe that an ultrasound examination is an obligatory part of prenatal care. To some extent this can be explained by the way in which ultrasound diagnostics have been treated by the press. A new exploration shows, however, another interesting change: There is reason to believe that the pregnant women of today prepare themselves for the ultrasound examination in a more serious way than earlier. Many women think through the risk of finding malformations and what to do if that happens. Many also discuss this theme with their partner in advance of the examination (Saetnan, this volume). It seems natural to interpret this finding as mainly a result of the media presentation in the 1990s.

Who has been invited to participate in the media debate about ethics? For the first time it seems like anybody can present their views of the ultrasound technology: various political parties, parents, scientists, organizations for the handicapped, etc. The media, and the national broadcasting channel in particular, have emphasized the point of "objectivity" or "balanced presentation." Usually this means that both eager defenders and convinced opponents are given the opportunity to present their views.

The scientists and practitioners have, in media appearances, often acted as if they were the only ones who knew how best to use technology for social benefit. This tendency also characterizes some of the scientists within prenatal testing. Sturla Eik-Nes has not acted like this. Despite his conviction that ultrasound screening is an important tool for pregnant women, and despite the fact that his staff has been performing late abortions, he has not concealed that the ethical dilemmas are uneasy. An engaging public debate in progress is a condition for a defensible practice within this field, Dr. Eik-Nes says. In this way he becomes a spokesperson not only for a scientific community but also for the common ethical doubt that has characterized the whole public Norwegian discourse on fetal diagnostics. This humble way of discussing the dilemmas has not made it easy for the adversaries of ultrasound screening to confront him in the media, because, as their main "target" in the public sphere, he bids their critical reflections welcome. This can be seen as an illustration of how the media in their homogeneous technological presentations late in the 1980s have had certain side effects on the ultrasound discourse later, through the personification of the (good) ultrasound news. Dr. Eik-Nes's authority as a public figure in the debate was in part built on those presentations, and he carries this authority with him into today's more humble debates on ethics.

The starting point for these years of ethical discussions was the Parliament's handling of the select committee report on humans and biotechnology. One might wonder why ultrasound diagnostics came to be so central in the media presentation of this work, while for example the politics of offering amniocentesis to all women older than thirty-eight years in order to discover Down's syndrome got far less attention. One explanation for this may be the quantity of the practice. This is not because quantity determines the importance of ethical dilemmas, but because the mass media might have emphasized the subject relevant to the largest proportion of their readers. However, whether it was the journalists themselves, the politicians, or for example organizations for the handicapped who made the ultrasound discussion so central is a question for further research.

REGIONAL VARIATIONS

So far I have treated the three largest newspapers as one unit. This is possible for several reasons. There is a high degree of harmony between the three newspapers' presentations. They often use the same news agency, and there is some cooperation between them in the sense that they to some extent share the same material and articles (*Adresseavisen* and *Aftenposten* in particular). However, a close study of the media material shows some small but interesting variations in information, subjects, and modalities.

The newspaper which has been most patriotic and uncritical of the technological development and practice is—not surprisingly—*Adresseavisen* from Trondheim, where the ultrasound laboratory is located. More than the others, this paper has maintained an enthusiasm for the technology and its clinical possibilities. There may be several reasons for this. In media research, it is common to find that newspapers are less critical of local activities than of more distant events, and they are more loyal to local people and spokespersons. Another factor here is that Trondheim, where the Norwegian Institute of Technology is located, tries to present itself as "the Technological Capital of Norway"— and the main newspaper in the region has followed up this attempt. This has led to a situation where the leading environment for the changes in maternity care in Norway, namely, the ultrasound laboratory, for a long time enjoyed free access, so to speak, to one of the largest newspapers in the country.

The largest of the regional newspapers, *Aftenposten* from the Oslo region, does not differ much from *Adresseavisen*. This is the only subscription newspaper that attempts to be a national paper (through both subscriptions and contents). The *Aftenposten* has a rather high profile in presenting science and technology, not least concerning medicine. This has implied considerable page space also for the ultrasound developers and defenders. On the other hand, *Aftenposten* gives room for debaters, in particular well-known people, and the combination of science/technology presentations and the public debates conveys the impression of giving proper presentation of the field—although neither paper has given much room for opinions from "outside" the already established actors.

Another regional newspaper, *Bergens Tidende* (*BT*) from western Norway, has presented the subject with somewhat more distance and ethical doubt (at least not uncritically to technology and practice). For example, this newspaper has given more room for articles about choice and alternatives to abortion as therapy. Due to *BT's* rather small and recent database, the present material contains mainly articles from the 1990s, when the ethical discussions took place all over the country. But still there are articles characterizing *BT* as different from the others. One example is that *BT* is the only one of the three papers to have interviewed one particular figure in the debate—a midwife who left the ultrasound laboratory in Trondheim after several years because she found her job too technical and because she felt that they were looking for malformations only. Another example is from when the second largest TV station in Norway made a documentary program on discoveries of Down's syndrome at the eighteenth-week ultrasound examination. The program showed how many of these cases lead to late abortions in the form of induced premature deliveries after which the children were left aside to die. *Bergens Tidende* was the only one of the three to give publicity to this program and to follow up with several articles on that subject. A third example is that *BT* only as late as 1991 found reasons to write about the technical advantages of ultrasound as being without pain or known risks for the patient. Several examples therefore show a kind of presentation significantly different from that of the other two newspapers.

How can we interpret these differences? One relevant factor may be the same as with *Adresseavisen:* nearness to (or, in the case of *BT,* distance from) the events. Bergen has a regional hospital, as has Trondheim, but the Bergen hospital is in the forefront in fields other than ultrasound and fetal medicine. The Bergen area is so to speak on the outskirts of the exciting events and developments in this field. Another reason may be the interpretation of *BT's* circle of readers. Although a small country, Norway is divided into several distinct cultural settings. In western Norway there are strong Christian puritanical traditions and ties. This may have affected *BT's* way of writing, both directly and indirectly. Indirectly because many of the journalists probably come from this region, and because the editorial staff may have an interpretation of what the readers want and accept. Directly because not a few of this theme's appearances in the newspapers come from readers who are self-identified Christian people around Bergen.

These differences between the newspapers are in one way just shades of variation on the same theme; but by comparing articles from different origins over several years, a structure of differences in rhetoric and use of language, headlines, and photos becomes visible. There might be several reasons for these regional differences, reasons that hardly can be examined without going into each newspaper's management and editorial office.

SUMMARY

This analysis is from a period of history where the term *media society* already sounds a bit old-fashioned but where the media seem to have more power than ever. This short presentation of ultrasound in the mass media is a story of how the media act in relations with the techno-medical developments to perform a discourse on what this is all about. The framework of "making news," combined with an understanding of ultrasound as an important health issue, accounts for some of the "design" of the media presentations. There are different opinions on what makes "good news," but the story of ultrasound diagnostics somehow seems to fill the various criteria anyway. Events have been close in both time and space, and development has gone so fast that it has been possible to maintain a continued interest among journalists, because there has often been something new to report on. This does not mean that the mass media has followed every step within the medical community; several discussions and happenings reported in the medical journals have not appealed that much to news journalists. But the combination of new technology and fetal diagnostics (as pregnancy is a condition of interest for a great deal of the readership) gives an a priori understanding of having news value, which has given the issue considerable attention through the media.

The national perspective (and patriotism) represent some kind of geographical closeness, although the patriotic tendencies have been most visible in the newspaper from the city Trondheim, where most of the developments have taken place. But probably more important for the media interest have been the long-lasting controversies surrounding ultrasound practice. Although both the focus and many of the arguments in the debate have changed, there has throughout been a struggle among medical professionals and between professionals and lay people. Such controversies are well known as a criterion for good news. In addition, the fact that the Norwegian ultrasound expertise over these years has been a rather small group has made the personification of the subject (and of one part in the controversies) quite easy.

At the same time this study shows how multiple and changeable the presentations may be due to time, place, and medium. The media presentation of ultrasound has gone through different, rather distinct, phases. The introductory phase 1982–86 was characterized by general discussions mainly on a statistical basis. From 1986 to 1990, presentations of new technological possibilities in a very excited and positive way had virtual hegemony in the newspapers. Since 1990, attention has been given mainly to ethical problems and doubts. A tendency during all these years has been that the media's power and independence have been used in a rather servile way. In this matter, as in many other cases of an exciting technological development, it is obvious that the mass media have not represented a critical voice regarding societal changes and medical practice until they were forced to do so. For instance, the ethical aspects weren't given proper attention (hardly any attention at all) until the political authorities put them on the agenda. On the other hand, if we interpret media merely as information channels (as media and not actors), this tendency can be seen as a mirror of the political and cultural way of assessing the dilemmas due to fetal diagnostics. Norwegian legislation and political discussions about prenatal testing have been characterized by some unwillingness, doubt, and bad conscience. This characterizes the whole discourse. We want new technology for therapeutic purposes, to help expectant parents and their children, but we don't like to see the dark side of this progress. This ideological and moral dilemma has led to a sort of ambivalent practice, where the Norwegian solution has been to give the main responsibility to the pregnant women themselves and their primary care physicians.

The discourse, and also the media's handling of it, deal with two levels of assessments. There is a social, general level, and there is an individual one. There is a dualism between these two levels, which has also marked the media talk. At a general level, the main question is whether the current use of ultrasound technology is positive or negative for society as a whole and for pregnant women in particular. There is still no scientific agreement about this question.[23]

At the individual level, there are pros and cons, too. But the media presentations are almost exclusively positive, and the way of presenting sunny individual stories has probably impressed the readers more than both general reports and the few negative individual stories. This can be seen in the use of front-page headlines, big photos of beautiful babies, and other indications of positive modalities. This has been one of the main problems for the critics of ultrasound screening: They lack the individual touching stories, and it is therefore more difficult to engage the public—and the journalists. This problem of catching public and journalistic attention affects both the scientists and practitioners concerned about health economics, and the feminists with their principled discourse on "technological" versus "natural" pregnancies and on issues of patient autonomy and the unproven safety of the practices. This may help explain why ultrasound defenders have prevailed in the media discourse. To what extent this "victory" also affects the pregnant women and their families is another question.

NOTES

1. This is a main approach for the project led by Saetnan, mentioned above.
2. About positive and negative modality (although not in the mass media in particular), see Latour 1987, chap. 1.

3. *Adresseavisen* Feb. 17, 1983; June 10, 1983; Jan. 19, 1984; Jan. 21, 1984; Sept. 14, 1984; June 13, 1985; Nov. 26, 1985, Aug. 28, 1986. *Aftenposten* Jan. 18, 1984; Jan. 20, 1984; Feb. 1, 1984; June 20, 1984; Sept. 29, 1984; Oct. 1, 1984; June 12, 1985; Oct. 22, 1985; July 31, 1986; Aug. 28, 1986; Aug. 29, 1986.

4. See also *Adresseavisen* Feb. 17, 1983. The perinatal period is defined as beginning at twenty-six weeks gestational age and ending one week after birth.

5. *Aftenposten* Jan. 18, 1984; *Adresseavisen* Jan. 19, 1984.

6. *Aftenposten* Jan. 20, 1984; *Adresseavisen* Jan. 21, 1984.

7. *Aftenposten* Aug. 29, 1986.

8. One argument against this policy has been that the voluntary status of the examination is illusory: to refuse an offer of an ultrasound examination makes the mother more responsible for her child's health (Schei 1992).

9. Interviews done by Ann R. Saetnan, presented in Saetnan 1995a.

10. *Adresseavisen:* letter to the editor from district medical officer Harald Kamps, Bjugn, June 16, 1983; article based on interview with Dr. Østensen, general practitioner, Nov. 26, 1985.

11. This account of events is what appeared in the mass media. Other accounts have also been given, implying conflicts both among physicians and among midwives. For instance, some midwives saw routine ultrasound work as a threat to the broader tasks and competencies of midwifery. See Saetnan 1996 for a discussion of one such account.

12. *Adresseavisen* Mar. 8, 1989. In Norway, education within sonography did not exist.

13. Exceptions: *Aftenposten* June 11, 1986, *Adresseavisen* June 21, 1986 and Mar. 8, 1989.

14. *Adresseavisen* June 5, 1986; Dec. 15, 1987; Jan. 23, 1988; June 18, 1988; Dec. 24, 1988; Aug. 12, 1989; Nov. 18, 1989; Feb. 9, 1990, Aug. 23, 1990; Oct. 25, 1991; *Aftenposten* Dec. 8, 1984; Apr. 7, 1987; Apr. 19, 1988; June 18, 1988; Dec. 24, 1988.

15. One exception is a letter to the editor, *Aftenposten* Apr. 8, 1987, by the female (and feminist) doctors Åsa Rytter Evensen, Janecke Thesen, Kirsti Malterud, and Reidun Førde, in which they criticized Dr. Eik-Nes.

16. *Adresseavisen* Nov. 29, 1985; Oct. 15, 1987; Dec. 22, 1988; Nov. 11, 1989; Nov. 22, 1990 and more.

17. *Adresseavisen* Nov. 29, 1985; Nov. 11, 1989; Nov. 22, 1990, and many articles in *Adresseavisen* 1993.

18. Stortingsmelding 25 (1992–93): *Om mennesker og bioteknologi,* presented by the government Mar. 12, 1993; Parliament discussion June 10, 1993.

19. *Aftenposten* July 18, 1989; July 19, 1989; Dec. 3, 1990; Apr. 27, 1991; Nov. 24, 1991; Feb. 23, 1992; Feb. 26, 1993; Mar. 16, 1993; Mar. 18, 1993; Apr. 1, 1993; Apr. 17, 1993; Apr. 18, 1993; Apr. 21, 1993; Apr. 24, 1993; May 23, 1993; June 10, 1993; June 17, 1993; June 20, 1993; July 5, 1993; Feb. 6, 1994; Feb. 16, 1994; Feb. 18, 1994; June 6, 1994; June 20, 1994; July 10, 1994; Feb. 1, 1995; Feb. 24, 1995; Feb. 25, 1995. *Adresseavisen* July 18, 1989; July 20, 1989; Nov. 10, 1989; Feb. 17, 1990; Aug. 8, 1990: Dec. 3, 1990; Jan. 22, 1992; Dec. 8, 1992; Mar. 13, 1993; June 10, 1993; Dec. 21, 1993; June 11, 1994. *Bergens Tidende* Oct. 2, 1990; Jan. 25, 1992; Mar. 11, 1992; Mar. 30, 1992; Apr. 9, 1992; Apr. 15, 1992; Mar. 10, 1993; Feb. 7, 1994; Feb. 11, 1994; Feb. 14, 1994; Apr. 20, 1994; June 14–15, 1994; Feb. 28, 1995; Mar. 1, 1995; Mar. 2, 1995.

20. For example, front-page headlines in *Verdens Gang* Jan. 24, 1996.

21. One unofficial estimate is that about half of those receiving a "serious or lethal" diagnosis choose to abort (Eik-Nes, personal communication), but estimates depend on how cases are categorized as well as on which hospital practice forms the set of experiences on which the estimates are based.

22. However, as this book goes into press, the abortion debate in Norway has hardened further, and lately (1999) there are tendencies to villainize the once-heroes of ultrasound.

23. For a presentation of the ongoing debate in medical journal literature regarding the scientific evidence for this practice, see Saetnan 1995b.

REFERENCES

Allern, Sigurd:

1992   *Kildenes makt: Ytringsfrihetens politiske økonomi* [The power of sources: The political economy of freedom of speech]. Oslo: Pax.

Backe, Bjørn, and Harald Buhaug (eds.):

1986   *Konsensuskonferansen 27–29/8, 1986: Bruk av ultralyd i svangerskapet* [The consensus conference Aug. 27–29, 1986: Use of ultrasound in pregnancy]. Report 8/86. Trondheim: NIS.

Høyer, Svennik:

1989   *Små samtaler og store medier* [Small conversations and large media]. Oslo: Scandinavian University Press.

Larssen, Karl-Erik, Leiv S. Bakketeig, Per Bergsjø, Per H. Finne et al.:

1982   *Vurdering av perinatal service i Norge 1980* [An evaluation of perinatal service in Norway, 1980]. Report 7/82. Oslo: NIS.

Latour, Bruno:

1987   *Science in Action: How to Follow Scientists and Engineers through Society.* Milton Keynes: Open University Press.

Norske Avisers Landsforbund [Norwegian Newspapers' National Association]:

1991   "Aviskatalogen" [Newspaper catalog].

NOU [Norwegian Public Analyses]

1984   *Perinatal omsorg i Norge: Helsearbeid blant svangre og fødende kvinner samt nyfødte barn* [Perinatal care in Norway: Health services among pregnant and delivering women and newborn children]. Presented June 19, 1984. NOU 1984: 17.

1991   *Mennesker og bioteknologi* [Humans and biotechnology]. NOU 1991: 6.

Saetnan, Ann:

1995a   Command Performance: A Sign of Success or Failure for Norway's First Consensus Conference? Paper presented at joint annual meeting for the Society for Social Studies of Science and the Society for History of Technology, Charlottesville, Va., Oct. 19–22.

1995b   To Screen or Not to Screen? Science Discourse in Two Health Policy Controversies. In *Just What the Doctor Ordered? A Study of Medical Technology Innovation Processes,* 115–56. Report no. 25. Trondheim: Center for Technology and Society.

1996   Speaking of Gender . . . : Intertwinings of a Medical Technology Policy Debate and Everyday Life. In Merete Lie and Knut H. Sørensen (eds.), *Making Technology Our Own? Domesticating Technology into Everyday Life,* 31–63. Oslo: Scandinavian University Press.

Schei, Berit:

1992   Gynekologen—på hellig grunn? [The gynecologist on holy ground?] In Agnes Andenæs et al., *Epler fra vår egen hage* [Apples from our own garden]. Report no. 4/92. Trondheim: Center for Women's Studies.

12

Thirteen Women's Narratives of Pregnancy, Ultrasound, and Self

Ann Rudinow Saetnan

PREAMBLE: COMPETING EXPERT NARRATIVES

What is the meaning of routine obstetric ultrasound? How does it impact on pregnant women? on their identities as women? on their place in the social structure? on their experience of pregnancy? The answers you get depend on whom you ask or who volunteers to voice an opinion. Until recently, medical experts and feminist critics of medical technology have been the most vocal, almost the only, proponents of answers to these questions.

These experts do not agree. According to one such expert, routine ultrasound is a source of information and empowerment both to medical personnel and to women themselves:

> *Expert 1:* If you ask, "What is modern ultrasound diagnostics?" . . . Well, we
> have moved the moment of information from the time of birth to twenty-
> two weeks ahead of that time. That's what we've done. For all those millions
> of years, information about the product of pregnancy has been at birth. And
> now in the course of a decade we have moved that moment twenty-two
> weeks ahead to eighteen weeks gestation, with possibilities for taking the con-
> sequences and making choices.

According to a feminist general practitioner, routine ultrasound is an imposition on women, usurping their own self-knowledge and subjugating them to unnecessary medical control:

Expert 2: This brings us back to the question of informed consent, and also to the issues that concern me from the feminist research perspective—things like: Do we empower women to take charge and trust their own resources? Are they to feel the baby kick inside them and experience that as something positive in itself? Or do we teach them that it isn't relevant, that they have to see it on a screen for it to be real? Are we to give them the information they need to make valid choices in their own lives? Or do we decide what's good for them and what's not? And there are basic philosophical differences in the population here, where [Expert 1] and I probably belong to different camps.

A third expert questions the accuracy of the information ultrasound providers claim to produce and the health benefits they claim ensue from that information:

Expert 3: I think [Expert 1] and company are going to have major problems defending themselves in that debate, because they have too weak a documentation of what's so splendid about their method of determining due dates. So let's say they're really left with just the discovery of a few malformations and terminating those pregnancies. Do you think something will happen with public opinion then? Take the women themselves up to the year 2000, who will be facing the consequences of the way one can be left to go on recklessly within obstetrics with this technology. What do you think? Is it conceivable that women's organizations and feminist groups might react more on an ethical-moral basis against that sort of a practice? That's the only thing I can see that could stop this.

The first expert responds to these critiques by invoking the voices of pregnant women themselves. According to this expert, it is women themselves who value the information that ultrasound provides and the decisions that ultrasound opens for them to make:

Expert 1: Over the years I've been through diagnostics on many hundreds of women with [fetuses with] lethal aberrations, and I can only remember a few who did not want to terminate the pregnancy when they received the information that they had a lethal aberration. And those who chose not to, they were women who for the most part due to some religious conviction or another wanted things to proceed on their natural course. And all of them, all those who wanted things to proceed on their natural course, they all request to come back for repeated ultrasound checkups so that they can receive information on the negative development of the fetus that we have predicted. They also ask to come back for ultrasound in their next pregnancy, even if they say, "We won't take the consequences of your findings then either and terminate the pregnancy. But we want to know." And then there's my impression of all the hundreds who have been through the diagnostics and received a diagnosis that there is a lethal aberration, and who chose to abort . . . all of whom say that they think it was positive that it happened that way. So I feel that we're headed for a period where we are on solid ground. Because the women who are subjected to this diagnostic, I feel that I know what *they* want.

These experts are all speaking of, and for, the same technological practice—that of examining all pregnant women with ultrasound. They are also all speaking of, and for, the same population of women. And although the above quotes are taken from private interviews,[1] these same experts have made similar statements about, on behalf of, and not least aimed at the same technological practice and the same population in various high-visibility public forums on numerous occasions.

I have previously argued that the narrative contests in which these experts have participated are a key mechanism through which the technology and its users take on sociotechnically gendered forms and meanings. Through this discourse the technology is constructed as a female-friendly or female-oppressive technology in the same instant as women are constructed as interested in or opposed to the technology. For instance, in Expert 1's narrative, pregnant women are implied to be opaque both to their health care providers and themselves: A pregnant body is a body in the way of knowledge; a pregnant woman is an anxious woman in search of knowledge; ultrasound is a technology through which a medical expert can provide her with that knowledge, which she cannot provide for herself even though it resides within her own body. To Experts 2 and 3, on the other hand, pregnant women are, however imperfectly, knowledgeable about their bodies. Ultrasound, then, is a technology that oppresses women in part by devaluing their knowledge, in part by providing them with unnecessary, uncertain, and unwelcome knowledge in its place.

Pregnant women have been massively exposed to these alternative views of themselves and of ultrasound technology. However, pregnant women's own voices have not, at least until recent years, played a significant role in the public debate concerning the practice of routine ultrasound in pregnancy. This article presents work in which I have sought out the voices of pregnant women.

THEORETICAL REFERENCE POINTS

"Do artifacts have gender?" ask Anne-Jorunn Berg and Merete Lie (1995), and answer that yes, they have. Borrowing from Sandra Harding's (1986) parsing up of gender as a social construction, we can argue that artifacts—technologies—have gender in the sense that they are entered into a culture's gendered symbol system. They have gender in the sense that they are sites for the negotiation of a gendered structure of relationships, such as a gendered division of labor. And they have gender in the sense that they are included in or excluded from individuals' gendered identities.

Borrowing from Haraway (1989) as well, I have previously looked at how these aspects of gender are achieved through contests among narratives. Specifically, I analyzed gender aspects of narratives in Norwegian public debates over the routine use of ultrasound in pregnancy (Saetnan 1996a, 1996b). The narratives I analyzed at the time were those of four types of activists in that debate—the Leading Expert, the Skeptical Specialists, the Midwife, and the Feminist Doctors. All were health professionals, and all took positions as spokespersons (Latour 1987) on behalf of both the technology and its users (pregnant women, fetuses, expectant fathers, technology operators, etc.). Remarkably, until very recently the public debate has not included the voices of women themselves (Kvande, this volume). Instead, the voices of pregnant women—as well as those of mothers and fathers, of fetuses, of the handicapped, of the public in general—have been represented in the debate by self-appointed spokespersons, especially health professionals.

The spokesperson role is at once both powerful and risky. On the power side of this equation, a spokesperson speaks with the volume of more than one voice. A spokesperson claims to speak on behalf of—and thereby with the enhanced authority of—a multitude of individuals, groups, natural phenomena, and/or artifacts. On the other hand, a spokesperson runs the risk that this multitude will not act as the spokesperson has claimed, thus damaging the spokesperson's credibility.

As we have seen in the preamble, the case in point involves several spokespersons making competing claims regarding the nature of both ultrasound and pregnant femininity. This rests on, and thereby also confirms, the ability of both technology and gender to support various interpretations—i.e., their *interpretative flexibility* (Pinch and Bijker 1987).

However, it does not necessarily follow that the existing spokespersons capture the full range of that flexibility. Some interpretations may not be spoken for and may thereby be missing from the public debate. Interpretations situated in interests in conflict with those of more vocal spokespersons are likely to be ignored (left unspoken or even unseen) by those spokespersons. Some interpretations lack spokespersons of their own because the individuals or groups holding those interpretations are poorly organized or otherwise disenfranchised. As Clarke and Montini (1993) have previously shown, this may not least be the case for lay women users (consumers) of medical technologies.

Lay users' interpretations may also be different from but compatible with those of more visible spokespersons such as health care providers. This too can contribute to the invisibility of lay interpretations, as there is no apparent need for lay users to publicly contradict their provider spokespersons. In fact, lay persons seeking medical treatment may find it in their interests *not* to contradict their providers and would-be spokespersons because they see themselves as dependent on these providers for services. For instance, Cussins (1996) shows how the interpretations of infertility treatments held by women seeking pregnancy and by providers at fertility clinics may differ and yet be, apparently harmoniously, "choreographed" together. Nonetheless, it is of both theoretical and social/political interest to make these lay interpretations visible, as Cussins has also demonstrated.

Different interpretations of gender and/or technology are not only socially positioned contingent to interests. They are also culturally and historically contingent. Cultural contingency and the importance of (local) users' interpretations have been shown by, among others, Andersen (1988) for numerically controlled tools, by Akrich (1992) for solar generators, and by Kirejczyk (this volume), Press and Browner (1994), Browner and Preloran (this volume), Gupta (this volume), and others regarding various technologies of human reproduction. Sorge and Warner (1986) state as a matter of principle that technologies *necessarily* will prove variable because they must be integrated (or embedded) into each new local cultural context where they are implemented.

Thus, the lay women's interpretations of fetal diagnostics found by Rapp (1988) among people of various ethnic backgrounds in New York, or by Press and Browner (1994) and by Browner and Preloran (this volume) among Mexican-Americans and non-Hispanic Americans in California, or by Morgan (1996, this volume) in Ecuador may, in addition to being different from one another, be very different from those I encounter in Norway.

It is on the basis of these theoretical reflections that I set out to listen to Norwegian women's narratives about their encounters with ultrasound diagnostics in pregnancy. Those narratives (thirteen interviews, each lasting about one hour) touched on a broad spectrum of themes including all three aspects of social gender: symbol, relational structure, and identity. In this essay I will concentrate on the ways these women describe gendered aspects of their experience with ultrasound. More specifically, I will concentrate on how their experiences with ultrasound intertwine with two sets of relations—the relationships of women to their health providers and to their conjugal partners—and how these relationships in turn intertwine with the women's views of themselves. Regarding the women's relationships to their health providers, I am interested in how the ultrasound exam is engaged in (re)negotiations of relationships of power and authority. Regarding their partners, I will examine how the women engage the ultrasound exam in (re)negotiations of relations of solidarity. In each instance, these (re)negotiations both build on and modify women's views of themselves as knowledgeable or unknowledgeable, competent or incompetent, isolated or socially supported during pregnancy.

METHODOLOGICAL REFLECTIONS

Ironically, here I too am placing myself in a spokesperson position on behalf of pregnant women—thirteen of them, to be precise. With what credentials? And why? Do we need other channels to access women's voices on this subject? Do women need other channels to make their voices heard? And if so, in what sense is my own research a different channel from those which already exist?

The fact that existing spokespersons have been self-appointed, and that they have made radically different representations of the interests of women, does not necessarily mean that they are wrong. Health professionals have claimed the authority of their ongoing contacts with the affected lay public through clinical encounters. (For example, "Over time I've been through diagnostics with hundreds of women carrying a fetus with a lethal abnormality. . . . So I feel we are on safe ground here, because the women who are subjected to these diagnostics, I feel I know what *they* want.")[2] However, any encounter bears the imprint of the relationship between the parties involved. What a pregnant woman says to a physician known to be enthusiastic about ultrasound and what she says to a physician known to be a feminist critic of ultrasound may be two different things. Furthermore, which of these physicians she chooses as her doctor may well be related to which opinions she herself holds on health matters. This may explain how activists in the debate can make such radically different representations of women's viewpoints, and yet each can reasonably claim the authority of their many contacts with women patients.

What a woman says on the subject to someone in charge of her antenatal care, and what she says to someone outside the medical care system (such as myself) may also be two very different things. But is one version necessarily more correct than another? There are arguments for believing that the latter version will be more nuanced and more complete. In the former type of encounter, the woman is in a position of dependence on the physician for her health care. She is likely to avoid arguing with her physician on matters of technology policy. If she strongly disagrees, she is more likely to seek out a different physician. She is also aware of limits on the physician's time and has a number of other issues to discuss that are likely to take precedence over a technology policy debate within the time available. Her encounter with me, on the other hand, is with a person with no direct influence on care provision, a person with no clear position in the policy debate, and a person willing to listen for however long the woman wishes to speak on this subject and however the woman herself defines the boundaries of the subject. Thus my authority as a spokesperson builds in part on the length and depth of the narratives of the women who have spoken to me.

On the other hand, my authority is weakened by the small number of women who chose to do so. Being outside the care provision system, I had no routine contact with pregnant women nor any legitimate access to names and addresses of pregnant women. Therefore, I could not draw a random or strategic sample of pregnant women through which to represent the pregnant population as a whole. Instead, I had to seek a means of distributing an invitation to women to contact me.

As over 99 percent of all pregnant women in the hospital district where I live do opt to attend for the sonogram which they are offered as a matter of routine at about eighteen weeks of pregnancy, and since the sonograms are provided by a single clinic, the most practical way to seek contact with these women is via that clinic. It was arranged that the clinic would insert an invitation letter from me and a postage-paid reply card addressed to me together with the letter that the clinic sends to inform women of their sonogram appointment. I then contacted women who sent me the reply card. Of the 120 invitations sent out, I received 12 replies. In addition, I interviewed one woman whom I happened to know who had declined the offer of a routine sonogram.[3]

Admittedly, this is an extremely low response rate. Were I attempting to reach a representative sample, I would have had to speculate long and deeply as to why women chose to respond or not respond to my invitation and how this might affect the distribution of narratives they presented to me. In all likelihood, I would have had to discard all the material as tainted in terms of validity and reliability. However, I could not have attempted representativity in any case as my respondents are self-selected. These women can, as several of them put it, "speak only for themselves." Speculations as to the bases and consequences of their self-selection decisions are therefore as unnecessary as they are unfruitful. Experiences and viewpoints reported by these women can be taken to exist within the population as a whole in at least the numbers (as opposed to the proportions) in which I encountered them in these thirteen narratives. Any further generalizations regarding the pregnant population as a whole must be based on theoretical reasoning rather than on mathematical distributions among the narratives.

About half of the interviews were conducted immediately after the sonogram exam, including two instances when I was invited to attend the exam itself. These interviews were conducted at an office I borrowed two blocks from the clinic. Due to holiday interruptions and the like, the remaining interviews were conducted at the nearest mutually convenient time following the exam.

This was anywhere from one week to several months later. The one woman who had declined a routine sonogram was interviewed six months after delivering her baby. All these interviews were conducted at the woman's home, at my office, or at an office I borrowed for the occasion near the ultrasound clinic—whichever the woman herself chose.

Interviews tended to last about an hour and were loosely structured according to a conversation guide. The guide reminded me to cover six questions relating to claims spokespersons had emphasized regarding pregnant women's opinions and interests, and three open questions to invite other themes that the women themselves might suggest.

Interviews were taped except in two instances—one when the tape recorder failed and one when a woman objected to the recorder. Those two interviews were reconstructed immediately following the interview on the basis of written notes. I then transcribed the tapes in anonymized form, which is to say that names and individual peculiarities of wording and pronunciation were "sanitized" from the transcripts. The transcripts constitute the raw materials for this essay. An earlier version of this essay was written in Norwegian and distributed to the thirteen women narrators. Their comments have been incorporated into this version of the essay. On this basis—the length and depth of the interviews, the fact that these women chose voluntarily to speak through me, and the fact that I have invited them to comment on my use of their narratives—I dare to take on the role of their spokesperson.

SELF-KNOWLEDGE VERSUS PROFESSIONAL AUTHORITY

One of the themes in the ultrasound debate has been whether ultrasound is a source of increased knowledge about the fetus—both for medical personnel and for the expectant parents—or merely a means of moving the ownership of knowledge from lay to expert hands. Have both women and their antenatal care providers been empowered by an increase of knowledge about the fetus? And if so, does pregnancy seem more real and immediate to women after a sonogram? Or has the balance of power shifted in that where care providers were once dependent on women for information about the state of their pregnant health, women are now dependent on ultrasound operators to "show" them their baby? And if the latter, does this move the experience of pregnancy "outside" the body, making it more distant and abstract? For instance, one feminist critic of ultrasound screening said to me in an earlier interview: "This is in part what concerns me here from a women's research point of view. Are women to be empowered to master and trust their own resources? Are they to feel the baby kick inside them and experience this as something positive in itself? Or are they to be taught that this isn't valid, that they have to see it on a screen for it to be real?"

Another critic was insulted on women's behalf that a due date estimated via ultrasound should be considered more reliable than one based on the woman's own knowledge of her menstruation dates and sexual history:

> These tables [i.e., the ones used to compute due dates on the basis of ultrasound measurements] were made on the basis of women who have reported a reliable due date. That's how they were constructed. So those men trusted *those* women. Why then can't they trust women *since* then who say, "I'm absolutely sure when I had my last period; I know when it was." There's just as much reason to trust these women as those who participated in making the basis for the tables for ultrasound estimation. But suddenly a woman's word isn't good enough. . . . And what we experience in practice is that midwives[4] sit there and change due dates by one or two days and the answer we get back is "March 19? No, March 21." And then you ask yourself, "What the hell?" Excuse me. It makes me so aggressive that I actually say "hell." What right do they have to sit there and do that? It's an insult! And I have to laugh a little, too. I think it's comical also.

A supporter of ultrasound, on the other hand, says that ultrasound increases knowledge about the fetus and that women themselves seek this knowledge: "As we learn more and more about ultrasound diagnostics and consequences, learn more about what we can find and the meaning of what we find, and learn to take the consequences of our investigations, then it will be more and more. . . . Yes, it will come to be more and more accepted and seen as necessary. Because of the information it provides."

What do the thirteen women I spoke to say? Do they feel that the ultrasound scan brings them new knowledge or that it displaces knowledge they otherwise possessed? Does it make the pregnancy seem more real to them, or more abstract? Does knowledge about the pregnancy become more embodied, or disembodied?

"Now I Have Proof!"

For some—all of them women going through their first pregnancy and who have not yet felt "quickening," the onset of that stage of pregnancy when one can feel the baby move—the ultrasound does seem to carry more authority than all other clinical tests and experienced pregnancy symptoms. For these women, we could say that the ultrasound displaced knowledge they already in some sense possessed but also that it made the pregnancy seem more real to them. The following interview excerpt can serve as an example:

It was a great moment actually. Because I didn't identify with being pregnant before. I haven't any . . . The only thing I can see is that I've put on some weight on my behind, but that's nothing to do with the fetus in a way. So now I'm finally sure there's something in there, and seen the heartbeat, and seen it move. So it was sort of . . . well, I had something of a revelation. I'd been looking forward to it, to the ultrasound, since the pregnancy felt so distant even though I was so far along. I haven't begun to feel it move, you see. So therefore I was quite excited. This has to do with the impression that you're only pregnant once you can see that belly. But as long as you don't have a belly, you're not really pregnant even if you have all the other symptoms. So I was having trouble identifying with it.

[Me: But now you feel pregnant?]

Yes, now so! Now I have proof!

However, for those who had felt "quickening," the sensations from within their own bodies took precedence over the images on the sonogram screen, making quickening a more important milestone in pregnancy than the ultrasound exam. For two of the thirteen, these two events coincided: "It was probably the biggest thing that has happened to me in relation to the baby I'm carrying, because it all became so real. It suddenly became an image for me, and I saw its face and saw it move, and it wasn't just a lump on my belly, right? And I had just begun to feel it move. But it was still early in the pregnancy, so I wasn't quite sure whether it was indigestion or the baby kicking. But now I saw it kick, and I felt a sort of a 'dip' in my belly and like 'Wow!'"

It is no surprise that the visual images on the sonogram screen are a powerful signal. However, they do not seem to have pushed aside the signals these women felt from within their own bodies. In Norway, where an ultrasound screen is positioned for the mother-to-be (and any guests she chooses to bring with her) to view, and where the operator makes an attempt to explain the images to her, it would seem that the ultrasound images can function as a supplement to and reinforcement of, rather than a replacement for or usurper of, the embodied experiences of pregnancy.

"The Point Wasn't to Show Me"

However, for the ultrasound to serve as a supplement to rather than usurper of knowledge based on the woman's embodied experience requires that woman being examined can relate the images on the screen to the sensations of her body. This was not always the case among the women I interviewed:

It was very strange to see the kid and what it was doing. Because the midwife told that it was standing there and covering its eyes with its hands, and waving its hands, and . . . almost as if to say something. But it was . . . it was so strange, because it was . . . I know it's happening inside me, but it was strange anyway. [laughs] Because it looks more like it's happening *out*side. And then . . . I can't understand that that picture I saw could be going on inside a belly no bigger than mine.

There's something about distancing yourself, whether you manage to think that it's something which is inside your belly.

[Me: Did you manage that?]

Yeesss . . . I don't know if I did. Because it's incredible that you should be seeing it on a screen. It really is. But luckily you get Polaroids to take home with you so you can look at it again. But . . . I suppose I did manage it. I think. At least my second pregnancy.

Furthermore, making this translation from screen image to bodily sensation seems to entail subordinating oneself to medical authority. Only one woman reported relying on her own interpretation of the images as much as on that of the midwife. For this woman, the fetus's level of activity—which she could observe for herself—was sufficient to confirm that it was healthy: "I was actually quite calmed by the ultrasound. Because I saw that the kid was kicking, and then I said to myself, 'My world, it just has to be healthy.' Because it looked so lively."

But for most of these women, the images were not intelligible without the explanations of the ultrasound operator. In fact, the midwife's ability to communicate an interpretation of the images seemed at times more important for this translation than the quality of the images themselves. For instance, one woman going through her second pregnancy compared the two ultrasound experiences as follows:

The first time she [the midwife] was a foreigner. She didn't manage to explain to me what was happening and what I saw. I didn't understand her and she didn't understand me. But this time she [another midwife] was tremendously good at explaining. So now I got all the little details about what we saw and how and why she did things.

[Me: Were the images the same? Were they as you had expected?]

Oh no! Last time the kid was lying so we saw a profile very clearly, fingers and toes and all that. And then the belly isn't the same, now that I've given birth before . . . as the midwife explained. There are more folds and wrinkles in between. So the images weren't as clear.

And as one woman pointed out, the examination is aimed not at showing the woman her baby but at various medical goals such as diagnosing abnormalities and estimating due dates. Thus, the woman is subordinated not only to the operator through her dependence on the operator for interpretation of the images but also to the operator's understanding of the scan's purpose:

> It wasn't all that difficult after a while to see what was a leg or a head. But since most of the scan was for them to do an examination for themselves, to see that everything was in order, then it was more difficult to follow what they were doing. Because the point wasn't to show me, "This is your baby, and here's what it looks like." It was just for them to measure, like.

Nevertheless, most of these thirteen women were able to maintain, to some extent, an interpretation of the scan as an opportunity to "see the baby," even as they recognized that the sonogram operators worked from other understandings of the scan's role. None of these women were confronted with a situation where a malformation was diagnosed, a situation that might force a confrontation between the two types of goals for the scan.[5]

"Ha, Ha! I Was Right!"

On the other hand, all but two had come away from the scan with revised due dates.[6] Did they feel their own self-knowledge to be contested? Were they insulted by this? Did it somehow impinge on their experience of the scan in terms of their own goals for it? In most cases the due date was postponed. The fetus was found to be smaller, and therefore registered as younger, than a due date based on the first day of the last menstruation would seem to indicate. Did it occur to any of these women that this might mean the baby was growth retarded? Did they find the change in due dates in any way alarming?

The answer to this last question is no. None of the women expressed the thought that the change in due dates might indicate that something was wrong with the baby or the pregnancy. Neither did they give any direct indication that they were insulted by the change in due dates, although some were disappointed: "Huff, yes! That [i.e., receiving a later due date] wasn't any fun. I pretty much knew when it was, because I'm absolutely regular with 28 days between. And this is a planned baby, so I'm pretty sure when it was conceived. But I had a little hope that maybe it had happened before, that they might move the due date three weeks forward. Three days more isn't so much, but when I have pelvic pains already now . . ."

In fact, one woman was quite triumphant in reporting that the ultrasound had confirmed the due date she had held to all along, calculated from when she knew she had had unprotected sex, but which her GP had "corrected" on the basis of her menstruation dates:

First I had calculated November 25. But now it's December 4, which is somewhere in the same vicinity.

[Me: Were you sure of the 25th?]

No. I had said December 4 or 5 myself. Ehhhm . . . I don't know
whether I had counted right, but I know we were at our cabin. [laughs!] So
I had a little suspicion that something happened then. But then the doctor
had calculated from my last menstruation and come to another date. But
now I got it confirmed that the date I had figured for myself was right. So
that was kind of fun, I think. Like "Ha, ha! I was right!" [laughs again]

Her triumphant laughter can indicate that some women do feel a certain
pride in knowing best when they got pregnant and that, as a corollary, they
might be a bit insulted to receive a different ultrasound-based due date. Although none of those I spoke with explicitly voiced any insult, some did hold
to their own calculations in spite of the ultrasound result or paid the ultrasound
result little mind:

It was a week shorter than we had thought. Because the due date we had
before was November 29, whereas we got December 5 when we were at the
ultrasound.

[Me: What do you think about that?]

Well, it's just a due date. But nobody knows whether it will be before
or after that date. It's just to have something to relate to. It could be two
months early. Nobody really knows. But I guess it's good to have a date to
look forward to.

Some had strengthened their own confidence vis-à-vis the ultrasound-
based due date by garnering support from the medical debate over the basis for
calculating dates from ultrasound:

Yes. It was moved—two weeks longer. Or . . . ten days, I guess it was. I had
. . . I was quite sure it was December 4, and then I got the 13th. Yes, nine
days, then. And I have very regular periods, so I was that sure about [laughs]
when it happened, so to speak. So it came as a big surprise.

[Me: So what do you think now?]

Somewhere in between, I hope. [laughs] See, I talked to my doctor
about it, and as he said, they're not entirely in agreement. Because some doctors say that all fetuses grow at the same rate around those weeks, and that
they've come just as far. *All* fetuses. But there are others again who don't
agree, who say that there can be some differences.

All in all, it would seem that these women have met a technology-based practice which is presented to them as more knowledgeable about their bodies than they themselves are. When the women are not insulted by this, it may in part be because they are not forced to accept the knowledge claims based on the technology. They manage—at least to some extent—to stick to their own claims in spite of being confronted with contesting claims from the ultrasound scan, and in spite of those latter claims being accepted by the ultrasound operators and other medical personnel. All this accumulation of authority need not be conclusive for the women themselves. There need be no open conflict between the various interpretations of the technology's purpose and authority.

Or rather, there need be no open conflict until such time as a medical decision needs to be reached on the basis of the due date. Come the day when, for instance, the woman herself claims to be two weeks post-term while her doctor maintains that the ultrasound shows she'll have to wait another week before labor can be induced, then a conflict between two views on the authority of the technology may arise. But until such a day, the doctor can maintain that the ultrasound is the more reliable source of information on how long the woman has been pregnant, while the woman can maintain her confidence in her own knowledge of her body; until such a day, the technology remains interpretatively flexible on that count.

The Worst-Case Scenario: "One Can Never Say with 100 Percent Certainty"

Another point of dispute over the ultrasound screening program has been the question of whether it does (or should, for that matter) relieve women's anxieties during pregnancy, or on the contrary, whether it engenders them. In other words, is knowledge unveiled by the ultrasound welcome? Does it improve the experience of pregnancy?

The competing claims can be summarized in the following four diagrams, each representing a hypothetical trajectory of anxiety level through pregnancy. The ultrasound scan is marked with a caret (^) below the time line. Figure 12.1 shows a situation in which anxiety is at a constant level, unaffected by the ultrasound scan. Figure 12.2 shows anxieties running high until relieved by a negative ultrasound (i.e., an ultrasound that shows no signs of malformation or disease in the fetus). Figure 12.3 depicts a situation where anxieties are elevated in anticipation of the ultrasound and thereafter remain at a higher level. Figure 12.4 shows a "surge" of anxiety engendered in anticipation of the ultrasound, relieved by a negative result, and thereafter returning to a stable level for the remainder of pregnancy.

To the extent that the thirteen interviews in this study can be taken as a "test" of these hypothetical alternatives, they offer most support for alternative 4. I find this support in the observation that several of the women reported a

Figure 12.1 Anxiety level unaffected by sonogram

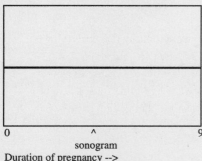

0   ^   9
sonogram
Duration of pregnancy -->

Figure 12.2 Anxiety level decreased by sonogram

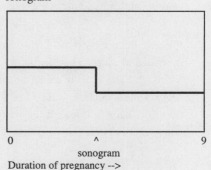

0   ^   9
sonogram
Duration of pregnancy -->

Figure 12.3 Anxiety level increased by sonogram

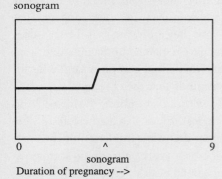

0   ^   9
sonogram
Duration of pregnancy -->

Figure 12.4 Sonogram releases a burst of anxiety, which it then alleviates

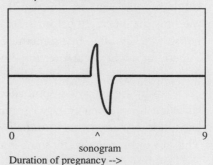

0   ^   9
sonogram
Duration of pregnancy -->

troublesome level of anxiety in the hours immediately preceding their scan. They then said that the scan relieved their worries almost as soon as they saw the first images on the screen, but in the course of the interview they later said, "Of course, the ultrasound can't show everything," that they still had no guarantee of a healthy baby. For instance, twelve minutes passed from "I dreaded it" to "I relaxed right away" to "Of course, things can still happen" in the interview quoted below:

> [Me: How did you experience the ultrasound?]
> Oh, I dreaded it! There was some excitement, but at the same time I felt that . . . that it's a judgment, you see, that now I'll really hear what I'm carrying inside me and if there's anything wrong or . . . My sister has been through quite a bit. One child was born without kidneys. So that sort of thing, then, that something was defective and now I would get to know. But once I was inside and lying there I thought it was just wonderful to see the little body

345

moving about. So then I relaxed right away. But I was restless in the corridor waiting area. Ooohhh! Pacing back and forth, back and forth.

[Twelve minutes later] So I felt that if only we're so lucky that everything is normal and we get a healthy baby . . . I'm still a bit anxious about that, although I was actually quite calmed by the ultrasound. Because I saw that the kid was kicking, and then I said to myself, "My world, it just has to be healthy." Because it looked so lively. And then too, I'm getting to be so far along that I'm over the worst now. Of course, things can still happen, but . . .

Others told of nightmares or sleeplessness the night before their scan. As with the woman quoted above, these women reported that they were calmed by the scan results, and then—only minutes later—they mention that they still have some worries. Not that they lose sleep over them any longer—that was only the one night before the scan—but they are aware that the scan does not show everything, that something may have remained undiagnosed, or that something might occur later in pregnancy that could compromise the health of the fetus. This is clear enough in their minds that they brought these concerns up in the interview spontaneously, without prompting from me. And although the women emerged from their scan quite elated, these fears were back in their narratives within half an hour after the completion of the scan. Thus it would seem that for some number of women the ultrasound scan serves as a "lightning rod" for anxieties concerning fetal health. It gathers these anxieties toward it, concentrating them and then releasing them for a time, after which they again build up to some more or less stable level.

This pattern was not evident for all the women I spoke to. Two reported that the scan did not represent a calming factor for them. One said that having been through four previous pregnancies, she was not much worried about health problems at all. She said this in spite of having lost one baby to SIDS (sudden infant death syndrome, or "cot death"). For her, the signals from her own body were sufficient to convince her that the baby was healthy:

There are many who feel safer after they've been to the ultrasound and seen. Maybe they feel unsure. Maybe especially first-time mothers. But I wouldn't have cared much if I weren't offered an ultrasound. Not now. But I chose to do it because I felt it was nice to see the baby.

[Me: This feeling that it's nice to see the baby, does it have anything to do with your having lost one child to cot death?]

No, I don't think so. Because I can feel it's alive. It's only *after* the baby's born that I'm scared, that my anxieties come.

Another chose not to have the routine scan because she felt it was as likely to increase her anxiety level as to decrease it. For one thing, she viewed a modicum of uncertainty regarding pregnancy outcomes as a natural and unavoidable condition from which it was unnecessary to seek refuge through prenatal diagnostics. For another, the scan could provide sufficient information to force her to make a choice and yet insufficient information on which to base that choice.

> My partner and I discussed it and found out that we saw no reason to take
> the ultrasound. And the reason for that . . . I just saw no point in it. And at
> the same time, I know that some receive the news at the ultrasound that
> there may be something dangerously wrong with the fetus, or some damage
> to the fetus. And I also know that one can never say with 100 percent cer-
> tainty how great that damage is. Nor can one say with 100 percent certainty
> that there is any damage. It's more of a "tendency" type of diagnosis, maybe,
> and we're talking about a 10–20 percent margin of error. Maybe more. I don't
> know. And I, or we, held the view that having a baby entails some risk. And
> that's a risk you have to calculate with when you choose to have children.
> And at the same time I have to say that there are no hereditary diseases in the
> family. We have no handicaps. So I didn't have that sort of reason to . . .
> Then I might have felt otherwise about the ultrasound. But I was in good
> shape. All the tests that are taken routinely were in order. So I saw no point
> in it. [. . .] And I felt that . . . well, my main argument was that: What if
> I'm told that there's an 80 percent chance that your child has spina bifida.
> What then? I wasn't interested in going through the rest of my pregnancy
> knowing that! One can't, with some of these major malformations, determine
> what the practical consequences will be. And another thing—because that's
> another thing they said [to convince me to take the exam], that I would be
> better prepared to receive a child with a malformation—and I completely dis-
> agree with that, because one is totally unprepared regardless, unless maybe
> one already has someone in the family with the same handicap. So I felt that,
> for me, the technology presented me with choices that I feel that I . . . well,
> I shouldn't take them. I should be spared having to make such choices.

Both by those women who were to some extent, for some (brief) period, calmed by the ultrasound and by the one who decided against an ultrasound in part because she saw it as a source of stress, the knowledge provided by the ultrasound was regarded as *inconclusive.* This too would logically make the ultrasound less authoritative, less capable of usurping the women's self-knowledge—at least in their own eyes. Again, that self-image probably becomes more difficult to maintain from the moment the ultrasound operator claims to have found something wrong with the fetus. However, these thirteen women had not experienced such a moment. For these women, it was possible to maintain their self-image as competent and autonomous knowers—as competent integrators of embodied and technology-based knowledge and/or as competent critics of technology-based knowledge—even in the face of the ultrasound laboratory's claims to superior knowledge of the fetus.

"IT'S YOU, YOUR HUSBAND, AND THE BABY IT'S ALL ABOUT"

The previous section examined (re)negotiations of the doctor-patient relationship in pregnancy in connection with the routine use of ultrasound. This section will focus on (re)negotiations of relationships between the pregnant woman and her partner.

"It's Good Not to Have to Be There Alone"

One point some have made regarding ultrasound is that this is one occasion in pregnancy when the expectant father can have the same access to information about the fetus as the mother. As is the case for health personnel, the mother's partner, friends, relatives, and previous children are otherwise at one remove from her embodied knowledge. Their access to her pregnancy experiences is indirect, via her narratives and at her discretion. Ultrasound images, on the other hand, can be experienced equally by both partners. Some see this as one of the advantages of ultrasound, that it provides an opportunity for the father to experience some of the "thrill" of pregnancy directly. Some see this as one of its disadvantages, in that it can shift power relations in the partnership on one of the few occasions when the woman otherwise has a power advantage.

About half the women I spoke with brought up this point. They too saw it as important that this was an occasion when their partner had almost as direct access to a pregnancy experience as they themselves. Those who took up this issue pointed it out as one of the advantages of pregnancy, but from a slightly different vantage point than mentioned above. It was discussed as an advantage not for the partner but for themselves. Being pregnant was in some ways a lonely experience. Sharing part of this more equally with a partner made it less so. Attending the ultrasound alone, especially considering the anxieties involved, would have made it more so.

In light of this, it is noteworthy that four of the women had been to ultrasound examinations for clinical reasons (e.g., bleeding, acute pain, suspected multiple pregnancy) either earlier in the current pregnancy or in some previous pregnancy—a situation even more susceptible to anxieties. On none of these occasions had their partners been present. In one instance, the woman states in the interview that her partner was refused admittance to the examination room although she requested his presence.[7] Another woman states that it wasn't convenient for her partner to accompany her on two previous occasions, which were due to their participation in a program for assisted fertilization. In the other two cases, it is clear that the women were alone, but they offered no explanations as to why.

According to staff members at the ultrasound clinic, the letter to women that informs them of their appointment time for the routine scan includes an invitation to bring along their partner or other person(s) they might wish to have along. No such invitation is sent in connection with a clinical examination due to symptoms of pathology; however, if a woman does bring someone with her to such an exam, the accompanying person will not be refused admittance to the examination room.[8]

One woman summed up the issue of partner participation particularly clearly:

> I think it's really fine, the way it is now, that you can have along with you . . . the father. Because . . .
>
> [Me: Was he with you also that first time (a clinical examination due to acute pains in the second month of pregnancy)]?
>
> No. Then I was alone. And I felt a little . . . because this pregnancy wasn't planned. And I've felt that I've been very much alone, to put it that way. I don't feel that he has completely understood what I'm going through. Or also, I've felt that he's been cheated of some of what I'm going through. So in that sense I think it's really fine that he got to come along now and see the same as me, so that we have something more in common to talk about. And so that we think of it as a baby already now, and not first after it's born.

Note that she constructs ultrasound as a family-building technology in several ways: It is an occasion for her partner to be supportive of her feelings, which in turn would alleviate her sense of loneliness. It is also an opportunity for her partner to partake more equally in the thrill of pregnancy. And it is an opportunity to start thinking about the baby as a family member.

In extending an invitation to the women to bring their partner and/or other family members or friends to the eighteen-weeks sonogram, the clinic lends support to this construction of the routine sonogram as a family-building occasion. Similar invitations are not normally extended to adults making appointments for medical examinations. As we have seen, sonograms offered on the basis of clinical symptoms are handled in this sense as ordinary medical appointments.

"Finally He Realized That I Needed to Talk about It"

I asked all the women who had taken the routine scan whether they had decided beforehand what they would do should they come away from the scan with a diagnosis that something was seriously wrong with the fetus. All the respondents answered that not only had they reached such a decision[9] but that they had reached it through discussions with their partners.[10] The one woman who had declined to take the routine scan had reached *that* decision (not to take the scan) together with her partner. Thus it is not only the experience of the scan itself but also the anticipation of a scan in the near future, or the question of whether or not to take such a scan, which these women took as an opportunity to involve significant others in the pregnancy.

In a few cases, the respondent's narrative indicates that gaining this involvement was the result of a conscious effort on her part:

[Me: Had you discussed this?]
Oh yes! Ho! It was embroidered on from one end to the other. He realized
that I wanted to talk about it. He didn't want to talk about it himself,
because he felt it was sort of an unpleasant topic, but finally he realized that I
needed to talk about it. And then it turned out that we had exactly the same
thoughts about it.

Thus routine ultrasound becomes constructed as a social technology, a family-building technology, both through sharing the experience of the scan and also in advance of the scan itself. Had I allowed myself space in this essay, I could have explored other aspects of this construction. For instance, according to some of the narratives, the scan is also an occasion for mobilizing and renegotiating relationships between the woman and her mother. The same applies to relationships between the parents, the new baby, and older children. Some of the narratives also mention the deployment of snapshots from the scan to establish the baby as a family member before its birth. And a broad spectrum of family and friendship networks are taken into consideration when agonizing over the hypothetical situation of coming away from the scan facing an abortion decision.

CONCLUSIONS: GENDER FLEXIBILITY . . . WITHIN LIMITS?

For about two decades now, Norwegian women have been confronted with—have in fact been a prime target group for—various constructions of the relationship between gender and obstetric ultrasound: of what pregnant women are like, what expectant fathers are like, what medical professional men and women are like, and why all of these groups should or should not be interested in ultrasound. Some of these constructions have been particularly powerful in that they have captured media attention. Of those, one has been even more powerful in that it has formed the basis for the ultrasound services which women are offered and which the vast majority of women encounter as a material reality when they attend for their routine scan. One might, therefore, expect that women's own narratives would reproduce these constructions.

Making Technology (and Pregnancy) Our Own

Not so. As we have seen above, these thirteen women created their own alternative constructions of gender, pregnancy, and ultrasound. While these constructions sometimes echoed elements of those of their self-appointed spokespersons in the debate, and while these elements may have been imported from that debate, in the women's own narratives they were integrated into different and original wholes.

For instance, the women who attended for a routine scan did not allow its results to usurp their embodied self-knowledge. On the other hand, neither did they reject the ultrasound results entirely when these conflicted with their previous self-knowledge. Instead, they found various ways of integrating the two while regarding neither as conclusive. We have also seen examples from the women's narratives where the gender impact of the partner's presence at the scan is interpreted in ways that are not depicted/predicted in the narratives of the various self-appointed spokespersons.

From this small, self-selected sample of women, it is not possible to say how typical these constructions are of the population as a whole. They are, however, present in that population; they are, therefore, possible.

When Interpretations Collide

And yet I am also left with a grounded suspicion that there might be abrupt limits to women's scope for interpretative flexibility of the gender-and-ultrasound nexus. These women either declined to attend for a routine scan or emerged from their scan with no indications of fetal or maternal pathology. Although most had their due date changed, they were not yet at a stage where the due date formed a basis for medical decisions and where disagreement over the due date might form a basis for conflict between incompatible constructions of the reliability of ultrasound as a source of information. But what if such a situation did arise?

And such a situation is almost inevitable currently in Norway. None of the thirteen women I interviewed mentioned any thoughts about their upcoming pregnancy leave, but eventually they will reach that stage of their pregnancy. Pregnancy and maternity leave are mandated in Norway, and they are separate entities. If a mother has been employed, she is entitled to twelve months of paid maternity leave after delivering her baby. She is also entitled to three weeks of paid pregnancy leave prior to delivery. Pregnancy leave may commence no sooner than three weeks prior to one's official due date, and any time left unused as of delivery is "forfeited." It may not be converted into maternity leave. If a woman has had her pregnancy dated with ultrasound, then the ultrasound due date is the official due date. This is the rule in connection with pregnancy leave, regardless of how the woman herself may view that due date. Since the majority of ultrasound due dates are later than the dates arrived at by other means, and since this appears to result in an increase in mature but pre-term births (Backe 1994), a routine ultrasound exam is likely to "cost" women a portion of their pregnancy leave. Although, as stated above, none of the women I interviewed mentioned this, it has been brought up since by several women who have heard me present earlier versions of this article.

Or—less frequently but more dramatically—once a diagnosis has been made, I suspect that it will prove difficult to maintain a lay construction of the meaning of ultrasound. At that point, the woman and her fetus will be placed much more firmly into a patient role, and in that role the medical-professional construction of reality rules hegemonic.

This is not to say that no interpretative flexibility will remain. As Browner and Preloran (this volume) have shown, women still can, and sometimes do, opt off the medical "conveyor belt," declining further diagnostics and/or the offer of an abortion when a test has shown suspicious results. There are also ways of recouping one's "lost" pregnancy leave, for instance, if one can convince a GP to prescribe sick leave toward the end of a pregnancy. It remains to be seen how Norwegian women respond to these types of situations.

NOTES

1. See Saetnan 1996a or 1996b for a more complete presentation of these interviews and interviews with several other experts active in the debate. The three experts cited here are (1) an internationally renowned gynecologist and expert on obstetric ultrasound who is also the driving force for routinization of obstetric ultrasound in Norway, (2) a feminist general practitioner who has been a member of several national committees on ultrasound services and similar health policy issues, and (3) an internationally renowned perinatal epidemiologist.

2. Excerpt from my interview with Norway's leading expert on obstetric ultrasound diagnostics.

3. According to the head of the clinic, only two women out of approximately five thousand pregnancies in the clinic's catchment area that year declined the offer of a routine ultrasound.

4. In Norway, routine sonograms are generally carried out by midwives at the nearest hospital obstetrics department. Some GPs carry out their own sonograms. All follow-up so-

nograms in cases where a tentative diagnosis has been made are carried out by specialist physicians at a designated ultrasound clinic.

5. I hope later in this project to interview women who have received such a diagnosis.

6. One had not taken the routine scan at eighteen weeks. The other had to return for a second scan to check for due dates, as the fetus had been positioned so that some of the measurements could not be obtained. She was instructed to walk around for a couple of hours and then return for a second attempt. The interview was conducted during this break in the examination.

7. She was sixteen and unwed at the time and was obliged to have an ultrasound to date the pregnancy in connection with an abortion application. This was in a previous pregnancy, and the exam was carried out at another clinic than the one which was the basis for my interviews.

8. This was confirmed over the phone by the clinic chief's secretary and by the head midwife.

9. In two instances the decision was to "cross that bridge if they came to it." The other ten had reached a hypothetical decision either to take an abortion if offered or continue the pregnancy. Sometimes that decision was elaborated in terms of conditions for the one choice or the other.

10. The one woman who was not living with the child's father mentioned discussing these issues with her mother and with friends.

REFERENCES

Akrich, Madeleine:
  1992 The De-Scription of Technical Objects. In Wiebe E. Bijker and John Law (eds.), *Shaping Technology/Building Society: Studies in Sociotechnical Change,* 205–24. Cambridge: MIT Press.
Andersen, Håkon With:
  1988 Technological Trajectories, Cultural Values, and the Labour Process: The Development of NC Machinery in the Norwegian Andersen Shipbuilding Industry. *Social Studies of Science* 18: 465–82.
Backe, Bjørn:
  1994 *Studies in Antenatal Care.* Trondheim: Tapir.
Berg, Anne-Jorunn, and Merete Lie:
  1995 Feminism and Constructivism: Do Artifacts Have Gender? *Science, Technology, and Human Values* 20(3): 332–51.
Clarke, Adele, and Theresa Montini:
  1993 The Many Faces of RU486: Tales of Situated Knowledges and Technological Contestations. *Science, Technology, and Human Values* 18(1): 42–78.
Cussins, Charis:
  1996 Ontological Choreography: Agency through Objectification in Infertility Clinics. *Social Studies of Science* 26(3): 575–610.
Haraway, Donna:
  1989 *Primate Visions: Gender, Race, and Nature in the World of Modern Science.* New York: Routledge.
Harding, Sandra:
  1986 *The Science Question in Feminism.* Ithaca: Cornell University Press.

Latour, Bruno:
  1987   *Science in Action: How to Follow Scientists and Engineers through Society.* Milton
         Keynes: Open University Press.
Pinch, Trevor J., and Wiebe E. Bijker:
  1987   The Social Construction of Facts and Artifacts; or, How the Sociology of Science
         and the Sociology of Technology Might Benefit Each Other. In Wiebe E. Bijker,
         Thomas P. Hughes, and Trevor Pinch (eds.), *The Social Construction of Technological
         Systems,* 17–50. Cambridge: MIT Press.
Press, Nancy A., and C. H. Browner:
  1994   The Meaning of Prenatal Diagnostic Testing for a Group of Pregnant American
         Women. Paper presented at the 1994 annual meeting of the Society for the Social
         Studies of Science, the History of Science Society, and the Philosophy of Science
         Association.
Rapp, Rayna:
  1988   Moral Pioneers: Women, Men, and Fetuses on a Frontier of Reproductive Technol-
         ogy. In Elaine H. Baruch, Amadeo F. D'Adamo Jr., and Joni Seager (eds.), *Embryos,
         Ethics, and Women's Rights: Exploring the New Reproductive Technologies,* 101–16. New
         York: Haworth Press.
Saetnan, Ann Rudinow:
  1996a Ultrasonic Discourse: Contested Meanings of Gender and Technology in the Nor-
         wegian Ultrasound Screening Debate. *European Journal of Women's Studies* 3(1):
         55–75.
  1996b Speaking of Gender . . . : Intertwinings of a Medical Technology Policy Debate and
         Everyday Life. In Merete Lie and Knut H. Sørensen (eds.), *Making Technology Our
         Own? Domestication Technology into Everyday Life,* 31–63. Oslo: Scandinavian Uni-
         versity Press.
Sorge, Arndt, and Malcolm Warner:
  1986   *Comparative Factory Organisation: An Anglo-German Comparison of Management and
         Manpower in Manufacturing.* Aldershot: Gower.

13

Magic and a Little Bit of Science: Technoscience, Ethnoscience, and the Social Construction of the Fetus

Lynn M. Morgan

An advertisement for an ovulation predictor kit in *Good Housekeeping* magazine (U.S.) shows a fuzzy blue orb penetrated by an electric-yellow sperm (see fig. 13.1). The caption reads, "Another satisfied customer." The fine print pushes the product: "Getting pregnant takes magic, and a little bit of science." The "science" here is a $27 kit designed to tell a woman when she is ovulating, thereby identifying the opportune time to conceive. The accompanying picture is obviously designed to depict fertilization, which in modern scientific discourse has come to be widely acknowledged as the beginning of pregnancy.

The advertisement depicts the central "fact" of modern scientific reproduction as understood in cosmopolitan cultures around the globe: fertilization is the beginning of life. Fertilization sets gestational development into motion, and gestational development results in new human life. Fertilization is thus both magical (in that it results in a brand-new person) and, increasingly, scientific (in that it is susceptible to scientific explication, manipulation, and enhancement). The power of this advertisement depends on a shared assumption among readers that science is the foremost system of knowledge capable of understanding, explaining, and assisting the reproductive process.

Scientific explanations of the "facts of life" are widely promulgated. They are codified in international health guidelines such as those developed by the World Health Organization to register fetal deaths, stillbirths, and live births (see Jewkes and Wood 1998). The fertility enhancement industry commodifies scientific understandings when it markets ovulation predictor kits and other conception techniques. Intracytoplasmic sperm injection (ICSI), for example, one of the latest techniques to become available, is used to inject a sperm

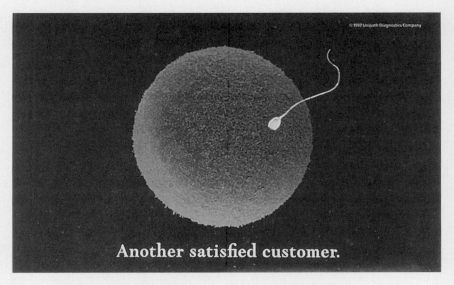

Another satisfied customer.

Figure 13.1 Advertisement for ClearPlan Easy Ovulation Predictor, © 1997 Unipath Diagnostics Company. Reprinted by permission.

directly into an ovum (and thus offer genetically related offspring to infertile men). Scientific explanations of reproduction are hegemonic in the sense that many people accept them as unassailable truths unmediated by cultural under-standings or assumptions.

As globalization brings disparate cultures into greater contact, it is impor-tant to remind ourselves that many societies subscribe to altogether different explanations of reproduction. In societies where the ethnophysiology of preg-nancy and intrauterine development are built upon different premises, for ex-ample, people may acknowledge no "moment" of fertilization that marks the inexorable beginning of new life. In fact, during the early months of pregnancy they may acknowledge only the most inchoate, incipient, and liminal forms of life. This essay reports on ethnographic research conducted in the highlands of Ecuador, where scientific explanations compete with localized knowledge about pregnancy. I will argue that the meanings attached to accepted "facts" of human reproduction—such as fertilization, fetal growth, and birth—are culturally produced, not only in "traditional" societies but in modern techno-scientific societies as well (see Clarke 1998; Franklin 1998).

The examples I present here could be used to reinforce the ethnocentric assumption that there is a wide disparity between technoscience (i.e., "our" modern, western "knowledge" based on scientific method) and ethnoscience (i.e., "their" premodern, nonwestern "beliefs" based on traditional worldviews) (Good 1994). Modernist theorists often assume a posture of technological and scientific superiority. They expect that, with time, modern scientific knowledge will replace "traditional" or "superstitious" views of reproduction in the non-industrialized world. But I will argue instead that technoscientific understandings of reproduction are also produced and hence "ethnoscientific"; that is, they are based on historically and culturally particular understandings of fertilization, gestation, and birth.

Technoscientific practices are as much products of cultural assumptions and values as are "non-modern" beliefs (Harding 1998; Latour 1993). "We" (the relatively elite, cosmopolitan, privileged) may imagine ourselves as more enlightened, knowledgeable, and modern than people in far-away places with their exotic beliefs. In comparison with "them," "we" imagine ourselves above the influence of culture, or we imagine ourselves immune from culture entirely (Rosaldo 1989). And yet, I will argue, technoscience is invariably affected by cultural peculiarities and idiosyncracies. Technoscientific practices rely on their own kind of magic. They do this, for example, when they conjure up images on the ultrasound screen and translate the "signals from beyond" into the language spoken by today's pregnant women (Mitchell and Georges 1997). They do this when they take a vague collection of data points (as in prenatal testing) and use them to predict definitive outcomes (Browner and Press 1995). As the wealthy and well-educated members of industrialized societies embrace technoscientific interpretations of assisted reproduction, it might be useful to remember the humility and ambiguity associated with the beginnings of life in other parts of the world.

THE TECHNOSCIENTIFIC IMAGINARY

As reproductive imaging technologies provide more concrete ways of knowing the fetus, the stories told about fetal development grow more elaborate and laced with intricate, scientifically sophisticated detail. The stories (and the fetuses they depict) appear in numerous formats, including posters on the obstetrician's office wall, popular films, pregnancy how-to books, pop-up picture books for children, a CD-ROM version of Lennart Nilsson's "The Miracle of Life," and the "birth stories" that parents tell their children. Young people today are exposed to multiple versions of the story, each of which begins, predictably, with conception: "Once upon a time, an egg was fertilized by a sperm" (Martin 1991). From there the story follows an unwavering, linear trajectory dominated by the language and imagery of physiology and developmental biology (Hahn 1995).

If fertilization is the beginning of the story, birth provides its "happily ever after" ending. Stories of pregnancy rarely mention miscarriage (although an estimated 20 percent of pregnancies end in miscarriage), nor do they mention induced abortion, Down's syndrome, cerebral palsy, HIV, or stillbirth (Ginsburg and Rapp 1999; Layne 1990, 1992, 1997). Pregnancy is today framed in scientific rather than religious or mystical language, although even scientific language ignores the empirical verity that many pregnancies do not result in live birth. The story must end with birth, because birth is the pinnacle of achievement. Lennart Nilsson's 1966 book of photographs of intrauterine development was entitled *A Child Is Born.* The original as well as subsequent editions are designed to convey the impression that the photographs represent the development of a single child from conception to birth. Yet this impression is not accurate. Claes Wirsén, one of Nilsson's physician collaborators, writes in his preface to the Swedish edition of 1976: "Our knowledge of human fetal development is based, now as before, on observations which can be made when a pregnancy for some reason or another is ended. These are not easily made observations—years of patient waiting twenty-four hours a day for the right cases and highly developed technical skills in treating the materials during the first precious minutes lie behind a work such as this." [Translated from the Swedish by Ann Saetnan. The English versions from this period are less explicit regarding the sources of the images.]

The narrative of inexorable progress from fertilization to birth is thus revealed as a carefully constructed fiction. It does not admit that pregnancy might be tentative or ambiguous, or that anything other than a full-fledged child or fully formed person might be the outcome. Thus we see that the technoscientific image of human reproduction is not an inevitable consequence of the data but a culturally produced, selective interpretation of those data.

The lived experience of pregnancy and birth is often steeped in uncertainties: When will the baby arrive? What will it look like? Will it be healthy? What kind of person will it grow up to be? Prenatal surveillance techniques attempt to allay uncertainty by providing additional information to prospective parents prior to birth. Testing procedures such as ultrasound and amniocentesis can, presumably, render pregnancy less tentative and make parents more informed and thus more confident (Rothman 1986). Tests focus on specific indicators such as age and size of the fetus, detection of specified chromosomal anomalies, and location of the placenta. The very act of testing implies scientific validity, hence test results are often interpreted as more definitive than is warranted by epidemiologic criteria. The climate of technoscientific certainty makes it difficult to imagine why some societies would tolerate ambiguity in their worldviews.

FERTILIZATION AS METAPHOR

What happens when we try to "separate the 'facts' of biological reproduction as scientific truth, from their operation as forms of cultural knowledge" (Franklin 1997, 51)? In keeping with my original example at the beginning of this chapter, let us imagine that fertilization operates as a metaphor, an example of how culture shapes our interpretations of the "raw facts" of biology. The *Good Housekeeping* advertisement depicts fertilization as an undisputed biological fact. Fertilization can be "seen" (with the aid of an electron microscope) and thus presumably "known." Yet cultural theorists note "that 'seeing' is a thoroughly situated and mediated activity" (Hartouni 1997, 3). The cultural particularity of how we view fertilization becomes obvious if we step outside the technoscientific "sitings/sightings" of fertilization to show how other cultures view it. This exercise in cross-cultural contrast reveals some of the technoscientific premises and assumptions about fertilization.

It is well known among anthropologists that the study of reproduction can provide insights about the organization and cultural logic of a society. In the late 1960s, the anthropological journals were brimming with debates over "virgin birth." The term referred to the supposed ignorance of the "facts" of physiologic paternity among the aboriginal peoples of central Australia. Yet, as Sarah Franklin points out in her lucid review of the topic, the debate said as much about "conception among the anthropologists" as it did about conception among so-called primitive peoples (1997, 17–72). For a long time, Franklin notes, anthropologists unreflexively projected their own cultural assumptions about biological facticity onto the debate. Gradually, however, some anthropologists and cultural theorists began to emphasize "the role of biological science in shaping the presumptions that are brought to bear on cultural interpretation" (66). Once we acknowledge the cultural imprints on our own assumptions about fertilization and gestation (see Morgan 1999), other local logics can become more comprehensible.

Many nonindustrialized societies understand pregnancy to be the result of sociological rather than biological factors. Anthropologists describe many societies in which the child-to-be is described as the literal instantiation of existing relationships. The Wari' Indians of Rondônia, Brazil, for example, "believe that conception occurs when a quantity of semen accumulates after multiple acts of sexual intercourse close together in time" (Conklin and Morgan 1996, 670; see also Jennaway 1996). Pregnancy cannot therefore be a mistake, because it is both the result and the evidence of a committed relationship between a man and a woman. In the Trobriand Islands, a woman becomes pregnant when a spirit child (waiwaia) enters her body. Weiner describes this as a reflection of Trobriand matrilineal ideology, which holds that each infant must be linked to her matrilineal ancestors (1988, 54–55). Paraphrasing Marilyn Strathern, the focus in such societies is not on the conceptus (or fetus or child) per se but on offspring as icons of already existing social relationships (1992, 61).

There is plenty of ambiguity inherent in these ethnographic accounts of conception and gestation; informants were reportedly uncertain about how to respond to the anthropologist's questions, or they disagreed with one another, or they invoked "folk" beliefs in certain situations but not others. But perhaps ambiguity is an understandable feature of societies that do not pin pregnancy to biological "facts." There can be no certainty, no absolute verity, no guaranteed outcomes, no dependable tests when pregnancy is thought to be contingent on the frailties and vagaries of human character or the unpredictable whims of supernatural spirits. Fertilization and gestation are thus as ambiguous, ambivalent, and unpredictable as the social and spiritual relationships they embody and exemplify.

In contrast, the technoscientific renditions of fertilization begin to look remarkably devoid of social content. The seed-and-soil metaphors of fertilization and generation traditionally associated with monotheistic, agricultural societies (Delaney 1991) are giving way in the industrialized West to metaphors and images dominated by the technological assist ("a little bit of science"). Fertilization (like gestation) is now increasingly depicted as occurring outside of women's bodies. Gametes are extracted from human bodies (off screen) and combined in petri dishes (on screen), where fertilization can be videotaped for spectators who watch this most intimate magical-and-scientific moment. Fertilization is filmed, edited, and given center stage in magazines, on television screens, and in the movies. It is portrayed as a finite event that happens at a precise moment in time, rather than as a long, uncertain process. The visual depiction of fertilization allows the viewer to shift her thinking; whereas the "moment of creation" may once have been amorphous, unknowable, and magical, it can now be considered a technoscientific fact. Visual images of fertilization depict it as an unambiguous achievement: boy (sperm) meets girl (ovum), boy gets girl, and together they live happily ever after (Martin 1991). As Franklin says, "Technological assistance is increasingly part of the production of new persons" (1998, 106). Spectators are not shown, would not want to see, the missed conceptions or miscarriages (for there is no magic in those). Increasingly, fertilization is a symbol of technological assistance, the commodification of life, and the achievements of science.

THE AMBIGUITY OF LIFE IN SAN GABRIEL DE CARCHI, ECUADOR

The following examples are drawn from the agricultural town of San Gabriel (population 10,000), province of Carchi, in northern Ecuador, where I conducted thirty ethnographic interviews in 1988. One woman told me that when she had miscarried after about two months of pregnancy, she was not sure what to do with the remains. She did not want to throw them away without ceremony [*botarlos*], for fear that the spirit (if there was one) might wander. Nor did she feel comfortable burying them in the children's part of the cemetery where dozens of pale blue crosses dotted the hillside. She finally decided to put the remains (*restos*) in a box and to bury the box just inside the cemetery, not very deep, along the fence. After much reflection, she had decided to bury this not-yet-child in sacred ground, but decidedly on its outer edge.

There were many manifestations of the liminality of the unborn and newly born in the rural Andean highlands of San Gabriel. Walking at night along steep, narrow roads, some women had heard the mournful cries of the *aucas,* the night-wandering spirits of aborted and unbaptized babies. The *auca* (the word also means "heathen" or "uncivilized" or, pejoratively, "lowland Indian") would wail in sorrow because it could not be admitted to heaven (Morgan 1997, 1998).

The attributes of personhood as described to me in San Gabriel contained room for a character not often found in the industrialized West: the liminal, incipient, semi-, or quasi-person. This "not-yet" figure may have a corporeal existence (which in the case of miscarriage is sometimes just blood, or "a chunk of meat with one eye"), but its moral status remains ambiguous and uncertain until it is baptized into the Catholic Church. For that reason, parents in San Gabriel would rush to baptize infants who showed the slightest sign of sickness. In the words of one fifty-nine-year-old woman, the veteran of twenty-two pregnancies, "as *auquitas* [little *aucas*] God and the angels don't accompany the child. It dies in darkness. God said we have to baptize them so they can be with Him and the angels, so they can accompany them. And if not, well, the *auca* is the devil, then. That would be painful and sad."

One priest in Quito told me that birth [*alumbramiento;* literally "bringing to light"] was an important dividing line in the transition to personhood, because it marked humanity [*hominización*] and permanence. But according to many of the women I interviewed in San Gabriel, birth did not resolve the status ambiguity of young quasi-persons; babies, they told me, remained vulnerable until they were baptized. When I asked about the function of baptism, one city-educated woman in San Gabriel told me, "My in-laws say that baptism keeps the devil [*cuco*] from carrying the child away. Sometimes the devil comes and kills it, and whatever. Once they are baptized you can leave them, you can go out wherever you want, but if they aren't baptized you can't leave them." If birth marks the physical separation of mother and child, baptism demarcates the spiritual separation of mother and child.

The social separation of mother and child was marked, at least in the memories of the older women, by yet another local custom. Years ago, women would remain secluded behind a *toldo* throughout the postpartum period. The *toldo* was a sheet hung over the bed to prevent dangerous "airs" from reaching the vulnerable new mother and child. Postpartum seclusion of mother and child from the rest of society is quite commonly found in the ethnographic literature as a classic feature of birth rites. Seclusion marks the liminal time during which new mother and child move from one status to another. While secluded, they are particularly vulnerable to supernatural threats and to mortal illness; the status of both mother and child is ambiguous and uncertain.

As the days pass after birth, both mother and child become more securely rooted to their new identities, although the routes of transition are different for each. Mothers should observe the *dieta,* a forty-day postpartum rest period during which they eat certain foods and refrain from housework, bathing, and sexual relations. Newborn children must be sheltered from wind and dew and from supernatural threats posed by storms, "evil hour" (6 A.M., noon, 6 P.M., and midnight), and local illnesses such as *colerín* (which is caused by a mother's jealous rage at an unfaithful husband) and evil eye. The older women in San Gabriel explained that the liminal period is shorter now than when they were young. Progress, they implied, carries danger, whereas the open acknowledgment of ambiguity in earlier times ensured that new mothers and children would be better guarded from harm.

Ambiguity seemed especially and inevitably vexing when I asked women about the fate of the unborn who die before birth. Do they become *aucas*? Does a miscarried fetus carry original sin if it has not yet suckled at its mother's breast? How could God see fit to deny entrance into heaven for a little innocent, who died according to God's will, after all? Could a miscarried or stillborn fetus be baptized? These are the questions the women asked me as I pressed them to say whether a miscarried or aborted fetus would become an *auca.* Many said frankly that they didn't know. Nevertheless, it was clear to me that the *auca* functioned to remind them of the fragility and spiritual ambiguity of young human life and of the importance of baptism.

Most of the women (as well as several clergy) I interviewed did not consider the ambiguity surrounding the beginnings of life to be a moral problem. Coming from the United States, where reproductive ethics debates are exceedingly polarized, I found it hard to accept this ambiguity at face value. Slowly, though, I realized that they accepted ambiguity with humility. Ambiguity was, for them, an inherent feature of social life rather than as a philosophical or policy conundrum to be resolved. They found liminality problematic only in specific, pragmatic situations, such as what to do with the issue of a miscarriage, or whether to baptize a stillborn infant, or whether to mourn an unbaptized child "with dancing" (*con baile*) or without. Those instances required a decision to be made, but the decision was often admittedly arbitrary. Neither a burial place nor a name bestowed nor the sprinkling of holy water could erase the ambiguity surrounding the fate of the soul.

But ambiguity was not restricted to the rural highlands. In the capital city of Quito, women who were unquestionably more familiar with scientific explanations of fertilization and gestation also countenanced ambiguity. Ambiguity characterized the gestating fetus, which was not personified or individualized as fetuses are, increasingly, in the United States.

ULTRASOUND AND AMBIGUITY IN QUITO

Routine ultrasound is fast becoming common in industrialized countries. In the United States, the more frequent use of ultrasound has coincided with a popular willingness to see the fetus as a "baby" and to use ultrasound to visualize the womb's inhabitant. Ultrasound offers a window onto the womb, a way to observe voyeuristically the secrets under the skin. (It is also, as Barbara Duden [1993] puts it, a way to "disembody women" by focusing on the fetus.) Middle-class American women imagine ultrasound images to be "real," the literal "in-sight" that science has provided. Under these conditions, ultrasonography is interpreted as "the benign face of science, assisting in an apparently natural process, promoting the conditions under which 'nature' will happen" (Strathern 1992, 49). The widespread availability of a technological device, however, tells us little about how it is interpreted or used. Rapp (1990) has described disparate reactions to ultrasound by women with different backgrounds in the United States. In 1992, I observed about thirty ultrasound examinations in a social security hospital in Quito, Ecuador. These observations were not exhaustive or conclusive, and I did not interview many of the patients. Nonetheless, my observations in the clinic offer a number of clues about the construction of the ambiguous fetus there.

Compared to the women I had interviewed in San Gabriel, the women in Quito might have been expected to share some of my technoscientific assumptions about this form of testing. They were mostly married, university-educated, middle-class, insured women living in the country's cosmopolitan capital. Each had been referred to a specialty clinic for ultrasound scanning because her obstetrician suspected a problem with the pregnancy (e.g., small fetal size for gestational age, or a suspected placenta previa). In the United States, the technician or physician conducting a routine ultrasound would likely have included the patient as a participant in the exam. The patient would have expected to watch the monitor throughout the exam, and the technician would have pointed out relevant features and movements. Yet the clinical encounters I observed did not follow this script, which indicated to me that patients and providers did not share the notion—so common in the United States—of the personified fetus-as-baby (see Mitchell and Georges 1997).

The exams I observed in Quito were anxious and tense, as each woman awaited a verdict about the fate of her pregnancy. As each patient revealed her belly and lay down on the table for the examination, she watched the doctor's face. He conducted the exam with the ultrasound monitor oriented away from her; she could not see the shadowy, crackling image on the screen. The physician said little during the exam, nor did he "read" the image aloud to the woman by pointing out sex or body parts or size or activity levels of the fetus. He printed images from the screen to clip into the woman's medical chart; she did not ask for or expect to be given a "fetal photo" for her scrapbook. During the exam she watched the physician's face (rather than the monitor), rarely asking a question. (The doctor explained to me that women are now learning that ultrasound can determine sex, so they ask him about that more often than they used to.) There is an air of anxiety in the room, as she waits to be told whether her pregnancy is at risk.

In the United States, ultrasound has become a tool in the reification of the fetal subject. As Donna Haraway points out, "The sonogram is literally a pedagogy for learning to see who exists in the world" (1997, 177). Ultrasound is interpreted as a test that can provide objective evidence of fetal subjectivity and personhood, even while it is simultaneously a practice that produces those qualities (Hartouni 1997, 19). In the Quito hospital where I worked, however, where there was no autonomous fetal subject, the purpose of ultrasound was not to introduce the mother-to-be to her "baby" but to determine whether the pregnancy was advancing normally. The focus was more on maternal health and on the embodied and potentially pathological dimensions of pregnancy. Elective induced abortion was not an option for the patient in Quito, even if the ultrasound showed fetal death. The physician sometimes told the patient that the pregnancy had not advanced and that a uterine evacuation would be required, but this was defined as dilation and evacuation, not as abortion. Furthermore, this would be the physician's determination rather than the woman's decision. This small case study from Ecuador demonstrates how the same technoscientific practice can be interpreted differently according to the medical circumstances (routine ultrasound versus diagnosis of pathology) and according to cultural context (personification of the fetal person versus emphasis on the pregnant woman).

Technoscientific practices such as ultrasound acquire and confer meaning only within given social contexts. In the United States, ultrasound has become a tool in the reification of the fetal subject; it provides objective evidence of fetal subjectivity and personhood while it is, simultaneously, a practice that creates those qualities. In Quito, however, where there is no autonomous fetal subject, ultrasound is about authoritative medical knowledge and patient subordination and quiescence, about the scientific control over access to modern technologies, and about the stratification inherent in who gets access to these modalities.

DENATURALIZING THE FETAL SUBJECT

This chapter has juxtaposed technoscientific representations of reproduction with alternate interpretations found in the highlands of Ecuador. Putting these contrasting interpretations into dialogue reveals a great deal about each society. In Ecuador, the genesis and birth of each new child remains inherently ambiguous and aloof from human control. Meanwhile, the industrialized West creates and fosters the presumption that technoscience will provide ways to understand and manipulate the production of new persons.

Philosophers and anthropologists have argued that the dichotomy between western rationality and primitive magical thinking is indefensible (Good 1994; Harding 1998). This chapter has adopted and extended that critique to western technoscientific renderings of reproduction. Wistful, perhaps, for the rational certainties of the modernist era, people in the technoscientific West still like to imagine that our truths might bear a closer resemblance to reality than "theirs," especially when our truths can be supported by technoscientific evidence. When advertisers feature fertilization as an event of monumental significance, they invite observers to think of it as fundamentally a biological (and not a social) process. They encourage readers to reify fertilization and to glorify the technologies that can identify and enhance it. When technoscientific procedures such as ultrasound portray the unborn as "child," observers are emboldened to ignore the tenuousness and uncertainty that might otherwise inform their understandings of pregnancy, miscarriage, birth, and young human life and death.

REFERENCES

Browner, Carole H., and Nancy Ann Press:
  1995 The Normalization of Prenatal Diagnostic Screening. In Faye D. Ginsburg and Rayna Rapp (eds.), *Conceiving the New World Order: The Global Politics of Reproduction*, 307–22. Berkeley: University of California Press.
Clarke, Adele:
  1998 *Disciplining Reproduction: Modernity, American Life Sciences, and the "Problem of Sex."* Berkeley: University of California Press.
Conklin, Beth A., and Lynn M. Morgan:
  1996 Babies, Bodies, and the Production of Personhood in North America and a Native Amazonian Society. *Ethos* 24(4): 657–94.

Delaney, Carol:
1991 *The Seed and the Soil: Gender and Cosmology in Turkish Village Society.* Berkeley: University of California Press.

Duden, Barbara:
1993 *Disembodying Women.* Cambridge: Harvard University Press.

Franklin, Sarah:
1997 *Embodied Progress: A Cultural Account of Assisted Conception.* London: Routledge.
1998 Making Miracles: Scientific Progress and the Facts of Life. In Sarah Franklin and Helena Ragon (eds.), *Reproducing Reproduction: Kinship, Power, and Technological Innovation,* 102–17. Philadelphia: University of Pennsylvania Press.

Ginsburg, Faye, and Rayna Rapp:
1999 Fetal Impressions: Reflections of Two Feminist Anthropologists as Mutual Informants. In Lynn M. Morgan and Meredith W. Michaels (eds.), *Fetal Subjects, Feminist Positions.* Philadelphia: University of Pennsylvania Press.

Good, Byron:
1994 *Medicine, Rationality, and Experience: An Anthropological Perspective.* Cambridge: Cambridge University Press.

Hahn, Robert A.:
1995 *Sickness and Healing: An Anthropological Perspective.* New Haven: Yale University Press.

Haraway, Donna:
1997 *Modest-Witness@Second-Millennium. FemaleMan-Meets-OncoMouse: Feminism and Technoscience.* New York: Routledge.

Harding, Sandra:
1998 *Is Science Multicultural? Postcolonialisms, Feminisms, and Epistemologies.* Bloomington: Indiana University Press.

Hartouni, Valerie:
1997 *Cultural Conceptions: On Reproductive Technologies and the Remaking of Life.* Minneapolis: University of Minnesota Press.

Jennaway, Megan:
1996 Of Blood and Foetuses: Female Fertility and Women's Reproductive Health in a North Balinese Village. In Pranee Liamputtong Rice and Lenore Manderson (eds.), *Maternity and Reproductive Health in Asian Society,* 37–60. Australia: Harwood Academic.

Jewkes, Rachel, and Katharine Wood:
1998 Competing Discourses of Vital Registration and Personhood: Perspectives from Rural South Africa. *Social Science and Medicine* 46(8): 1043–56.

Latour, Bruno:
1993 *We Have Never Been Modern.* Trans. Catherine Porter. Cambridge: Harvard University Press.

Layne, Linda:
1990 Motherhood Lost: Cultural Dimensions of Miscarriage and Stillbirth in America. *Women and Health* 16(3): 75–104.
1992 Of Fetuses and Angels: Fragmentation and Integration in Narratives of Pregnancy Loss. In David Hess and Linda Layne (eds.), *Knowledge and Society,* 29–58. Greenwich, Conn.: JAI Press.
1997 Breaking the Silence: An Agenda for a Feminist Discourse of Pregnancy Loss. *Feminist Studies* 23(2): 289–316.

Martin, Emily:

1991   The Egg and Sperm. *Signs: A Journal of Women, Culture, and Society* 16(3): 485–501.

Mitchell, Lisa, and Eugenia Georges:

1997   Cross-Cultural Cyborgs: Greek and Canadian Women's Discourses on Fetal Ultrasound. *Feminist Studies* 23(2): 373–401 (reprinted in this volume).

Morgan, Lynn M.:

1997   Imagining the Unborn in the Ecuadoran Andes. *Feminist Studies* 23(2): 323–50.

1998   Ambiguities Lost: Fashioning the Fetus into a Child in Ecuador and the United States. In Nancy Scheper-Hughes and Carolyn Sargent (eds.), *Small Wars: The Cultural Politics of Childhood.* Berkeley: University of California Press.

1999   Materializing the Fetal Body; or, What are Those Corpses Doing in Biology's Basement? In Lynn M. Morgan and Meredith W. Michaels (eds.), *Fetal Subjects, Feminist Positions.* Philadelphia: University of Pennsylvania Press.

Rapp, Rayna:

1990   Constructing Amniocentesis: Maternal and Medical Discourses. In Faye Ginsburg and Anna Lowenhaupt Tsing (eds.), *Uncertain Terms: Negotiating Gender in American Culture.* Boston: Beacon.

Rosaldo, Renato:

1989   *Culture and Truth: The Re-Making of Social Analysis.* Boston: Beacon.

Rothman, Barbara Katz:

1986   *The Tentative Pregnancy.* New York: Viking.

Strathern, Marilyn:

1992   *After Nature.* Cambridge: Cambridge University Press.

Weiner, Annette B.:

1988   *The Trobrianders of Papua New Guinea.* New York: Holt, Rinehart & Winston.

14

Para Sacarse la Espina (To Get Rid of the Doubt): Mexican Immigrant Women's Amniocentesis Decisions

C. H. Browner and H. Mabel Preloran

Recent attention has focused on the processes implicated in the medicalization of U.S. childbirth, particularly the significance of technological advances in driving the thrust toward hegemony. Physicians began attending home deliveries in the middle of the eighteenth century, attracting patients away from midwives with the promise of technical expertise in the areas of pain control, the use of forceps, and surgical intervention. The movement from home to hospital deliveries led to further consolidation of physicians' authority as women gave birth under conditions determined not by women themselves but by physicians. At the same time, women, particularly those from middle- and upper-class backgrounds, facilitated these medicalization processes by actively seeking physician-assisted hospital deliveries, which they felt to be safer, less painful, and less arduous (Leavitt 1986; see also Borst 1992). By 1950, 88 percent of all U.S. births were in hospitals with physicians in attendance (Devitt 1977); today the number has reached 99 percent (Jordan 1993).

The intent of obstetrical technologies began to change after World War II as new understandings of human physiology emerged. The "machine" metaphor, which had defined the parameters and principles of biomedical paradigm since the Industrial Revolution, was replaced by an ecological one. In this view, the body is "an open system of communication interacting with the exoteric cosmos and its ecological processes" (Destounis 1972, 68–70, quoted in Arney 1982). Physicians came to regard the body as less a mechanical entity than as a system composed of other systems that were articulated at many different points and levels. At the same time, the organizing concept in obstetrics shifted from "confinement" to "surveillance" (Arney 1982). And as birth became something to be managed rather than something to be attended or dominated, technical advances moved away from efforts to control or influence the course of the reproductive process and toward its monitoring.

Unlike childbirth technologies, which were hailed as progress by both women and physicians, the consequences of the growing use of fetal diagnostic, monitoring, and surveillance technologies are more ambiguous. While obstetricians claim that the "new" obstetrical technologies reduce anxiety during pregnancy and make childbirth less frightening, social scientists have shown that these technologies may produce their own anxieties (Green 1990; Kolker and Burke 1994; Marteau et al. 1989; Rothenberg and Thomson 1994) and that they increase the likelihood of obstetrical intervention, such as cesarean deliveries (Haverkamp and Orleans 1982; Leveno et al. 1986). Many women now regard pregnancy as a risky endeavor and doubt their ability to give birth without technological assistance (Davis-Floyd 1992; McClain 1983, 1988).

Therefore, few U.S. women reject obstetrical diagnostic and monitoring technologies out of hand (Hubbard 1986; Press and Browner 1997). Believing that the health of their fetus rests largely in their hands, they want to do everything they can to bring about a healthy birth (Browner and Press 1995). They also want those around them to know they are doing all that is possible in the hope this will lead to less guilt and blame should the worst occur. One pregnant woman, when asked her intentions about fetal testing, said, "I'm not sure I know what's available. I know I won't have amnio because I'm too young for that, but I want whatever else they have to offer" (Browner, field notes, 1995).

This uncritical acceptance of any and all obstetrical technologies is most common among well-educated, middle- and upper-class European American women. The picture for poor ethnic minority and immigrant women is more complex. They are significantly less likely to use the new obstetrical technologies, particularly those for fetal diagnosis (Nsiah-Jefferson 1994; Press and Browner 1997; Rapp 1993). This may be a matter of access and the fact that they are not as likely to be offered them. But there may also be profound cultural reasons why less educated ethnic minority and immigrant women are less often drawn in the "new" reproductive technologies for fetal diagnosis.

Here we consider this issue. We present preliminary data on the reasons a group of recent Mexican immigrants decided whether or not to accept amniocentesis after they had been told they were at high risk for bearing a child with a birth defect based on the results of a blood screening test. We hypothesized that women in this population would be more likely to decline amniocentesis because they were less fully tied to the view that medical interventions are essential for a healthy birth. Specifically, we thought that women who felt confident in their ability to bear a healthy child would be more likely to refuse fetal diagnosis.

THE CALIFORNIA AFP PROGRAM FOR PRENATAL SCREENING

Because this research was carried out within the context of California's state-administered program for fetal diagnosis, a brief introduction to California's alpha-fetoprotein (AFP) program and the choices it offers pregnant women will help orient the reader to our results. We considered California a propitious place to explore the relationship between ethnicity and the use of obstetrical technologies because the state program was designed to provide all pregnant women access to fetal diagnostic services regardless of their ability to pay for them.

In 1986, California became the first state to legislatively mandate that all pregnant women who begin prenatal care before the twentieth week of gestation be offered AFP screening for neural tube defects and Down's syndrome. Screening is conducted at the woman's normal site of prenatal care through a routine blood test, with the analysis performed at one of the approved laboratories located throughout the state. By 1996, 68 percent of all pregnancies underwent screening (Thompkinson and Roberson 1996).

The program is funded like an insurance pool. A single fee (reset from $40 to $115 in 1995 and generally paid for by private insurance or MediCal, California's Medicaid program) covers the costs of the blood screening test, plus genetic counseling, ultrasonography, and amniocentesis at a state-approved prenatal diagnosis center should a woman screen positive.

Women who screen positive are offered genetic counseling and further testing at a state-approved prenatal diagnosis center. Counseling, by a master's level genetic counselor, generally lasts between forty-five and sixty minutes. The significance of a positive screen is explained at this time, and a family and reproductive history is taken so that the woman's risk can be more precisely assessed. The role of the genetic counselor is to provide information that could help a woman reach a decision about whether or not to have amniocentesis, but in theory s/he does not have to offer an opinion as to whether or not the woman should be tested.

Between 8 and 13 percent of women screen positive low or positive high (Burton, Dillard, and Clark 1985; Evans et al. 1987; Greenberg 1988); the rest screen negative. A positive low screen indicates increased risk for Down's syndrome and other chromosomal abnormalities; positive high suggests the possibility of neural tube defects (anencephaly or spina bifida), intestinal, kidney, liver, or placental problems, or other poor birth outcomes including fetal demise. Some genetics counselors show their clients photos of children with the birth defects that the fetus is at risk for. Yet because most conditions detected through fetal testing vary substantially in severity and have uncertain courses, the risk assessment a genetic counselor can provide any individual patient is necessarily imprecise.

Women are offered a Level 2 high resolution ultrasound at the close of the genetic counseling session. Like routine ultrasound, this test visualizes the fetus using high-frequency sound waves and appears to carry no iatrogenic risk. Only rarely does a woman refuse the Level 2 ultrasound. About half the time, this ultrasound reveals a benign explanation for the positive screen, most often a misdated pregnancy. In these cases, the woman is reassured that the pregnancy appears normal and is sent home. Occasionally, the ultrasound reveals a gross problem such as anencephaly or some other structural disorder. If ultrasonography does not explain the reason for the abnormal AFP test, the woman is generally offered amniocentesis.

Amniocentesis is a surgical procedure in which a physician inserts a 3½" hollow needle through the mother's abdomen into the uterus to remove about one to two teaspoons (30cc) of amniotic fluid. In California, amniocentesis is performed through the twentieth week of gestation. Cells and fluid are sent to a laboratory for analysis, which takes from ten days to three weeks. Complications from amniocentesis are uncommon, but include cramping, bleeding, infection, and occasionally fetal injury or miscarriage.[1]

Unless the pregnancy is very far advanced, a woman does not need to decide on the spot whether or not to have amniocentesis. Yet some counselors do urge women to make an immediate decision, and some women prefer to take advantage of being at the hospital to get the procedure over with. If a woman seems ambivalent or inclining toward amniocentesis refusal, the counselor generally suggests that she go home to think over her options. Women who do not immediately accept the amniocentesis, however, are highly unlikely to return for the procedure (Preloran and Browner 1997).

Most women who have amniocentesis receive normal results. Women who test positive are informed as to the treatments that may be available for the type of defect found. They are also offered an abortion, which in California may be performed through the twenty-fourth week of gestation.

METHODS

These results are part of a larger study about Mexican-origin couples' decisions about amniocentesis, but only findings from women who were recent immigrants and none from male partners are presented here. Couples were recruited from the state-approved prenatal diagnosis centers at three public hospitals in southern California. All women had tested positive on the AFP-screening blood test, and all were offered amniocentesis. Of 355 potential participants,

Table 14.1 Sociodemographic characteristics of Mexican immigrant women offered amniocentesis

	Accepted (N = 26)	Declined (N = 17)
Mean age (years)	31.1	28.9
Education (primary or less)	56.7%	40.2%
Household income (< $20,000/year)	84.6%	75.0%

Note: No significant difference between groups.

defined as women with Spanish surnames who were offered genetic counseling following AFP testing, 43 (12%) fit our criteria that at least one member of the couple be of Mexican origin and be willing to be interviewed.[2]

For this pilot phase of the research, we conducted semistructured, face-to-face interviews lasting one to several hours with forty-three women. In some cases the data were obtained in a single interview session, while in others we made repeat visits. Interviews were conducted after women had decided whether or not to have amniocentesis, but some were still waiting for the results. All interviews were conducted in the participant's language of choice by one of the investigators or a trained bilingual interviewer. Most were conducted in participants' homes; additional data were sometimes subsequently obtained by telephone.

The fact that the research design required both members of the couple to agree to a lengthy interview may have biased the sample in the direction of couples in which the men were more involved with their families and with their wives' reproductive health care. However, our data show that women made most of the amniocentesis decisions and that when they did not it was because they wanted their husband to decide in order to limit their own burden of responsibility (Browner forthcoming). We believe, therefore, that recruiting only couples in which both partners were willing to be interviewed had no significant impact on our findings.

RESULTS

Sixty percent (*N* = 26) of the 43 women agreed to the amniocentesis following a positive AFP test, and 40 percent (*N* = 17) declined. We found no significant differences between groups in age or household income, amount of schooling, score on a standardized acculturation instrument (Marín et al. 1987), or length of time in the United States (see tables 14.1 and 14.2).

The two groups' reproductive histories also revealed no significant differ-

Table 14.2 Immigration background of Mexican immigrant women offered amniocentesis

	Accepted (N = 26)	Declined (N = 17)
Marín Acculturation Score	18.3	20.8
Years in United States	9.8	7.9

Note: No significant difference between groups.

Table 14.3 Religiosity of Mexican immigrant women offered amniocentesis

	Accepted (N = 24)	Declined (N = 16)
Mean religious practice[a] (range: 0–3)	.35	.27
Increased church attendance during decision	29.2%	47.1%

Note: Three women were not Catholic. No significant difference between groups.
[a]Mean sum of responses to questions (0 = no, 1 = yes): Do you attend mass every Sunday? Do you confess and take communion? Do you perform any activity for the Church?

ences. The mean rate of induced abortion, although low in both groups, was similar, and there were no notable differences in the number of pregnancies, miscarriages, or children who had died. Those who accepted amniocentesis were somewhat more likely to have had children born with birth defects and a family history of birth defects, but the differences were not large enough to be significant.

It is commonly believed that amniocentesis acceptance rates are lower in Latinas than in many other groups due to their strong adherence to Catholicism, which teaches that abortion is murder. In our study, no such links were found (see table 14.3). Although all but three women were Catholic, few were particularly observant. We measured religious observance by asking three questions: Do you attend mass every Sunday? Do you confess and take communion? Do you perform any activity for the Church? Contrary to expectation, we found that women who agreed to the amniocentesis scored slightly higher on religious practice than those who declined, although the difference between groups was not significant. Those who declined were more likely to indicate that they had attended mass more often than usual when making their decision, although again the difference did not reach statistical significance.

Also contrary to expectation, abortion attitudes did not predict test decisions. A larger proportion of those who declined described themselves as

Table 14.4 Abortion attitudes in general of Mexican immigrant women offered amniocentesis (%)

	Accepted (N = 24)	Declined[a] (N = 16)
Strictly opposes abortion in all circumstances	26.9	43.8
Abortion should be up to the individual	30.8	37.5
Abortion acceptable in "extreme" circumstances	42.3	6.3
Don't know	0	12.5
Total	100.0	100.0

[a] N is less than 26 for women who accepted and 17 for women who declined owing to missing data.

Table 14.5 Views on abortion for themselves personally among Mexican immigrant women offered amniocentesis (%)

	Accepted (N = 26)	Declined[a] (N = 16)
Abortion personally unacceptable in all circumstances	53.9	81.1
Abortion personally acceptable in "extreme" circumstances	30.8	18.8
Abortion personally acceptable in less than "extreme" circumstances	11.5	0
Don't know	3.8	0
Total	100.0	100.0

[a] N is less than 17 owing to missing data.

"strictly opposed" to abortion for other women (table 14.4). Yet large proportions of both groups could be described as tolerant on the subject, saying either that they regarded abortion for others as acceptable in the event of "extreme" circumstances or that the decision should be left to the individual. However, despite these generally tolerant views, the majority of both groups said they would never personally consider an abortion, nor would they abort their current pregnancy under any circumstances (table 14.5).

We found support for our hypothesis in sharp and statistically significant

Table 14.6 Views associated with amniocentesis of Mexican immigrant women offered amniocentesis

	Accepted (N = 26)	Declined (N = 16)	Significance
Trusts own intuition about pregnancy	56.5%	87.5%	$p \leq .05$[a]
Worried when offered amnio (range 0–3)	2.28	1.29	$p \leq .05$[b]

[a] Based on χ^2.
[b] Based on t-test.

differences between groups in the feelings the women reported about the pregnancy and their reactions on being offered amniocentesis (table 14.6). Women were asked, "Do you feel you can tell if the baby is fine?" Although the majority (69%) of both groups said yes, far more women who declined than who accepted amniocentesis did so. The sources of their knowledge included feeling fetal movement, the absence of pain, feeling the same as they had in previous pregnancies, and simply "intuition." Women who declined also reported significantly less worry on being offered amniocentesis than did those who accepted the procedure. We asked participants to rate their level of worry on a four-point scale: not at all worried, a little, somewhat, extremely. The mean score for women who accepted was quite high: 2.3 out of a maximum of 3 (s.d. = 1.3). It was nearly a full point lower (mean = 1.3; s.d. = 1.5) for those who declined.

WHY REFUSE AMNIOCENTESIS?

"It's just not necessary—and it's a risk!"
—*Zoila Gonzales*

Our open-ended interviews offer insight into the factors behind amniocentesis acceptance and refusal for the women in this study. While a small proportion of those who refused said they did so because they would not abort the pregnancy under any circumstances, this was not the sole or the most important factor motivating most who declined the test.

Most who declined (as well as many who accepted) considered the risks of amniocentesis so formidable as to not be worth the purported benefits of informing physicians and reassuring patients. While women everywhere express anxieties about the prospect of amniocentesis, they were especially strong in this study population. Women found the idea of amniocentesis extremely frightening. Nearly all also held the erroneous belief that the needle is inserted through the navel, a thought they, not surprisingly, found unnerving. Even after genetic counseling, several concluded that the amniocentesis is "like a small operation." Others refused in part because they feared that they would go crazy or even die from the complications.

Several women recounted highly detailed stories, some based on hearsay, about the dangers of amniocentesis, which from what they said they heard ranged from the unnecessary stress of a false positive through severe physical or emotional consequences to miscarriage. Others were fearful that the fetus would be injured, specifically blinded by the needle, or born with other problems because, as Cristina Dominguez explained, "The baby isn't totally formed. It's just beginning to form, and so they could have taken out a hand or a foot that hadn't formed or something like that." But even more acute than fears about injuring the fetus was the fear of miscarriage. Seventy-one percent of women who refused amniocentesis characterized the procedure as either "rather" or "extremely" risky for the fetus; 46 percent of those who accepted agreed with this assessment ($\chi^2 = 2.47$; difference between groups not significant).

But these perceived dangers of amniocentesis were only part of the reason why women declined. More important, most who declined said they saw nothing in their reproductive histories or current reproductive experiences to warrant the concern raised by providers based on the woman's screening test result. Isabel Lopez, for example, who refused amnio, explained her reaction on being told she had tested positive: "I didn't pay attention. I said to myself, 'Bah, this low, and what?' I thought that because I was eating little because I had been vomiting, that was why the protein was low." Others who refused were also not worried, either because they had previously tested AFP-positive or knew others who had done so and subsequently given birth to healthy babies. Still others were reassured by the detailed ultrasound they were given at the genetics clinic. Elena Jimenez explained, "They said that the AFP result was low but that the ultrasound gave a result that everything was fine. So I said, if everything is fine, why do they want to continue excavating [escarbando]?" In fact, amniocentesis is offered in precisely such cases when ultrasound does not explain the reason for the positive AFP test, but Elena saw little value in more information.

Others who refused amniocentesis bolstered their refusal by drawing on previous reproductive success. Asked, for instance, about her reaction to testing AFP-positive, Dolores Fermin replied, "They said that I had low blood. . . . I didn't give it much importance. I have three girls and everything was always fine. In one pregnancy, I lost it, but that was a long time ago." In Dolores's mind, her reproductive history is normal despite the early miscarriage, and so she viewed the current positive test result as inconsequential.

Still other women drew on "intuition" to question the value of further testing. As Elena Garcia said, "They say, look, better to know, better to be informed. But I have my daughters and I know. . . . I feel that everything is going fine. . . . Mothers feel if their child is well or sick. I feel it's fine." Fernanda Moya similarly explained, "I have to be sincere. I hope I don't seem arrogant, but I know I'm fine. I don't know how to explain it. It's like a security that I don't know where it's coming from." Patricia Solís also questioned the value of further intervention when she said, "The road to hell is paved with good intentions. I believe doctors and nurses want the best for us [pregnant woman]. But if your womb is telling you that your baby is fine, why should you listen to other [voices]?"

In sum, the positive AFP test did not seriously challenge the confidence most who declined had that the pregnancy was normal. They dismissed the test result as insignificant, drawing on their own "embodied" knowledge, experience, or intuition to justify their refusal. They therefore saw no need for the reassurance a negative amniocentesis could provide. Those few who had serious doubts about the health of the fetus said they were unwilling to abort it even if those doubts were confirmed, so they, too, saw no value in being tested. The simple wish "to know"—often nearly overpowering among those from European American backgrounds (Press and Browner 1997)—held little importance for this group.

WHY ACCEPT AMNIO? *PARA SACARSE LA ESPINA*

We previously indicated that 54 percent of those who accepted amniocentesis said they would never abort a pregnancy. Thirty-one percent said they would consider abortion "only under the most extreme circumstances," such as their own life being in danger. Only 12 percent said they would definitely consider aborting the fetus if a serious birth defect were found. With opposition to abortion so significant, why, then, did they agree to amniocentesis?

"[The doctors] know what to do and you don't know all that. When you go to a doctor, it's because you're going to pay attention to what he says. . . . They're the ones to make that kind of decision, because they're the ones who know what the problem is" (Ernestina Zambrano). Those who agreed to amniocentesis did so in part in deference to medical authority. They accepted the clinical view that the positive AFP test meant that there might be a problem, and they did not want to live in uncertainty for the remainder of the pregnancy. Several drew on the Mexican metaphor of *una espina clavada en la corazon* (to be pierced through the heart with a thorn, or to have a doubt cast) to explain how they felt on hearing they had screened positive. Asked to elaborate, one woman explained, "It's like you want to get rid of it and, like a doubt, it eats at you; it only grows [worse]." These women believed amniocentesis would provide reassurance, that it would help them get rid of the doubt (*sacarse la espina*) or remove the thorn of uncertainty.

Women who accepted exhibited a very strong faith in physicians and medicine, particularly U.S. medicine. They found the prospect that doctors could steer them wrong almost, if not entirely, inconceivable. Rebeca Suarez's view was typical: "I trust [doctors]," she said. "They have always helped me, especially in this country. Why would they recommend this if I didn't need it?"

While all recognized that the amniocentesis was not mandatory, they nonetheless perceived it as strongly advised. Susana Telles explained, "She [the genetic counselor] never *told* me to do it [that is, to have the amnio]. She said, 'If you want to, that's fine.' But I knew they wanted me to do it, and if they told me to do it, I wanted to." Juana Negro expressed a similar view when asked why she had agreed to testing. "It had to be done. There was no question," she said, regarding it as part of the larger package of prenatal care.

For these women, agreeing to amniocentesis was based less on a desire for diagnostic information than on a wish to be good, compliant patients. "We did the test to help the doctors," explained Angela Palma, "because the doctors were confused and so were we." Yet those who accepted amniocentesis were not simply acceding to medical authority. They found compelling reasons in their own reproductive experiences for agreeing to the procedure.

Although, as previously shown, there were no systematic aggregate differences in the two groups' reproductive histories, experientially a different picture was seen: Women who accepted amniocentesis often justified having done so on the basis of prior reproductive health problems. Their doubts were diverse, and no one particular type of problem emerged as most significant. Yet these reconstructed reproductive histories provided women an explanation for the positive screening test result and justification for further testing.

Laura Mora, for instance, had had multiple miscarriages and wanted desperately to bring a pregnancy to term. She found the genetic counseling session unsettling because she was asked many questions she could not answer about diseases in her husband's family that she thought the counselor implied could be the source of her miscarriages. Asked what had led her to agree to amniocentesis, she replied, "To tell you the truth, I think it was the fear. The people there [doctors, etc.] put a fear or a terror into you. . . . I thought better end this battle (*lio*), better to know one way or the other . . . because not knowing is terrifying."

Others said they, too, wanted amniocentesis because of worries about their fetus's health. Marta Gallardo had had two children born with disabilities, and she was fearful it would happen a third time. Nora Omar felt very vulnerable emotionally during her pregnancy because she had been assaulted on the street and thought the fetus might have been injured. Olivia Palma was alarmed by what was seen on the ultrasound exam. She explained, "They told me that the AFP had come out low and that [during ultrasound] they had seen something in the baby related to . . . Down's syndrome. Well, I didn't know what to say, 'related.' They said, 'There are two cysts on the brain, but these are here and not there. The baby could be fine, but because you came out low on the AFP, that's why we believe that it's better to do amniocentesis." She continued, "I'm one of those people that wants to know one way or the other . . . not to have that doubt [*la duda clavada*]. Why doesn't it move? Why is it moving so much? Because with the other baby, that one kept moving around, and this one I don't feel moving as much." These doubts led Olivia to want the reassurance that amniocentesis could provide.

In no instance was it easy for these women to agree to the amniocentesis. Many were fearful of the procedure and its known risks. Yet their faith in physicians and willingness to acquiesce to medical authority allowed them to put their fate in doctors' hands. Those who agreed, however, did not do so without careful reflection or, in their own minds, just cause. They carefully analyzed their prior reproductive experiences to convince themselves of their "need" for the test. They saw their providers supporting this decision. Although genetic counselors and other clinicians are trained to respect patient autonomy (Clarke 1991; Kolker and Burke 1994), women tended to feel they were following their providers' wishes when they agreed to the test.

DISCUSSION AND CONCLUSIONS

These recently emigrated Mexican women were more than twice as likely as European American women to refuse amniocentesis (Walker 1995).[3] We do not know whether the factors associated with acceptance and refusal would be replicated in a larger sample. Some of the differences that were not significant (for example, religious practice, abortion attitudes, individual or family history of birth defects) may in fact prove so when we have more data. We also need a better understanding of what is being tapped by the dimension we call "intuition." In our sample, it failed to correlate with lower levels of education, acculturation, or less time in the United States, variables which might be expected to lead women to regard amniocentesis as unnecessary. Yet our findings remain provocative even in this small sample because they offer a glimpse of medicalization processes as they unfold.

Technologies for the monitoring and surveillance of pregnancy have grown so common that many U.S. women insist on having them, even in the absence of any medical indication (Thorpe, Harker, Pike, and Marlow 1993). This is particularly true for ultrasound, but it is also rapidly becoming the case for other kinds of fetal diagnostic techniques, such as amniocentesis. Although abortion is the only intervention in the event of a serious birth defect, over half of the women in our study who agreed to amniocentesis said they would not abort under any circumstances. In our earlier research, the proportion was even greater: only 13 percent said that they would consider abortion if all the tests showed their fetus had a serious anomaly (Press and Browner 1997). How these women would react in the event of a positive diagnosis is unknown. Studies indicate that most women whose fetuses are diagnosed with significant birth defects do, in fact, end their pregnancies (California Dept. of Health Services 1990).

The desire of those who agreed to amniocentesis to please their clinicians was quite apparent. We do not know whether this desire to please a clinician, or the fear of saying no to one, could lead a reluctant or ambivalent woman to actually abort her pregnancy. The effects of pressure from health care providers—whether overt or subtle—on women with deeply conflicted views about abortion to end their pregnancies and the effects of such abortions on the women who have them remain unknown. Yet with abortion as contentious as it remains throughout American society, these issues are too important to be ignored.

Those who declined amniocentesis did so for two main reasons: most continued to believe that the pregnancy was normal despite the positive screening test result, and they feared the procedure could harm the fetus. Our data do not allow us to determine why this group remained so confident that the pregnancy was normal and the fetus was healthy in light of the positive screening test result. However, they do show that women who refused displayed varying degrees of skepticism about the accuracy and authority of medical information, along with far more willingness to trust their own more phenomenologically derived knowledge (Abel and Browner 1997). Yet despite their refusal to fully acquiesce to biomedicine's technological imperative, those who refused were in fact active consumers of prenatal medical care. They comfortably went along with those aspects of it that they believed would enhance fetal health and well-being, including monthly office checkups, blood tests, dietary changes, and prenatal supplements. Yet unlike those who accepted, they did not feel obliged to agree to everything that biomedicine had to offer. Instead, they drew on alternative sources of knowledge to reassure themselves that the fetus was in good health.

For many in this small group of recent Mexican immigrants, the risk of genetic disease did not seem particularly salient. More worrisome was that by consenting to amniocentesis, they could conceivably cause their fetus harm. Yet the views seen in this population may in fact be easily dislodged. Second- and third-generation Mexican-origin women are far more likely than recent immigrants to agree to fetal diagnostic testing, including amniocentesis. Future research will more fully explicate the processes by which Mexican-origin women come to accept the more mainstream American view that fetal diagnosis is imperative.

NOTES

We wish to thank UC-MEXUS and the UCLA Center for the Study of Women for helping fund this project. Earlier versions of this paper were presented at the University of California Conference to Highlight Research and Policy Initiatives in Chicano/Latino Topics, University of California, Riverside, on October 20, 1995, at a workshop sponsored by the UCLA Program in Cultural Studies in Science, Technology, and Medicine and the Center for the Study of Women on April 4, 1996, and the 1996 annual meeting of the American Anthropological Association. We wish to thank Maria Cristina Casado and Jeffrey McNairy for their help with interviews and Adele Clarke, Christine Morton, Susan Markens, and Arthur J. Rubel for constructive feedback on earlier drafts. Ann Walker, director of the genetics program at the University of California, Irvine, generously made available unpublished data.

Pseudonyms have been given to all study participants.

1. Rates of miscarriage following amniocentesis at the three participating hospitals ranged from 1/500 to 1/200 (authors' field notes, 1996).

2. Of the remaining 312, 3 percent refused to participate, 32 percent were Latino but not of Mexican origin, 30 percent could not be reached by phone, 26 percent were not offered amniocentesis, and 9 percent were interested but unable to participate for various reasons such as family illness, moving out of the area, etc.

3. Walker 1995. Analysis of 1994 data on amniocentesis acceptance rates at the University of California at Irvine Medical Center, Orange. Eighty-one percent of the 141 non-Hispanic women in this clinic who were offered amniocentesis accepted the procedure, as opposed to 60 percent of the 290 Hispanic women.

REFERENCES

Abel, E. K., and C. H. Browner:
  1997 Women's Selective Compliance with Biomedical Authority and the Uses of Subjugated Knowledge. In M. Lock and P. Kaufert (eds.), *Pragmatic Women and Body Politics.* Cambridge: Cambridge University Press.
Arney, William Ray:
  1982 *Power and the Profession of Obstetrics.* Chicago: University of Chicago Press.
Borst, C. G.:
  1992 The Professionalization of Obstetrics: Childbirth Becomes a Medical Specialty. In R. D. Apple (ed.), *Women, Health, and Medicine in America: A Historical Handbook,* 197–215. New Brunswick, N.J.: Rutgers University Press.
Browner, C. H.:
  Forth- Situating Women's Reproductive Activities. *American Anthropologist.*
  coming
Browner, C. H., and N. Press:
  1995 The Normalization of Prenatal Diagnostic Testing. In F. D. Ginsburg and R. Rapp

(eds.), *Conceiving the New World Order: The Global Politics of Reproduction,* 307–22. Berkeley: University of California Press.

1996   The Production of Authoritative Knowledge in American Prenatal Care. *Medical Anthropology Quarterly* 10: 141–56.

Burton, B. K., R. G. Dillard, and E. N. Clark:

1985   The Psychological Impact of False Positive Elevations of Maternal Serum Alpha-Fetoprotein. *American Journal of Obstetrics and Gynecology* 151: 77–82.

California Department of Health Services:

1990   A Report to the Legislature: Review of Current Genetics Programs. Genetic Disease Branch, California Department of Health Services. March.

Clarke, A.:

1991   Is Non-Directive Genetic Counseling Possible? *Lancet* 338: 998–1001.

Davis-Floyd, R.:

1992   *Birth as an American Rite of Passage.* Berkeley: University of California Press.

Destounis, N.:

1972   *Psychosomatic Medicine in Obstetrics and Gynecology, Third International Congress, London, 1971.* Basel: Karger.

Devitt, N.:

1977   The Transition from Home to Hospital Birth in the United States, 1930–1960. *Birth and the Family Journal* 4: 47–58.

Evans, M. I., et al.:

1987   Establishment of a Collaborative University-Commercial Maternal Serum Alpha-Fetoprotein Screening Program: A Model for a Tertiary Center Outreach. *American Journal of Obstetrics and Gynecology* 156: 1441–49.

Green, J. M.:

1990   Calming or Harming? A Critical Review of Psychological Effects of Fetal Diagnosis on Pregnant Women. Galton Institute Occasional Papers, 2d series, no. 2.

Greenberg, F.:

1988   The Impact of MSAFP Screening on Genetic Services, 1984–1986. *American Journal of Medical Genetics* 31: 223–30.

Haverkamp, A. D., and M. Orleans:

1982   An Assessment of Electronic Fetal Monitoring. *Women and Health* 7: 115–34.

Hubbard, R.:

1986   Eugenics and Prenatal Testing. *International Journal of Health Services* 16: 227–42.

Jordan, B.:

1993   *Birth in Four Cultures: A Cross-Cultural Investigation of Childbirth in Yucatan, Holland, Sweden, and the United States.* 4th ed. Prospect Heights, Ill.: Waveland Press.

Kolker, A., and B. M. Burke:

1994   *Prenatal Testing: A Sociological Perspective.* Westport, Conn.: Bergin Garvey.

Leavitt, Judith Walzer:

1986   *Brought to Bed: Childbearing in America, 1750–1950.* Oxford: Oxford University Press.

Leveno, K. J., et al.:

1986   A Prospective Comparison of Selective and Universal Electronic Fetal Monitoring in 34,995 Pregnancies. *New England Journal of Medicine* 315: 615–18.

McClain, C.:

1983   Perceived Risk and Choice of Childbirth Service. *Social Science and Medicine* 17: 1857–1965.

1988   Patient Demand for Repeat Cesarean Section. Paper presented at the annual meeting of the American Anthropological Association, Phoenix.

Marín, G., et al.:

1987   Development of a Short Acculturation Scale for Hispanics. *Hispanic Journal of Behavioral Sciences* 9: 183–205.

Marteau, T. M., et al.:

1989   The Impact of Prenatal Screening and Diagnostic Testing upon the Cognitions, Emotions, and Behaviour of Pregnant Women. *Journal of Psychosomatic Research* 33: 7–16.

Nsiah-Jefferson, L.:

1994   Reproductive Genetic Services for Low-Income Women and Women of Color: Access and Sociocultural Issues. In K. H. Rothenberg and E. J. Thomson (eds.), *Women and Prenatal Testing: Facing the Challenges of Genetic Technology,* 234–59. Columbus: Ohio State University Press.

Preloran, H. M., and C. H. Browner:

1997   Efectos de la informacion genetica en las costumbres del embarazo de mujeres mexicanas residentes en los Estados Unidos. *Revista Anual de Investigaciones Folkloricas* 12.

Press, N. A., and C. H. Browner:

1997   Why Women Say Yes to Prenatal Diagnosis. *Social Science and Medicine* 45: 979–89.

Rapp, R.:

1993   Accounting for Amniocentesis. In S. Lindenbaum and M. Lock (eds.), *Knowledge, Power, and Practice: The Anthropology of Medicine in Everyday Life,* 55–76. Berkeley: University of California Press.

Rothenberg, K. H., and E. J. Thomson (eds.):

1994   *Women and Prenatal Testing: Facing the Challenges of Genetic Technology.* Columbus: Ohio State University Press.

Thompkinson, Gwynne, and Marie Roberson:

1996   Expanded AFP Screening Program Status Report. *Genetically Speaking* 7(2): 5.

Thorpe, K., L. Harker, A. Pike, and N. Marlow:

1993   Women's Views of Ultrasonography: A Comparison of Women's Experiences of Antenatal Ultrasound Screening with Cerebral Ultrasound of Their Newborn Infant. *Social Science and Medicine* 36: 311–15.

Walker, Ann:

1995   Personal communication.

15

Cross-Cultural Cyborgs: Greek and Canadian Women's Discourses on Fetal Ultrasound

Lisa M. Mitchell and Eugenia Georges

For millions of women in North America, Australia, Europe, and increasingly elsewhere as well, at least one or two ultrasounds have become an expected and routine part of pregnancy. For physicians and sonographers, ultrasound represents a necessary, passive, and neutral technology, capable of providing, as one obstetrical text describes it, "a window of unsurpassed clarity into the gravid uterus . . . [and] exquisite detail regarding the fetus and the intrauterine environment" (Pretorius and Mahoney 1990, 1). The possibilities of seeing, we are told, are numerous: the state of fetal anatomy; growth and development; numerous fetal pathologies; the sex of the fetus as early as eleven weeks; and fetal sleep, rest, and activity patterns. There are even claims of witnessing fetal masturbation (Meizner 1987) and, as Lisa Cartwright (1993) has pointed out, enough fetal behavior for one psychiatrist to begin the practice of fetal psychoanalysis.

For women, ultrasound has become firmly lodged as a "normal" part of pregnancy, allowing a sneak preview of our baby's sex, age, size, physical normality, and possible personality. So convincing is the cognitive and sensual apprehension of the fetus via the electronic mediation of ultrasound technology that women may routinely experience a "technological quickening" several weeks before they sense fetal movement in their own bodies (Duden 1992). This article examines what we call the cyborg fetus of ultrasound imaging: the mode of knowing and feeling the fetus through the coupling of human and machine. As Donna Haraway (1992) has described it, the cyborg is a "co-construction" of humans and nonhumans. Thus any exploration of the cyborg fetus must dwell both on the distinctive features of the ultrasound technology and of the local cultural understandings and practices in which it is deployed. If, as Haraway (1991, 180) has also claimed for the cyborg, "the machine is us, . . . an aspect of our embodiment," it then becomes necessary to inquire into how the cyborg is inflected when "us" is situated in distinctive cultural contexts, with distinctive understandings and practices regarding persons, pregnancy, and technology.

Cyborgs have rarely been explored outside the Euro-American context. In celebrating its utopian potential, the ways in which the cyborg is culturally inflected may be overlooked and thus questions about "what is *not* shared in an emerging global culture of reproduction" obscured (Rapp 1994, 34, our emphasis). In this article, we draw on our separate studies of routine fetal imaging to explore how the cyborg fetus of ultrasound imaging is culturally configured through practice and discourse. It is based on fieldwork carried out in an ultrasound clinic at a Canadian hospital (by LMM) and a similar study carried out in a public hospital in Greece (by EG). Both studies draw on observations of scans and on interviews with sonographers, pregnant women, and their partners. We look at the cyborg fetus through a cross-cultural lens to highlight that which is culturally and historically specific to North American and Greek understandings of the cyborg fetus. A cross-cultural perspective is also crucial for "getting at the complexities of the way power operates in society" (Hess 1995, 14). As we will show, the couplings of body and machine, as mediated and translated by experts, are firmly embedded in culturally and historically specific scripts. Yet, even as these couplings are culturally shaped, they in turn shape the embodied experience of pregnancy in novel ways. We begin with an extensive discussion of ultrasound in the North American context, first showing how this coupling simultaneously dissolves women's bodily boundaries, undermines their experiential knowledge, and represents the fetus as an autonomous, conscious agent. We then illuminate how sonographers employ specifically North American cultural scripts about personhood, maternal altruism, and bonding to intervene in the physical and social relationships of pregnancy. Third, we discuss some of the ways in which North American women may use the "transgressed boundaries and potent fusions" (Haraway 1991, 154) of ultrasound's cyborg fetus to reflect on and rework their experiences of pregnancy. We then turn to ultrasound practices in Greece to examine the culturally specific production of fetal and pregnant subjects there. In both contexts, the cyborg fetus of ultrasound imaging is often represented alone, as if removing it from the body and life of the woman improved the chances of understanding it. Throughout this article, we try to resist this dis-location, by re-membering the cyborg and critically examining its production in the embodied and social coupling of woman, machine, and sonographer. In the conclusion, we reflect on the implications of our cross-cultural perspective for emerging understandings of cyborgs and the processes of cyborgification.

SONOGRAPHIC PRACTICE: SEEING THE (NORTH AMERICAN) BABY

Like all cyborgs, the cyborg fetus arises through the coupling of human and machine. As part of the "mechanics" of this coupling, a transducer is rolled over the woman's belly. If the ultrasound is done during the first twelve weeks of pregnancy, the transducer, phallic-shaped and sheathed with a condom, may be inserted into her vagina. Guided by the sonographer's hand, high-energy sound waves are projected from the transducer into her womb and the reflection of these waves produces an image of the uterus, placenta, and moving fetus on a televisionlike screen.

Ultrasound examinations of pregnant women labeled "high risk" and those with a "suspected anomaly" are generally carried out by a physician, usually an obstetrician, radiologist, or gynecologist. The much larger number of "routine" scans done each year in Canada are more likely to be done by lower-paid female ultrasound technicians. During each fifteen- to twenty-minute routine scan, sonographers search for a fetal heartbeat, note the position and number of fetuses, and assess fetal age, size, development, and the expected due date by measuring parts of the fetus. Using ultrasound to discover and know the cyborg fetus is, in Haraway's (1991, 164) terms, a problem of translation; sonographers must translate not only the physics of echoes into the landmarks of the fetal and maternal body but also the clinical and social meaning of those landmarks. The repetitive and routinized work of translating ultrasound's echoes into the cyborg fetus is fatiguing and the fear of missing fetal anomalies is stressful, yet sonographers strive to make routine ultrasounds pleasurable for expectant couples. Routine ultrasounds are often conducted in a relaxed and conversational tone as sonographer, pregnant woman, and other observers talk, share jokes, and clearly enjoy themselves.

The cyborg fetus is, however, often difficult to spot. Sonographers must be trained to see the grayish ultrasound echoes as distinctive uterine and fetal landmarks and structures that convey diagnostic information. Women and their partners, in turn, depend heavily on the sonographers' accounts of the image in order to see their little cyborg baby. As part of their role as gatekeepers, Canadian sonographers quickly and silently search for a fetal heartbeat and major anomalies. Once they believe that the fetus is alive and "normal" at this level, sonographers begin to do what they refer to as "showing her the baby." Describing the image for the woman includes some diagnostic information (usually fetal age, weight, and a statement that "everything looks okay"). Talk about the cyborg fetus by sonographers to expectant parents also includes statements about its (1) physical body, appearance, and activity, (2) subjectivity, (3) potentiality, and (4) social connections to kin and to sonographers. These statements resonate with sonographers and many pregnant women as signs of both humanness and selfhood and thus are integral to how the ultrasound image is made culturally meaningful as a "baby."

Sonographers' descriptions of the physical parts of the fetus pass through a cultural sieve, as they select out those parts which they believe are most appealing and reassuring for women—the beating heart, the skull and brain, "baby's bladder," and the hands and feet, especially the fingers and toes. Sonographers consider that the "weird" or "strange-looking" fetal face at sixteen to eighteen weeks may be alarming to women. Later in pregnancy, the rounded fetal nose, forehead, and cheeks often receive special comment, and sonographers like to include the face in a woman's own copy of the image. During the ultrasound, parts of the fetal body are often not simply named but are described in terms of fetal behavior, their "babylike" appearance, and their resemblance to the anatomy of other family members. Fetal movement seen during ultrasound may be referred to as "the baby moving." Often it is described as a particular kind of movement—an activity. Thus the fetus is described as "playing," "swimming," "dancing," "partying," and "waving."

Canadian women sometimes refer to the photographic images of the early fetus in their guides to pregnancy as "alien" or "E.T." However, what is called forth even during the earliest routine ultrasounds observed in the Canadian clinic is the image of an idealized infant, rather than that of a fetus or embryo with its distinctive appearance, uncertain subjectivity, and contested personhood. Even the term *fetus* is generally restricted to diagnostic matters and to discussions among sonographers, although there is considerable variation among Canadian hospitals on this point. It is rare to hear expectant parents use the term *fetus,* and some sonographers discourage women and men from using it. For example, during a scan that one of the authors (LMM) observed, a man looked at the ultrasound photograph handed to him by the technician. "Great!" he said. "Now I can put this on my desk and say, 'This is my fetus.'" The technician replied, "Your fetus? Ugh! Don't say that! It's your baby."

Uncertainty about fetal subjectivity is also erased in the cyborg. Awareness of surroundings and of being distinct from other selves, as well as intention, moods, and emotion on the part of the fetus are included frequently in the explanation of the image for parents. Fetal movement that impedes the process of conducting the examination may be described as evidence that the fetus is "shy," "modest," or "doesn't like" something. As sonographers attempt to visualize the fetus, they may comment: "He moves away when I try to take the picture," or "He's shy. He doesn't want his picture taken." They also refer to fetal shyness and modesty when visualizing the genitalia is difficult. Conversely, a clear, easily attained fetal image may be offered as evidence that the fetus is "being good" or "very cooperative."

The cyborg also demonstrates its potential, its ability to acquire elements of cultural competence such as language, a moral sense, or a role as a "productive" member of society. Just what kind of person the fetus will become (athletic, smart, wakeful, fast-moving, just like Dad) is revealed in the sonographers' explanation. Activity seen during the ultrasound may be described in terms of future behavior of the baby or young child: "Your baby is moving a lot. You're gonna be busy!" Sometimes such statements are gender specific: "What a big baby. It must be a boy!" "With thighs like that it has to be a girl."

The compelling nature of this cyborg is especially evident when sonographers see an image that they particularly like. Their postures, facial expressions, and voices change as they lean closer to the screen, often tilting their heads and smiling. Sonographers may even touch, stroke, and "tickle" the on-screen image, particularly the fetal feet, and create a voice so the fetus may "speak" to the expectant couple and communicate its "feelings." Expectant couples watch, delighted, as sonographers may wave to the image, speak to it, giving instructions, words of encouragement or reprimand, as in "Hold still, baby" and "Smile for the camera." Often these are instructions for the fetus to do something for the parents: "Say hello to Mama," or "Don't move, so Papa can see you." At these moments, sonographers and expectant couples closely resemble people admiring a baby in someone's arms.[1]

Personified in these ways, the cyborg fetus mesmerizes the viewer into forgetting that the embodied, conscious, perceptive actor of ultrasound is the woman. The distinction between the fetus inside the woman and the collection of echoes on-screen is blurred, creating what Sarah Franklin (1993, 537; see also Duden 1993) has called "bodily permeability," allowing the viewer to move "seamlessly from the outside to the inside of the woman's body." The erasure of their bodily boundaries and bodily knowledge passes unnoticed or without comment by many women, as they are captivated by the fetal image or distracted by the discomfort of the full bladder that some hospitals still insist upon. This bodily permeability may also be desired by many women. Their excitement about the "chance to see," their conviction that "seeing is believing," and their fascination with the printout of the fetal image—the "baby's photo"—that they take home all underscore the cultural valorization of the visual, a point to which we will return in our concluding discussion.

A few women express a sense of sadness that their intimate privileged knowledge of the fetus is lost during ultrasound. Some are startled to see fetal movement on-screen when they do not yet sense it. Seeing this movement prior to bodily quickening reinforces women's acceptance that ultrasound provides authoritative and distinctive information, but for some women it is unsettling.

> "It was like it [the fetus] moved for her [the sonographer], but not for me." (Christina, twenty-five, secretary)

> "It was neat and all that, you know, to see the baby moving. But, I don't know, I guess I thought the mother was supposed to feel it. Like that's when you know it's there." (Tina, twenty-eight, social services worker)

> "We could see it moving and I told her [the sonographer] I had felt it when I was taking the Metro. She said that wasn't it, that I couldn't feel it until a few more weeks. I thought for sure it was the baby moving, but I guess not." (Teresa, twenty-seven, business owner)

After listening to the sonographer lay claim to the fetus, some women, like Teresa, try to (re)assert the importance of their own bodily awareness in detecting fetal movement and knowing fetal age and gender. But contests over knowledge about the fetus are usually won by the cyborg, spoken for by the "expert" sonographer. For example, estimates of fetal age based on ultrasound measurements nearly always take precedence in physicians' reports over the estimates given by women. Sidelined into what some physicians call an "unreliable source" or a "poor substitute" for the ultrasound-generated knowledge, women are left trying to relocate the fetus in their own bodies, looking back and forth between the image on-screen and their own abdomens.

The fact that very few women express negative feelings or are critical of ultrasound while they are pregnant may also be due in part to their feelings of dependence on the technology. For many of the Canadian women interviewed, the first few months of pregnancy bring about a heightened sense of the possibilities of their own bodies. They talk at length about subtle changes in its shape and appearance and worry openly about its normality and potential for failure. Anxious about miscarriage and fetal abnormalities, many women hesitate to tell friends and extended family about the pregnancy or to signal their changing status by wearing (more comfortable) maternity clothing, effectively putting the pregnancy "on hold" until after they "pass" the first ultrasound examination. Their dependence on ultrasound diminishes somewhat by the second routine scan during the seventh month of pregnancy. By that time, a woman's own bodily knowledge, based largely on fetal movements, conveyed the message that "everything is okay." By postpartum, however, the appeal and persuasiveness of the cyborg was eroded, when women expressed disappointment and frustration with ultrasound's failure to accurately predict fetal size, long and difficult labors, or cesarean deliveries.

MUM, DAD, AND CY-BABY

Through these conditions of "bodily permeability" and the dis-location of the fetus onto an external monitor, women are simultaneously marginalized and subjected to increased surveillance. As they carry out the scan, sonographers mediate not only the bodily and physical connections between woman and fetus, but also their emotional attachment and social relationship. The cyborg fetus, as we discussed, emerges as a social being, a social actor with a distinctive identity—"the baby"—enmeshed in a social network where a pregnant woman and her partner are often referred to as "Mum" and "Dad" and family members who are present are encouraged to look at their "niece" or "grandchild" or "baby brother."

Linked to these identities and included in the sonographers' accounts of the fetal image are normative and culturally specific expectations about parental behavior. Implicit in these accounts is the idea that women who come for ultrasound, who avail themselves of the benefits of this technology, are doing what is best for their babies. The sonographers refer (among themselves) to certain women as "nice patients." These are women who, the sonographers believe, "care" about the fetus; that is, they show interest in the image and concern about fetal health but not too much interest in fetal gender. These women tend to receive detailed and personalized accounts of the cyborg, as described above. In contrast, abbreviated accounts of the image may be given to women believed to be disinterested in the image or more concerned about fetal gender than fetal health.

The sonographers' accounts of the ultrasound image are infused with a powerful cultural script on "natural" behavior for pregnant women and mothers. According to this script, women from certain groups, "different races" to use the sonographers' term, are assumed to be abnormal or "different" by nature: impassive, unemotional, or overly interested in the "wrong thing." Black women and First Nations women are sometimes said to be unexcited or unmoved by the prospect of having a baby and thus may receive relatively brief accounts of the fetal image. In the Canadian clinic, one of the authors (LMM) was told by sonographers that "some women just want to know the sex." East Asian and South Asian women, in particular, are said to be "overly" interested in knowing the fetal sex, and it is assumed that they want only male babies.[2] Women who appear to be particularly interested in learning the fetal sex are often told: "Finding out the sex isn't important. The most important thing is that the baby is healthy." If sonographers are concerned that a woman will be disappointed by the sex of the fetus, especially if they think she may seek to terminate the pregnancy, they may simply tell her that they are unable to see whether it is a boy or girl.

This discourse on motherhood is played out not only along lines of cultural or "racial" difference but also in terms of reproductive history, personal habits, and self-discipline. Women having their first child may be dissuaded from knowing the fetal sex with statements such as "This is your first? You don't want to know, do you? You can always try again." Women in their teens, women in their forties, women with more than four or five children may be asked about their decision to have a baby at this point in their lives. Women over thirty-six may be asked to give reasons if they mention refusing amniocentesis. Similarly, if they admit to smoking during pregnancy, women may be shown the image of the placenta and told, incorrectly: "We can see the smoke in it." Obese women, told that "it's hard to see," are thereby reminded that their bodies are an obstacle to prenatal diagnosis. Women are constantly monitored during ultrasound, not only for fetal anomalies or physical conditions that may complicate labor and delivery but also for their own shortcomings—failure to monitor their bodies and behavior, failure to be compliant and selfless—in short, for failing to be "good mothers."

Central to this discourse on maternalism is the notion of "bonding" or emotional attachment to the fetus. The idea of using ultrasound to modify women's sentiments and behavior toward fetuses first appeared in clinical journals during the early 1980s (e.g., Fletcher and Evans 1983). As one physician wrote to the *British Medical Journal,* ultrasound should help women to view the fetus "as a companion aboard rather than a parasite responsible for the symptoms of pregnancy" (Dewsbury 1980, 481). Once elevated to the status of "psycho-social benefit," bonding with the cyborg fetus during ultrasound quickly became a new area of ultrasound research.[3] Detailed explanations of the fetal image were said to stimulate "positive feelings" toward the fetus and the reaction of women to the image could then be re-presented as a gauge of their emotional commitment to the fetus. The power of the cyborg fetus to stimulate a woman's "natural" mothering response is now also assumed to reduce her anxiety and improve her compliance with such things as medical advice, regular dental care, and the avoidance of cigarettes and alcohol (Reading et al. 1982, 1988). As we discussed earlier, the cyborg fetus also serves to identify those women whose "nature" is different. The disciplinary response or corrective action for being different varies from the "silent treatment" observed in the Canadian clinic to the more draconian efforts of some American lawmakers to legislate mandatory viewing of ultrasound fetal images as a way of dissuading pregnant women from having abortions (Lippman 1988, 442).

The use of ultrasound to promote bonding follows a path similar to the "One-Two Punch of Birth in the Technocracy" as described by Robbie Davis-Floyd (1998). That is, once having mediated and helped effect the conceptual separation of pregnant woman and fetus, ultrasound later comes to be regarded as integral to the process of re-membering the two, that is, technologically "bonding" mother to fetus. Maternal attachment, formerly considered "natural," a ubiquitous "instinct," can no longer be left to nature and to women.[4] In recent years, the sonographer's objective has expanded to encompass fathers as well. As a new clinical niche, "family-centered sonography" has been promoted as a means of enhancing both maternal and paternal attachment to the fetus (Craig 1991; Spitz 1991). In the Canadian clinic, during the routine ultrasounds, male partners are encouraged by sonographers to "move closer" to the screen and to talk about the image; women who come alone to the examination are asked, "Your husband didn't come?"[5]

BOUNDARIES, FUSIONS, POSSIBILITIES

What "dangerous possibilities" do the "transgressed boundaries [and] potent fusions" of ultrasound hold for women in North America? Universal and comprehensive health insurance throughout Canada includes at least one prenatal scan, and many women now expect this technologically mediated introduction to the fetus. Although the vocabulary, idioms, and metaphors among women's accounts of the cyborg fetus varied, there are few markedly different voices.[6] It is clear that many of these women feel reassured and empowered by the cyborg-ification of the fetus. Hearing the sonographer say, "Everything is fine," and seeing the heart beat or fetal movement is eagerly accepted by most women as evidence that they will give birth to "a normal baby" and can publicize the pregnancy. The sonographers' re-description of the fetus in sentimentalized and personalized terms, a particular emphasis at the research hospital, also touches a chord with many women. They use what they saw and heard during ultrasound as both proof of the fetal presence (as opposed to merely "being pregnant") and a means of discovering their baby's gender and clues about its behavior, character, and family resemblance.

> "I know now it's gonna have my attitude. It was calm and slow moving.
> If it was more like my husband, the baby would move a lot more and pace
> around. I mean, my husband's a great guy, but I'm glad it's gonna have my
> personality." (Marie-Claude, twenty-seven, sales clerk)

"The first thing I saw, it's crazy I know, but this kid has my husband's legs. Everything about it was like my husband. Just the way it looked, the build, the bones, the proportions. It was incredible." (Sylvie, twenty-five, florist)

Notably, for a small group of women, recent immigrants to Canada and unfamiliar with both ultrasound and the North American discourse of maternal-fetal bonding, ultrasound is viewed as a diagnostic test rather than as a means of elaborating the social identity of the fetus.

The cyborg created and apprehended in this ritualized, technological, and public quickening appears to transform the social reality of pregnancy for some Canadian women. The dis-location of the fetus from women's bodies and from their experiential knowledge opens up a space with multiple possibilities for monitoring, controlling, and altering women's behavior during pregnancy. For more than a decade, Ann Oakley (1984, 185) and others have argued that ultrasound is one of "a long line of other well-used strategies for educating women to be good mothers." Women, however, are not passive recipients of ultrasound; they are attuned to the possibilities of using the cyborg fetus in the context of their own social relationships.

Ultrasound offers some women a means of re-scripting or validating their position in a network of family and friends. For example, one twenty-four-year-old woman, a business owner, gave an enlarged photocopy of the ultrasound image to her parents and in-laws, hoping to convince them that she and her partner were "really serious about each other." For some women, ultrasound holds the possibility of stimulating or engaging a partner's interest in the baby and testing his commitment to the relationship. "I want him to know that this is a baby. It's not going to go away. He just can't get it yet. I guess it's a physical thing. Men don't have all the changes in their body. . . . The ultrasound changes that. It's like a slap in the face for him! Now he's got to get serious about us and this baby" (Vicky, twenty-five, medical receptionist).

Among one-quarter of the women, those who had once miscarried or are particularly anxious about miscarriage, ultrasound echoes are especially and poignantly meaningful as reassuring "proof" that they *will* have a baby. A few are even willing to use the ultrasound as evidence to counter the opinions of their own doctors. Twenty-seven-year-old Marie-Claude, a sales clerk, said: "I was so excited after the ultrasound. I took my picture in to my doctor the next week and said, 'See, see. I told you this time it would be all right.' She's very cautious, always saying, 'Let's take it one step at a time.' But I feel great."

From these interviews, it is clear that some Canadian heterosexual, middle-class women may embrace the cyborg fetus as a means of confirming, strengthening, or testing their relationships with partners, kin, and friends and as a way of asserting the authority of their bodies and voices. The possibilities that the cyborg fetus holds for North American women of different medical traditions and birth philosophies, for women with disabilities, single parents, pregnant teenagers, and lesbians need to be researched.

SONOGRAPHIC PRACTICE: SEEING THE (GREEK) BABY

In the small city in eastern Greece that is the focus of this section, pregnancy is intensively monitored through monthly prenatal visits with obstetricians, in which fetal ultrasound plays a prominent role. Pregnancy and birth have only recently been redefined as technology-intensive medical events, however. Until a generation ago, home births attended by traditional midwives were still common, and many of the mothers of the young women interviewed had given birth in their homes. The medicalization of pregnancy and birth that has occurred throughout Greece is one manifestation of the widespread modernization that has occurred since World War II. Yet, although proceeding rapidly, the medicalization process remains uneven, and local knowledges of the pregnant body have not been entirely displaced by technological and biomedical discourses.

This prosperous city, a popular destination for tourists from northern Europe on whom its economy heavily depends, serves as the local hub for medical care. The vast majority of the region's births take place in the city's public hospital in which all interviews and observations were conducted. As part of the National Health System established in 1983 by the socialist government, the hospital provides low-cost antenatal care to about nine hundred women a year. In the mid-1980s, the hospital acquired its hand-me-down scanner from Athens, and soon fetal imaging became a routine procedure. By the 1990s, not only did no pregnancy go unscanned but women attending the hospital also typically had several more scans over the course of a normal pregnancy than did Canadian women. Most had four, but a few had up to seven. Normal pregnancies are scanned with ultrasound for various reasons, including confirming a suspected pregnancy, charting fetal growth, establishing due dates, ascertaining presentation of the fetus, and, surprisingly often, responding to a woman's request to "see the baby."[7]

As many pregnant women and their husbands explained, the public hospital is widely preferred to the city's sole private clinic as much for its stock of "machines" (*mihanimata, mihanes*) as for the high quality of its physicians, all of whom are male. As enthusiastic "consumers," women exerted a strong demand for fetal imaging that was, in part, a product of the machine's status as a metonym for the structural and symbolic superiority of modern medical science and technology in general. Additionally, ultrasound, the only "machine" routinely used in pregnancy and birth, deliberately conjoins the technoscientific to the visual—both important signifiers of the modern in western culture. Physicians, too, particularly those of the under-forty generation, explicitly identified ultrasound as indispensable to the practice of "modern" obstetrics. As one older obstetrician, who was critical of what he considered to be the younger physicians' overuse of the technology, observed: "There are few things my hands can't find that the ultrasound can. My hands are my eyes. . . . But patients think it's more modern to use a machine. They themselves wouldn't trust just a manual exam. The doctor needs to show that he's modern, too. That is, some will do an exam with a machine just because a woman will trust him more if he does." As a result of such associations between technology, medical progress, and modernity, some older hands-on methods still widely used in Canada, such as dating the pregnancy by measuring the height of the uterine fundus, have been completely replaced by ultrasound.

The association between fetal ultrasound imaging and modern visual technologies is explicitly acknowledged in Greek everyday usage. Ultrasound is most commonly referred to as "television" (*tileorasi*), and doing an ultrasound is referred to as "putting the baby on television" (*na valoume to moro stin tileorasi*). Television is an apt metaphor for fetal ultrasound imaging in Greece. In its ubiquity it provides a major vehicle for the dissemination of images of modernity, the West, and "modern" behavior (Handman 1983; McNeill 1978). The women interviewed were nearly all born around the time television was first introduced in Greece (1966), and they have thus grown up with its discursive conventions, not least of which is its "ability to carry a socially convincing sense of the real" (Fiske 1987).

As is the case in Canada, the ultrasound scan as performed in the Greek public hospital is a formulaic procedure that resonates with ritual overtones. The following description is of a typical session, which usually lasts about five minutes. For most women, it is replicated several times over the course of their pregnancies, with little variation and in near silence.

Toward the conclusion of the routine prenatal examination, the physician (or the woman) may suggest "putting the baby on television." The woman then follows the physician down the hospital corridor to a small room, lit dimly only by the shadowy gray light emanating from the ultrasound monitor. No other medical staff member is present during the session, but the woman may be accompanied by family members, usually her husband and possibly a small child. The woman lies on the examining bed next to the apparatus and, generally without being instructed to do so (because she has done this before), wordlessly pulls her skirt or slacks and underwear down below her abdomen. The physician squirts her exposed abdomen with a coupling gel and begins to probe its surface with the transducer.

The screen is generally turned toward the physician. The woman can view it by craning her neck, but her eyes are often directed toward the face of the physician, who quickly and silently scans the entire fetal image, then focuses on the genital area for a while. At this point, the physician may break his silence to announce "girl" or "boy"—unless the woman has already jumped in to tell him she doesn't want to know the sex. (This rarely happens, however.) Or the physician may tell the woman that the position or age of the fetus doesn't permit him to see the sex this time and that he will look again next month. Finally, the physician scans to the skull and freezes the image in order to measure the biparietal diameter (skull width). He checks a chart over the bed upon which the woman is lying and announces the age of the fetus in weeks and days. If the physician himself does not tell the woman at this point that "the baby is all right" (no anomaly was ever detected in the over eighty sessions observed), she will ask. Most often, this is the only time she speaks. The physician then wipes the gel from the woman's abdomen with a paper towel and leaves. If her husband is with her, as was the case with about one-third of the women, they may exchange a few quick comments in the corridor, usually about the fetus's announced sex.

Obviously, except for fetal sex, the doctor's terse announcements during the ultrasound procedures do not go beyond the most basic diagnostic information. Given the quite different performances in the two settings, it is striking that the great majority of the Greek women, like so many of the Canadian women, asserted that fetal imaging had given them a sense, often their first sense, of the "reality" of their pregnancies. For instance, Popi, twenty-four, a working-class housewife, said: "I didn't believe I had a baby inside me. When you don't feel it or see it, it's hard to believe. It's something that you can't imagine—how the baby is, how it's growing, how it's moving. . . . After I saw it on the screen, I did believe it. I felt it was more alive in me. . . . I had also seen it [a fetus] on television, but it's different to see your own." And Stavroula, twenty-five, a middle-class housewife, said that with ultrasound, "You have an idea of what you have inside you. I became conscious that it was a person. I hadn't felt it as much before. I had to see it first." As occurred among the Canadian women, the bodily permeability effected by ultrasound either passes without comment or is eagerly desired as the Greek women too are captivated by the fetal image. Many also move beyond the limited diagnostic information they receive to appropriate the fetal images for themselves, endowing them with qualities that are meaningful to them alone: "I became conscious that it was a person" or, as Stavroula went on to explain, "At that moment, you feel that it's yours, the only thing that's yours."

Also like the Canadian women, the Greek women depended on the ultrasound technology to assuage feelings of uncertainty associated with the unpredictability of pregnancy. Although awareness of certain kinds of "risks" to fetal health has been expanded and heightened by women's exposure to biomedical discourse, both physical and mental disabilities have historically been highly stigmatized in Greek culture (Arnold 1985; Blue 1993; Blum and Blum 1965; Velogiannis-Moutsopoulos and Bartsocas 1989). Disabilities are dreaded not only for their direct consequences for the affected individual, but also for the stigma they may bring to the entire family. Because they are often believed to be hereditary, they may affect the marriage prospects of other family members.

Not surprisingly, then, women commonly described feelings of "anxiety" (*anhos*), "anguish" (*agonia*), and "nervousness" (*trak*) just before the scan, which were put to rest once the physician announced that "the baby is all right." This statement by Maria, a twenty-five-year-old hairdresser, was typical: "I had a lot of anxiety before my first ultrasound, because you can't know what's inside you. Until then, you only see your stomach. After, I felt more sure. You see that all is well."

All of the women interviewed took the doctor's assurance that "the baby is all right" to mean that the fetus was physically integral or, to use the women's words, that the "baby had its hands and feet," "all its organs," and was "entirely limbed" (*artimeles*). What it could not reveal, the women agreed, was how these organs, including the brain, functioned. Thus, in both Greece and Canada, evidence of fetal personhood was read through signs of physical normalcy and fetal gender. However, in distinct contrast to the Canadian women, none of the Greek women felt that ultrasound could provide any information on fetal personality or other subjective characteristics. (In fact, asking this question usually provoked puzzled looks.)

Given its role in assuring women about fetal health and assuaging anxieties (some of which, ironically, are iatrogenic in origin) and in providing the first sensation of the reality of the pregnancy, it is also not surprising that the Greek women most often described strong feelings of pleasure on visualizing the cyborg fetus and that, as in Canada, almost none were critical of the technology. Indeed, the Greek women's descriptions of their experiences with ultrasound were enthusiastic, on occasion even ecstatic. For instance, Katerina, twenty, a middle-class housewife, explained, "The first time I saw the baby, I was crazy with happiness. It was a contact with the child. Every time I went to the doctor, I wanted to see the child again." Litsa, a twenty-eight-year-old shopkeeper, said, "After my first ultrasound, I felt like I did when I saw it after giving birth—that much happiness." And Zambeta, eighteen, a clerk in a bakery, exclaimed, "I had four ultrasounds, and that wasn't enough! When the doctor first suggested it, I couldn't wait to see it. I was so impatient, the minutes-long wait seemed like eons. . . . I thought it would be like on television, that I would see the little hands, like under a microscope. But I wasn't disappointed. I saw it move. I saw that it was healthy." Beyond the ability to reassure women, ultrasound images generate visual pleasures that appear to derive their impact and poignancy from the influence of television's realist conventions, as we discuss in greater detail in the following section.

CULTURAL CYBORGS

The cyborg fetus is a cultural rather than a natural entity. The Canadian cyborg fetus may display emotions and consciousness, a distinctive or potentially distinctive self, and be immersed in social relationships; however, in Greece it is clear that other cultural scripts are at work. In this section, we explore more fully the similarities and differences in the production of fetal and pregnant subjects through the couplings of machine and body. Although the sonographers' descriptions of the ultrasound image are very different in Greece and Canada, women in both countries regard the image as a powerful and objective glimpse of what is "really" happening inside their wombs. Ultrasound's persuasiveness is due in part to the circumstances of its production at the hands of authoritative white-coated medical professionals. The "truthfulness" and authority of the image are further reinforced through the dramatic ability of the cameralike apparatus to compensate for the deficiencies of the human eye—both the doctor's and the woman's (Crary 1990). In this regard, women's use of metaphors of other visualizing machines (television, camera, microscope) to refer to the ultrasound apparatus is revealing. For both Greek and Canadian women, a common early exposure to television may have socialized them to be "relatively flexible readers of images" (Condit 1990, 85) and thus prepared them to metaphorize the shadows that appear on the screen into "my baby." The sense that what is seen on the screen is "really real" also derives from the codes and conventions of visual realism that ultrasound shares with other visual technologies. Thus, for instance, ultrasound's ability to reveal fetal movements in "real time," like "live" television, imparts a feeling of "nowness" that promotes a sense of immediate contact with the fetus on the screen. As the impact of the mass media has become increasingly global, so too has the visual realism that is one of its most characteristic genres. In the process, boundaries of cultural difference may become blurred (Appadurai 1991, 205).

Other boundaries remain, however. Although many Canadian and Greek women appear eager and willing to accept the cyborg as an improvement over their own cultural understandings of the fetus, the ways in which they metaphorize the fetal blur indicate culturally specific understandings of ultrasound technology, pregnancy, and fetal personhood. Unlike the Canadian women, the Greek women never spoke of the fetus as an autonomous in utero subject, and attributions of fetal personality, agency, and potentiality were notable for their absence. According to the tenets of the Greek Orthodox Church, to which nearly all Greeks belong, the soul, and thus personhood, is acquired at conception. Yet, as translated into everyday cultural understandings, fetal persons, like persons generally, are constituted processually across time, and relationally, through their connections with others, most importantly with family members, and not as autonomous and separate units (Triandis 1988, 82). Here it should be emphasized that cultural categories of personhood should not be taken as monolithic, homogeneous, and static representations across time and context. Instead, we suggest, they are best understood as historically and culturally specific folk models, which may, and often do, exist alongside alternative and sometimes contradictory understandings (Becker 1995; Mageo 1995; Spiro 1993). For both the Greek and the Canadian women, relational and individualistic models coexist, but for each, one model tends to dominate. For example, although many of the young Greek women considered themselves "incomplete" without motherhood, other valued aspects of their experience, such as consumption, self-care, and waged work, point to the ascent of more individualistic models. Similarly, the Canadian women's talk about the fetus in terms of its relations and resemblance to family suggests that they also value the procedure for the connections it "showed."

Yet many of the Canadian women do think of the fetus as a separate individual. As Barbara Katz Rothman (1989, 114, 59) points out, the view of the fetus "not as part of its mother, but as separate, a little person lying in the womb" has deep historical roots in North American traditions of viewing individuals as "autonomous, atomistic, isolated beings." Moreover, during the last few decades, a significant rupture has occurred in the way the fetus is conceptualized, talked about, and acted upon. The fetus is no longer simply a separate entity but increasingly an agent in its own right. Representations in medical discourse (reflected in recent popular culture as well) have shifted from passive and parasitelike to active and independent (Franklin 1991, 193; Hartouni 1991). Thus the "feto-placental unit" is said to issue hormonal commands to the mother who, if she wants to do what's "best for baby," must learn to read her moods and bodily symptoms as evidence of fetal signals for nutritious foods, rest, and regular medical care. This notion of the fetus-as-agent is powerfully naturalized through the discourses of science and maternalism and reinforced in popular culture and anti-abortion rhetoric.

The North American fetus has become highly visible as a public figure, reflecting once again distinctive constructions of the person, as well as divergent historical and political contexts. Electronic and print media stories about fetal diagnosis and therapy, fetal rights, and the abortion issue appear frequently. Anti-abortion movements are undeniably better organized, more vocal, and more politically powerful in the United States, but Canadian women's understandings of pregnancy are infused with their personal reflections on the legal, ethical, and political controversy over fetal rights and abortion. For example, although only a few of the Canadian women interviewed describe themselves as "anti-abortion" or "pro-life," nearly all women avoided the term *fetus,* saying it reminded them of the abortion issue. The North American fetus is also a source of cultural entertainment, appearing in Hollywood films, in advertisements for telephone companies and cars, and in comic strips and novels (Taylor 1992). Through these diverse representations, North Americans have become accustomed not only to *seeing* the fetus but also to seeing the fetus as a *social actor.*

In Greece, however, there is no public fetus. Images of the fetus in the media are not frequent, and only an occasional poster in the public hospital exhorted women not to smoke during pregnancy. Aspects of local knowledge of pregnancy and the fetus that provide alternative interpretive frameworks persist alongside medical and popular-scientific discourses. In everyday contexts, the pregnant woman's body and its contents are less sharply demarcated than they become in the medical setting. Instead, they are embedded in more social understandings in which the well-being of both fetus and woman crucially depend on the intentions and actions of others. Two examples illustrate this more relational perspective. Because children are culturally highly valued (despite, or today, perhaps because of, one of the world's lowest birthrates), pregnancy is thought to incite the envy of others who can unintentionally cause harm. Thus pregnant women are considered to be especially vulnerable to the effects of the evil eye. In the past, pregnancies were hidden for this reason. Contemporary pregnant women protect against the evil eye by wearing beads and amulets, which they also secure immediately to the pillows of their newborns in the hospital. A second example is the social response to the strong food cravings that pregnant women are expected to display. Women are routinely offered morsels of food that they happen to smell, not only by their familiars (their husbands should be especially attentive to these cravings) but also by a neighbor or even the occasional street vendor, lest they be responsible for telltale birthmarks in the shape of the food withheld. Both of these practices suggest moral (and thus prescriptive) understandings of person and body that are crucially embedded in interpersonal relations and that stand as alternatives to the firm borders delineated by more individualistic models.

At the level of Greek public discourse, a particularly telling manifestation of the tendency to emphasize the relational over individualistic premises of fetal personhood can be found in anti-abortion discourse. Abortion is a much more common experience for Greek women than for North American women. Despite the teachings of the Greek Orthodox Church, which equates abortion with the sin of murder, church opposition to abortion remains relatively muted, and anti-abortion discourse in the public sphere is largely limited to the periodic lamentations of the press or of politicians lamenting the rapidly falling birth rate. In public discussion, Greece's high abortion and low birth rates are conceptually linked and are represented primarily as threats to Greece's geopolitical security and to the continuity of the Greek nation, the *ethnos,* or organic national whole, and of the Greek "race" and religion (Georges 1996, 510; Halkias 1995). The Greek context thus differs markedly from North America, where attention has overwhelmingly focused on issues of maternal choice and the fetal individual and its rights.

Not only are fetal subjects culturally constructed in symbiosis with ultrasound technology. So too are pregnant women. For the Greek women, actively consuming ultrasound technology can be read as one way of constituting oneself as a modern pregnant subject. Medical technology (like technology in general) can be seen as part of the "standard package" of European consumer goods that are desired (particularly by the newer middle classes of Greeks who flourish in the prosperous city studied by EG) less perhaps for their utility than for their symbolic value. "Europe" and "European" are tropes that carry particular rhetorical force in Greece today. Historically, the idea of "Europe" is closely related to what has been called a "perennial crisis" in Greeks' sense of identity (is Greece part of the East/Orient or of the West/Europe?). This conundrum has deepened in recent years as a result of Greece's "full" membership in the European Union, membership that Greece has actively embraced. In practice, however, Greece is often regarded by the more powerful EU states as a marginal, unruly, and "semi-Oriental" junior partner, whose capability of applying western values and institutions remains in doubt and whose principal merit, it would seem, is as a quaint and exoticized "pleasure periphery" for northern European tourists (Papagaroufali and Georges 1993, 236; Costa 1993, 38). In this ambiguous contemporary Greek moment, consumption, perhaps especially consumption of technology and expert knowledges, represents a significant means of identifying oneself as modern and, more to the point, a member of the New Europe. In such a context, the intensive and repetitive use of ultrasound technology can be interpreted as a ritual of consumption that facilitates the representation of oneself as modern and European. Ultrasound is thus both a metonym for modernity and a vehicle for constructing oneself as a modern subject, not only for mothers and fathers, who selected the public hospital largely for its "machines," but for the physicians as well, who regarded the technology as indispensable to the practice of "modern" obstetrics.

In contrast, a few of the Canadian women talked about ultrasound as an example of "medical progress" or "something our mothers didn't have," but most did not. Canadian women seem to regard the ultrasound primarily as a means of "doing what's best for baby" and relieving their own anxieties about anomalies and miscarriage. Rather than a metonymic connection to a modern identity, ultrasound in Canada is firmly embedded in an individualizing ideology of risk and maternal responsibility. Implicit in women's anxieties and actions is the belief that "good" mothers do not take risks and therefore should avail themselves of ultrasound (see also Quéniart 1992).

Differences in Greeks' and North Americans' constructions of the fetal and maternal person are further highlighted when we compare popular cultural translations of expert knowledge about pregnancy. One such important channel for the diffusion of scientific images and knowledge is pregnancy guides. As Barbara Katz Rothman (1986) observed, middle-class North American women typically "take pregnancy as a reading assignment." In fact, all of the Canadian women had read pregnancy guides, many of which contain Lennart Nilsson's famous photographs of the live fetus in utero. About half of the Greek women had used a pregnancy guide, and the majority had consulted the same book, *Birth Is Love* (Sikakai-Douka n.d.). The only guide written by a Greek, *Birth Is Love* includes reprints of Nilsson's images—in this case, the earlier (1965) photographs of autopsied fetuses. However, the Nilsson images in the guides read by the Greek and Canadian women are embedded in sharply contrasting rhetorical constructions. Instead of the soft-focus, vulnerable, solitary, pink, thumbsucking North American in utero "baby," the grainy black-and-white photos included in *Birth Is Love* are far from cuddly. Throughout the Greek text, attention is focused almost exclusively on the physical characteristics and development of the fetus. When fetal personhood is discussed, it is consistently described in processual and relational terms rather than as an either/or state. Thus the guide's author flatly asserts that in the earliest stages of pregnancy "the embryo doesn't have any human characteristics!" (Sikakai-Douka n.d., 20). Becoming human is described as a process that unfolds over a considerable period of time. Even at the end of pregnancy the fetus is characterized as "a complete newborn, if not however, a complete person. Another state begins . . . only after some years will its development, its flowering, be complete" (68). Eventually, the author asserts, the fetus "will grow into an admirable extension of ourselves" (60).

In contrast, the guides read by the Canadian women portray the fetus, even during the early weeks of pregnancy, as a sentient, active, and socialized individual, often engaged in purposeful activities, and they emphasize maternal-fetal bonding as a central and essential experience of pregnancy. In the Greek text, this discourse on prenatal bonding is conspicuously absent. Although maternalist assumptions remain strong in both Canada and Greece, the discourse of fetal individuality and separateness that prevails in North America helps foster the "need" to promote a "bond" between now conceptually divided individuals.

In *Birth Is Love,* despite its sentimental title, much less of the advice dispensed revolves around the fetus. The guide does devote a considerable amount of attention to advising women about consumption—of medical technologies (including ultrasound), maternity clothes, cosmetics, prenatal care, expert knowledge, and so on. Throughout the text, the specific behaviors and practices being promoted are routinely identified as "European," "American," or even, in one instance, "Canadian." On the one hand, this tagging represents a rhetorical strategy for establishing the authority and credibility of the expert advice being dispensed. On the other, the prescription to follow "European" or "western" practices can also be interpreted as advice on how to construct one's self as a modern pregnant subject. The guide also contains a lot of advice on how to be a proper patient, urging women to be prompt for appointments and precise and concrete in their reports to the physician, and to recognize that if they have complaints about their physicians, they themselves prompt some of the behavior of which they complain. Thus, in addition to encouraging women in their pursuit of a modern pregnant subjectivity, the guide also has a disciplinary program, attempting to instruct women on how to become modern pregnant *patients* as well. This disciplinary goal is virtually absent in the Canadian guides. Rather, Canadian women, presumably already disciplined and medicalized long before Greek women, can now be "rewarded" with maternal-fetal communication.

CONCLUSION

Conceived and widely regarded as the means to revealing what is natural, true, and common to all fetuses and pregnancies, fetal ultrasound imaging appears to lack culture, to be a universalizing technology. As we attempt to show in this article, the cyborg fetus emerging from this technology says as much about the cultural and historical conditions of its production as it does about "nature" (Haraway 1992, 304). Specifically, our article illustrates that cyborgification simultaneously reproduces and reconfigures understandings of and relationships with the fetus. In other words, it both shapes and is shaped by local understandings and global discourses. Thus the ultrasound apparatus may dramatically expand the sensual and cognitive apprehension of the fetus, but it does so within the constraints of dominant discursive formations. One advantage of the cross-cultural perspective we have adopted here is the possibilities it opens up for exploring the complex ways in which these powerful discourses operate in specific societies.

In Canada, ultrasound is about the separation and reconnection of individuals. Pregnant women expect that they will "meet their baby" on the ultrasound screen, and they are encouraged by experts to see in the image digitalized evidence of a gendered, conscious, and sentient fetal actor communicating its demands and needs. Caught in a complex and very public ideology of fetal risk and maternal responsibility, Canadian women embrace ultrasound as a means of demonstrating that they are "good mothers" who are willing to work at forging bonds with their unborn babies.

In Greece, the production of fetal and pregnant subjects is markedly different. Ultrasound's evidence of fetal physical normalcy is read as evidence of fetal personhood. However, fetuses remain relational beings whose personhood is constituted primarily through social networks. As the Greek women eagerly demand and consume ultrasound technology, they actively identify themselves as modern pregnant subjects and, by implication, symbolically affiliate themselves with Europe and the West.

Yet if the cyborg fetus collaborates in the reproduction of dominant discourses about personhood, motherhood, and modernity, it also helps reconfigure women's experiences of pregnancy. For if, as we noted at the beginning of this article, "the machine is us," the cyborgification that results expands and alters the bodily experience of pregnancy in significant ways. Through their intimate interaction with the ultrasound, both Greek and Canadian women have emphatically redefined the experience of quickening as occurring when they first see the fetal image on the screen. "Seeing the baby" and "putting the baby on television" are now what make the pregnancy feel "real." However, this reconfiguration is not a simple and automatic result of visualizing the sonographic blur. Rather, it is mediated by the codes and conventions of a visual realism embedded in the very design of the technology. Through the ultrasound apparatus, these mass-mediated codes and conventions, now globally familiar, have become part of the commonsense bodily experience of pregnancy for both North American and Greek women. In its reproduction and reconfiguration, the cyborg fetus is constructed of cultural understandings, both local and global.

NOTES

This article is reprinted from *Feminist Studies* 23, no. 2 (September 1997): 373–401, by permission of the publisher, *Feminist Studies*. We are grateful to Rayna Rapp for encouraging us to develop an earlier version of this article and to the editors of the journal for permission to reprint.

1. While ultrasound images in Canada may show consciousness, emotion, and intention as obvious and "natural" facts of the cyborg fetus, the varieties of ultrasound practices among Canadian hospitals point to the continual shaping and filtering of these fetal images by institutional agendas, professional contests, and personal styles. At one Canadian hospital, obstetrician-sonographers compare their ultrasound practices with those of radiologists, claiming that radiologists can obtain technically superior images and more precise measure-

ments but that they lack certain communicating skills. "Knowing how to talk to patients" during ultrasound, taking the time, that is, to "show women the baby" and personalize the fetal image is believed by the obstetricians to be an essential part of good prenatal care. At a second hospital, one of the sonographers dismissed queries about why her clinic discusses only the diagnostic elements of the ultrasound and does not "show the baby." "We're not in the entertainment or warm fuzzies business," she said bluntly. "All that talk is just stuff to make women feel better. We're using it [ultrasound] to look for problems, make diagnoses, and then we send them home."

2. In a recent article, Sunera Thobani (1993) shows how the opening of a sex selection clinic in the United States directed at South Asian women in western Canada reinforced racist and patriarchal assumptions about South Asian culture.

3. See, e.g., Garel and Franc (1980), Grace (1983), Kemp and Page (1987), Kohn et al. (1980), Milne and Rich (1981), Sparling et al. (1988), and Villeneuve et al. (1988).

4. See Eyers's (1992) analysis of the historical and social construction of mother-infant bonding.

5. For more on men's and women's differing responses to fetal ultrasound, see Sandelowski (1994).

6. At the time of the interviews, the 49 Canadian women were between the ages of 22 and 33 and living with a male partner. The women, awaiting the birth of their first child, had been labeled by their obstetricians as "low risk" for fetal anomalies or complications of pregnancy. Most of the women are Canadian-born, but they construct their identities along diverse cultural lines. They include, by their own terms, women who are "Lebanese," "Anglophone," "Italian-Canadian," Québécoise," "Jewish," "WASPS," and "just Canadian." They are also women from different religions, educations, and work worlds, but their lifestyles, homes, and incomes signal their middle-class status. Despite differences in their cultural and social locations, their narratives on the cyborg fetus are strikingly similar, indicative perhaps of both the pervasiveness of ultrasound in Canada and the particular emphasis the research hospital places on personalizing the ultrasound.

7. Such intensive monitoring of pregnancy is not a regional aberration, but reflects Greek obstetrical practice generally. Medical students in Athens are taught to do three scans per normal pregnancy, one in each trimester, and a recent survey of over five hundred normal pregnancies in Athens found that, in fact, 93 percent of women had had at least one fetal ultrasound scan, with about one-quarter experiencing two or more scans in the third trimester alone (G. Breart et al. 1992).

REFERENCES

Appadurai, Arjun:
  1991 Global Ethnoscapes: Notes and Queries for a Transnational Anthropology. In R. Fox (ed.), *Recapturing Anthropology*, 191–210. Sante Fe: School of American Research.
Arnold, Marlene S.:
  1985 *Childbirth among Rural Greek Women in Crete: Use of Popular, Folk, and Cosmopolitan Medical Systems*. Ann Arbor: UMI Dissertation Information Service.
Becker, Anne:
  1995 *Body, Self, and Society: The View from Fiji*. Philadelphia: University of Pennsylvania Press.

Blue, Amy:

1993   Greek Psychiatry's Transition from the Hospital to the Community. *Medical Anthropology Quarterly* 7(3): 301–18.

Blum, Richard, and Eva Blum:

1965   *Health and Healing in Rural Greece.* Stanford: Stanford University Press.

Breart, G., et al.:

1992   Pre-Partum Care in the EC Countries—Preliminary Results of a European Concerted Action. In J. G. Koppe et al. (eds.), *Care, Concern, and Cure in Perinatal Medicine.* Lancaster, U.K.: Parthenon.

Cartwright, Lisa:

1993   Gender Artifacts in Medical Imaging: Ultrasound, Sex Identification, and Interpretive Ambiguity in Fetal Medicine. Paper presented to the American Anthropological Association annual meeting, Washington, D.C.

Condit, Celeste M.:

1990   *Decoding Abortion Rhetoric: Communicating Social Change.* Urbana: University of Illinois Press.

Costa, Janeen:

1993   The Periphery of Pleasure or Pain: Consumer Culture in the EC Mediterranean of 1992. In Thomas Wilson and M. Estellie Smith (eds.), *Cultural Change and the New Europe.* Boulder: Westview.

Craig, Marveen:

1991   Controversies in Obstetric Gynecologic Ultrasound. In Mimi Berman (ed.), *Diagnostic Medical Sonography: A Guide to Clinical Practice.* Vol. 1, *Obstetrics and Gynecology,* 551–62. Philadelphia: J. B. Lippencott.

Crary, Jonathan:

1990   *Techniques of the Observer: On Vision and Modernity in the Nineteenth Century.* Cambridge: MIT Press.

Davis-Floyd, Robbie:

1998   Mutilation and Prosthesis: The One-Two Punch of Birth in the Technocracy. In Robbie Davis-Floyd and Joseph Dumit (eds.), *Cyborg Babies: From Techno-Sex to Techno-Tots.* New York: Routledge.

Davis-Floyd, Robbie, and Joseph Dumit (eds.):

1998   *Cyborg Babies: From Techno-Sex to Techno-Tots.* New York: Routledge.

Dewsbury, Anton:

1980   What the Fetus Feels. Letter, *British Medical Journal,* 16 February, 481.

Duden, Barbara:

1992   Quick with Child: An Experience That Has Lost Its Status. *Technology in Society* 14: 335–44.

1993   *Disembodying Women: Pespectives on Pregnancy and the Unborn.* Cambridge: Harvard University Press.

Eyers, Diane E.:

1992   *Mother-Infant Bonding: A Scientific Fiction.* New Haven: Yale University Press.

Fiske, John:

1987   *Television Culture.* New York: Routledge.

Fletcher, John, and Mark Evans:

1983   Maternal Bonding in Early Fetal Ultrasound Examinations. *New England Journal of Medicine* 308(7): 392–93.

Franklin, Sarah:
  1991 Fetal Fascinations: New Dimensions to the Medical-Scientific Construction of Fetal Personhood. In Sarah Franklin, Celia Lury, and Jackie Stacey (eds.), *Off-Centre: Feminism and Cultural Studies,* 190–205. New York: Routledge.
  1993 Postmodern Procreation: Representing Reproductive Practice. *Science as Culture* 3, no. 17, pt. 4: 522–61.
Garel, M., and M. Franc:
  1980 Réactions des femmes à l'écographie obstétricale [Women's reactions to obstetrical sonography]. *Journal of Gynaecology, Obstetrics, Biology, and Reproduction* 9: 347–54.
Georges, Eugenia:
  1996 Abortion Policy and Politics in Greece. *Social Science and Medicine* 42(4): 509–19.
Grace, Jeanne:
  1983 Prenatal Ultrasound Examinations and Mother-Infant Bonding. *New England Journal of Medicine* 309(9): 561.
Halkias, Alexandra:
  1995 When Talking about the Nation Means Talking about Babies: The Case of Greece's Demografiko and the Press' Portrayal of Abortion. Paper presented at the Modern Greek Studies Association meetings, Cambridge, Mass., November.
Handman, Marie-Elisabeth:
  1983 *La violence et la ruse: Hommes et femmes dans un village Grec.* La Calade, Aix-en-Provence: Edisud.
Haraway, Donna:
  1991 *Simians, Cyborgs, and Nature: The Reinvention of Nature.* New York: Routledge.
  1992 The Promises of Monsters: A Regenerative Politics for Inappropriate/d Others. In Larry Grossberg, Cary Nelson, and Paula Treichler (eds.), *Cultural Studies,* 295–337. New York: Routledge.
Hartouni, Valerie:
  1991 Containing Women: Reproductive Discourse in the 1980s. In C. Penley and A. Ross (eds.), *Technoculture.* Minneapolis: University of Minnesota Press.
Hess, David:
  1995 *Science and Technology in a Multicultural World.* New York: Columbia University Press.
Kemp, Virgina, and Cecilia Page:
  1987 Maternal Prenatal Attachment in Normal and High-Risk Pregnancies. *Journal of Obstetrics, Gynecology, and Neonatology in Nursing* 16 (May/June): 179–83.
Kohn, C. L., et al.:
  1980 Gravidas' Responses to Real-Time Ultrasound Fetal Image. *Journal of Obstetrics, Gynecology, and Neonatology in Nursing* 9: 77–80.
Lippman, Abby:
  1986 Access to Prenatal Screening Services: Who Decides? *Canadian Journal of Women and the Law* 1(2): 434–45.
McNeill, William H.:
  1978 *The Metamorphosis of Greece since World War II.* Chicago: University of Chicago Press.
Mageo, Jeanette:
  1995 The Reconfiguring Self. *American Anthropologist* 97 (June): 282–96.
Meizner, Israel:
  1987 Sonographic Observation of In Utero Fetal Masturbation. *Journal of Ultrasound in Medicine* 6 (February): 111.

Milne, L., and O. Rich:
  1981 Cognitive and Affective Aspects of the Responses of Pregnant Women to Sonography. *Maternal-Child Nursing Journal* 10: 15–39.
Oakley, Ann:
  1984 *The Captured Womb: A History of the Medical Care of Pregnant Women.* Oxford: Basil Blackwell.
Papagaroufali, Eleni, and Eugenia Georges:
  1993 Greek Women in the Europe of 1992: Brokers of European Cargos and the Logic of the West. In G. Marcus (ed.), *Perilous States: Conversations on Culture, Race, and Nation,* 235–54. Chicago: University of Chicago Press.
Pretorius, Jack Dolores, and Barry S. Mahoney:
  1990 The Role of Obstetrical Ultrasound. In David Nyberg et al. (eds.), *Diagnostic Ultrasound of Fetal Anomalies: Text and Atlas,* 1–20. Chicago: Chicago Year Book.
Quéniart, Anne
  1992 Risky Business: Medical Definitions of Pregnancy. In D. Currie and V. Raoul (eds.), *The Anatomy of Gender,* 161–74. Ottawa: Carleton University Press.
Rapp, Rayna:
  1994 Commentary on AAA panel "Reproducing Reproduction." *Anthropology Newsletter* 8 (November): 33–34.
Reading, Anthony, et al.:
  1982 Health Beliefs and Health Care Behaviour in Pregnancy. *Psychological Medicine* 12: 379–83.
  1988 A Controlled, Prospective Evaluation of the Acceptability of Ultrasound in Prenatal Care. *Journal of Psychosomatic Obstetrics and Gynecology* 8: 191–98.
Rothman, Barbara Katz:
  1986 *The Tentative Pregnancy: Prenatal Diagnosis and the Future of Motherhood.* New York: Viking Penguin.
  1989 *Reinventing Motherhood: Ideology and Technology in a Patriarchial Society.* New York: W. W. Norton.
Sandelowski, Margaret:
  1994 Separate, but Less Unequal: Fetal Ultrasonography and the Transformation of Expectant Mother/Fatherhood. *Gender and Society* 8(2): 230–45.
Sikakai-Douka, Aleka:
  n.d. *Birth Is Love.* Athens: Self-published.
Sparling, Joyce, et al.:
  1988 The Relationship of Obstetric Ultrasound to Parent and Infant Behaviour. *Obstetrics and Gynecology* 72: 902–7.
Spiro, Melford:
  1993 Is the Western Concept of the Self "Peculiar" within the Context of World Cultures? *Ethos* 21 (June): 107–53.
Spitz, Jean Lea:
  1991 Sonographer Support of Maternal-Fetal Bonding. In Mimi Berman (ed.), *Diagnostic Medical Sonography: A Guide to Clinical Practice.* Vol. 1, *Obstetrics and Gynecology,* 565–71. Philadelphia: J. B. Lippencott.
Taylor, Janelle:
  1992 The Public Fetus and the Family Car: From Abortion Politics to a Volvo Advertisement. *Public Culture* 4(2): 67–80.

Thobani, Sunera:

    1993   From Reproduction to Mal[e] Production: Women and Sex Selection Technology. In G. Basen, M. Eichler, and A. Lippman (eds.), *Misconceptions: The Social Construction of Choice and the New Reproductive and Genetic Technologies,* 138–53. Hull, Quebec: Voyageur.

Triandis, Harry:

    1988   Collectivism v. Individualism: A Reconceptualization of a Basic Concept in Cross-Cultural Social Psychology. In G. K. Verma and Christopher Bagley (eds.), *Cross-Cultural Studies of Personality, Attitudes, and Cognition,* 82. New York: St. Martin's Press.

Velogiannis-Moutsopoulos, L., and C. S. Bartsocas:

    1989   Ethics and Medical Genetics in Greece. In Dorothy Wertz and John Fletcher (eds.), *Human Genetics: A Cross-Cultural Perspective,* 209–34. Heidelberg: Springer.

Villeneuve, Claude, et al.:

    1988   Psychological Aspects of Ultrasound Imaging during Pregnancy. *Canadian Journal of Psychiatry* 33: 530–35.

16

Situating Fetoscopy within Medical Literature and Lived Experience: An Opening for Social Analysis

Deborah Blizzard

Since the early 1990s, a small network of obstetric, gynecologic, and perinatal physicians have been creating a "new generation" of fetoscopy, a reproductive technology that offers endoscopic access to the embryo-fetus. Given its abilities to view, sample, and manipulate the in utero environment, developments in fetoscopy may alter the current state of prenatal diagnosis and therapy and women's pregnancy experiences. Although fetoscopy development and use are occurring in relatively isolated research centers or clinics, the effects are far-reaching. To date, there is little social analysis on this process. It would be beneficial for social scientists from a variety of backgrounds and theoretical assumptions to analyze fetoscopy while it is developing and flexible.[1] As a newly developing reproductive technology, fetoscopy may both alter, and be altered by, the persons who design and use it.[2] Social scientists are uniquely positioned to investigate this process by analyzing the contexts in which social interactions occur. Such analysis will lead to better understanding of an emergent technology and its potential sociocultural effects.

This work identifies current fetoscopy development and use by analyzing medical journals and women's lived experiences. In their articles, some physicians use comparisons and analogies to draw from better-known tools to illustrate fetoscopy developments, bringing to light important similarities and differences. This practice not only helps physicians place the tool within their shared professional perspectives but may also prove useful for social scientists trying to better understand the tool. In particular, social scientists may use insights from existing social analyses of reproductive tools and experiences (e.g., amniocentesis, ultrasound, and open fetal surgery) to identify relevant issues for fetoscopy analyses. Just as physicians must "make sense" of fetoscopy, women undergoing procedures must also situate the tools within their reproductive and life experiences. It is useful to investigate whether patient experiences support or challenge criticisms of other tools. With such analysis, social scientists may help forge fetoscopy into a tool that is worthwhile in its present use and may minimize future criticisms.[3] Such analyses not only would be an intellectual project for social scientists but would also prove useful for the women, their companions, and physicians who struggle to make sense of the tool and its many implications.

METHODOLOGY

This analysis draws from eleven months of ethnographic fieldwork in a hospital and a nonprofit research organization that are creating fetoscopy (September 1997–July 1998), social science critiques of reproductive tools and experiences, and fetoscopy reports in medical journals. Many of the earlier published accounts of fetoscopy presented it as a primarily diagnostic tool; however, recently fetoscopy has developed into an operative tool. In this analysis I use accounts of both diagnostic and operative cases because much of the literature highlights fetoscopy as a diagnostic procedure and most of my fieldwork analyzed it as an operative procedure. The tool is still developing, and it is useful to consider both options as possible developmental outcomes.

The first part of this analysis describes the medical uses and risks associated with fetoscopy. To illustrate fetoscopy, I draw from the medical literature, highlighting comparisons and analogies with existing tools. Medical articles not only offer detailed descriptions of the tools and procedures but also situate fetoscopy within physicians' shared context and perspectives. Social scientists can take up these analogies, using them as starting points to further their own understandings of the tool. By so doing, current advances in fetoscopy may be considered in light of social analyses of other reproductive tools (for examples of comparisons for the diagnostic approach, see Reece, Goldstein et al. 1994; Reece et al., 1995a, 1995b; Quintero, Puder, and Cotton 1993; for comparisons for the operative approach, see Luks et al. 1994, 1996; Quintero, Puder, and Cotton 1993).[4]

The second part of this analysis draws from social science literature and ethnographic study to identify the contexts in which patients pursue fetoscopy. While comparisons help social scientists understand the tool, as sociocultural experiences the procedures are unintelligible without situating the lived experience of parent-patients.[5] While conducting my research, I observed eighteen fetoscopy procedures (two patients underwent two procedures). With patient consent, I observed the surgical team in the operating room, wore the required surgical scrubs, and followed aseptic technique. The cases were diverse, ranging from purely diagnostic assessments of the fetus to operative approaches that included shunting and biopsy. Beyond single fetuses, operative fetoscopy was also used in twin (and triplet) pregnancies when the fetuses shared blood disproportionately, leading to fetal distress and possible harm to or demise of one or more fetuses. When this occurred, operative fetoscopy was used to separate (laser) shared placental blood vessels, and in extreme situations (following ethical review), fetoscopy was used to tie off (ligate) the umbilical cord of a nonviable or dying fetus in an effort to save the other fetus(es) from harm.[6] During my fieldwork I formally interviewed sixteen women choosing to undergo fetoscopy and nine companions of these women (generally a partner or father of the fetus).[7] Beyond formal interviews, I had many informal conversations with the patients and their companions.[8] The interviews typically lasted thirty minutes to one hour, were conducted in their hospital rooms, and took place one or two days after the procedure (in two cases I interviewed informants before surgery and in two cases I interviewed informants shortly after they returned home). I used a semi-open-ended interview approach, asking them to tell me about themselves and their experiences with fetoscopy. With this approach I listened to their stories, including how and when they chose to begin and end it. At the conclusion of the interviews, many of the patients thanked me for my time and interest. During these final exchanges, some also expressed their concern over what they considered to be a general lack of knowledge by both medical and lay persons about their (and their fetus or baby's) conditions and potential treatments. Many wished to be interviewed in the hope that more people would learn about their situation and find it helpful in their own decision making.

DEFINING FETOSCOPY: CREATING COMPARISONS

Fetoscopy has evolved in a number of ways leading to some uncertainty as to the appropriate name for the tools (e.g., Quintero, Puder, and Cotton 1993; Ville et al. 1997; Simpson and Elias 1996). Although there is a growing medical literature surrounding new developments in fetoscopy, analysis of the articles shows that the exact names of tools vary. For example, in articles reporting on diagnostic uses, some physicians use the words *transabdominal* or *transcervical embryoscopy, endoscopy, embryofetoscopy,* or *fetoscopy* (other names and descriptors are also suggested) to refer to the in utero visualization and, in some cases, possible sampling of an embryo-fetus or uterine environment. Variations in name often reflect differences in the physical structure and use of the tools (e.g., construction of the scope, size of insertion, period of gestation, route of access, or how close the tool is placed to the embryo-fetus). Like diagnostic procedures, physicians pursuing in utero surgery also use multiple names to refer to their tools. For example, names suggested include operative fetoscopy, fetendo, and surgical endoscopy. The tools have not "stabilized" (Bijker, Hughes, and Pinch 1987). They are in flux and open to a variety of interpretations regarding their clinical use and therapeutic potential. While variations do exist within diagnostic and operative approaches (as evident in the multiple names), it is the similarities when compared with other tools that are useful for social analyses. Although the differences are important from a medical perspective, they are less critical in a social science framework that identifies general patterns to technology use and potential sociocultural implications. For the purposes of this analysis, I use *diagnostic embryofetoscopy* or *embryofetoscopy* as an umbrella term to represent early transabdominal endoscopic visualization and potential sampling of the in utero environment (including the embryo-fetus).⁹ I use *operative fetoscopy* as an umbrella term to represent in utero surgery. When citing medical journals, I keep the original term offered by the author(s).¹⁰

Fetoscopy can be considered a collection of tools that offer endoscopic access to the in utero embryo-fetus. Once inside, some tools may also draw samples from the uterine environment or deliver therapy through in utero surgery. Loosely, advances in fetoscopy may be separated in two ways:

1. It is a diagnostic technology used to visually identify (and in some cases sample) part of an embryo-fetus or uterine environment (diagnostic embryofetoscopy).
2. It is a therapeutic technology used to deliver in utero surgery (operative fetoscopy).

These classifications are broad representations of a flexible tool, and in some cases a fetoscopic procedure might fall within both categories. For example, in the operative cases that I observed, the physician moved between using a scope as a diagnostic tool that "viewed from afar" and as an operative tool that "worked on" the fetus or the in utero environment. I consider diagnostic and operative procedures as two avenues of fetoscopy, recognizing that this separation is not always clear or distinct. With their visual capabilities, both diagnostic and operative approaches are fundamentally diagnostic tools, yet they differ substantially in their ability to alter a pregnancy. To draw attention to one over the other or to hold one as the "preferred" fetoscopy is to miss the point: within the medical literature both are considered minimally or relatively less invasive tools that offer in utero access to an ongoing pregnancy with the intent of alleviating a problem. How this problem is defined, treated, and made meaningful is a project for social analyses.

CLASSIC FETOSCOPY: INSIGHTS AND TECHNICAL PROBLEMS

Although the first reported attempt to view an in utero fetus occurred in 1954 (transcervical access), it was not until the late 1960s, and continuing through the 1970s, that researchers began using a transabdominal approach in their attempts to view and sample the fetus and uterine environment (e.g., Benzie 1980; Quintero, Puder, and Cotton 1993; Reece 1999). These transabdominal procedures were used in the second and third trimesters of pregnancy and were eventually termed "fetoscopy" (e.g., Scrimgeour in Quintero, Puder, and Cotton 1993). Physicians could not only see the fetus but also photograph it, thereby inviting others to see as well (e.g., Grannum and Copel 1990; Simpson and Elias 1996; Oakley 1984; Duden 1993). Similar to amniocentesis, many physicians used ultrasound to determine the location of the fetus before inserting the tool. While access to the fetus aided some diagnoses, fetoscopy development was hindered by technical constraints. For example, the endoscope could not generate an image of the entire fetus (Quintero, Puder, and Cotton 1993; Duden 1993), and because of its size it required a trocar (larger needlelike instrument) through which it was passed. The relatively large size of the tool was potentially disruptive to pregnancies and, depending upon the operator, led to an estimated 5–7 percent rate of pregnancy loss (Grannum and Copel 1990). One group argues that in "experienced hands" the loss rate ranged between 2 and 5 percent, which was still "severalfold higher than those associated with amniocentesis" (Quintero, Abuhamad et al. 1993, 1556). The loss rate, in conjunction with limited access, yielded a "risk-versus-benefit . . . [analysis that] somewhat limited the use of fetoscopy" (Reece et al. 1992, 776).

It is misleading to assume that fetoscopy's "failure" to develop into a commonplace tool was only due to its technical constraints. Fetoscopy was also affected by improvements in reproductive ultrasound (e.g., Quintero, Puder, and Cotton 1993; Gannum and Copel 1990; Simpson and Elias 1996; Pennehouat et al. 1992; Ville et al. 1997). When sampling was not necessary, physicians could use ultrasound images to make diagnoses based on the physical appearance of the embryo-fetus. With refined, externally administered ultrasound, there was less medical need for the more invasive fetoscopy (e.g., Pennehouat et al. 1992; Ville et al. 1997). Yet some physicians did not abandon fetoscopy: "Despite its low profile throughout the last decade . . . fetoscopy has maintained its role as an alternative diagnostic and therapeutic tool for certain clinical situations" (Quintero, Puder, and Cotton 1993, 563). Although physicians continued to use fetoscopy for some diagnoses (in other words, development slowed but never stopped), in general the procedure retreated to the background of embryo-fetal diagnostics and never gained the widespread use of other reproductive tools such as amniocentesis or ultrasound.

A RESURGENCE OF FETOSCOPY

Constructing the Artifact

Advances in endoscopy and sampling techniques have led to new developments in fetoscopy (diagnostic embryofetoscopy and operative fetoscopy) that not only are gaining momentum in research groups but may offer new approaches to embryo-fetal diagnoses and therapies (e.g., Hobbins 1996; Reece et al. 1993; Quintero, Puder, and Cotton 1993; Reece 1999). Although durations vary, many reports indicate that embryofetoscopy generally lasts less than fifteen minutes and is commonly administered under local anesthesia.[11] An operative procedure is substantially longer, requiring either local or general anesthesia (all operative cases that I observed were conducted under general anesthesia with the average surgery lasting approximately two to three hours, depending on the particularities of the case, such as position of the fetus). Even though these tools show characteristics of "classic fetoscopy," they have particular and potential applications (Quintero, Puder, and Cotton 1993).

Diagnostic procedures offer visual access and potential sampling in the first and second trimesters. Unlike a sonographic representation of the embryo-fetus, the image is a magnified color picture, providing a more refined image than ultrasound (e.g., Quintero, Puder, and Cotton 1993). The clearer image gives the technique a "foot up" compared to other tools; the physician is able to see a clearer representation of embryo-fetal features before making clinical diagnoses or performing in utero surgery.[12] Also, recent developments have led to small diameter scopes, "thin gauge" (e.g., Quintero, Puder, and Cotton 1993) or "needle" (e.g., Reece et al. 1997) embryofetoscopy which, like amniocentesis, do not require a trocar and may be placed directly into the amniotic sac. With small-diameter access, some researchers argue that diagnostic embryofetoscopy may gain access to the embryo-fetus when the immune system is not fully developed, thereby making it amenable to certain therapies including genetic therapy (e.g., Quintero, Puder, and Cotton 1993; Reece 1997a, 1999). One physician reports, "Embryofetoscopy will make it possible to perform stem-cell transplantation or gene therapy during the first trimester of pregnancy, at a time when the fetus is immunologically naive and when the chances for engraftment are greatest. The new technology provides an opportunity for us to treat a variety of genetic disorders before their disabling effects are realized" (Reece 1997a, 119). However, it is not clear how early access must be to accomplish such a task (Hobbins 1996; Evans et al. 1994).

Also taking advantage of visual access, operative fetoscopy is another development in fetoscopy that offers in utero surgery. According to two proponents: "The key characteristics of this approach include the combination of two imaging techniques—endoscopy and ultrasound—making use of their individual advantages while allowing the performance of surgical procedures with minimal disturbance to the pregnancy [citation offered]" (Quintero and Evans 1995). Its ability to combine the benefits of seemingly dissimilar yet useful tools is exciting to physicians: "This still largely theoretical modality combines the familiar, but hitherto mostly diagnostic, technique of fetoscopy with the surgical freedom of open fetal operations and the claimed 'non-invasiveness' of endosurgery. Indeed, the line between old-fashioned fetoscopic sampling and modern-era endoscopic surgery is fading" (Luks and Deprest 1993, 1). Unlike a diagnostic approach, operative fetoscopy is used later in pregnancy after a diagnosis is made. The physician places a trocar transabdominally into the amniotic sac and then uses that same channel to insert miniature surgical tools such as scissors and forceps (if desired, the physician may use more than one trocar). Unlike amniocentesis or diagnostic embryofetoscopy, operative fetoscopy is a lengthy procedure that does offer therapy to a developing fetus. Although it is only used in a handful of cases, operative fetoscopy is diversifying, treating fetal conditions including amniotic band syndrome (the physician cuts constrictive "bands" that have attached to the fetus) and twin to twin transfusion syndrome (the physician lasers shared placental blood vessels through which identical twins share blood disproportionately) (on amniotic band syndrome, see Quintero, Morales, et al. 1997; on twin to twin transfusion syndrome, see Quintero, Romero, et al. 1996; Ville et al. 1995; DeLia 1996). In the former case, fetoscopy is used to save fetal limbs from amputation and deformity, while the latter case saves the fetus(es) from harm (including neurological damage or death). Operative fetoscopy's advantage lies in offering in utero surgery through relatively minimal points of entry.

While diagnostic embryofetoscopy and operative fetoscopy differ, they are also similar. Both may access the amniotic sac where they can draw off amniotic fluid for analysis. In this way, amniocentesis and classic fetoscopy appear to merge within these newly developing tools. Similarly, like ultrasound, physicians can visually target the tool on the embryo-fetus (or other in utero region, i.e., the placenta) to withdraw blood, tissue biopsies, or perform surgery. The ability to see the embryo-fetus clearly, and to sample from or potentially alter it and its environment through minimal points of entry, separates these tools from amniocentesis, ultrasound, open fetal surgery, and classic fetoscopy.

Constructing Risk

When constructing medical technologies, risk (in its many forms) is a consideration for physicians and patients alike. To illustrate risk, some physicians use comparisons to better known tools and procedures. For example, risk analogies to diagnostic embryofetoscopy may include amniocentesis. Operative fetoscopy is generally positioned in relation to open fetal surgery. In both cases, diagnostic embryofetoscopy and operative fetoscopy may be considered against the risk of "not knowing" or "not altering" the condition of the embryo-fetus or the pregnancy.

When compared with more routine reproductive technologies, diagnostic embryofetoscopy researchers do not have the comparable clinical experience or accompanying statistics regarding the safety of their techniques (Quintero, Puder, and Cotton 1993; Ville et al. 1996). To illustrate, before 1994, transabdominal thin-gauge embryofetoscopy (TGEF) procedures had only been performed on women electing to terminate a pregnancy (Quintero, developer of TGEF, personal communication).[13] Today, embryofetoscopy is used as prenatal diagnosis on continuing pregnancies, and physicians are designing the tool so that it is less likely to cause gestational disruptions, including fetal loss and amniotic fluid leakage.

Particularly worrisome is the potential for amniotic fluid leakage. "Because of its recent introduction, data on amniotic fluid leakage do not exist for TGEF, although we suspect the incidence will be similar to the 1.7 percent reported for early amniocentesis [citations offered]" (Quintero, Puder, and Cotton 1993, 573).[14] One group continues at length to try and identify a spectrum of statistical risk by considering the tool in the context of amniocentesis and classic fetoscopy:[15] "The technique . . . when performed expeditiously, is analogous to an early amniocentesis with an 18-gauge needle. . . . It is underscored that the technique is not analogous to second-trimester fetoscopy [citation offered], which carried a 3% to 7% fetal loss rate, because the trocar utilized in fetoscopy was 2.2 x 2.7 mm in diameter, which is significantly larger than an 18-gauge needle" (Hobbins et al. 1994, 549). The risks of early amniocentesis and diagnostic embryofetoscopy appear comparable; however, it is necessary to be clear at what time during the pregnancy the test is administered, how large the point of entry, and how soon thereafter a negative outcome may be attributed to a procedure.[16]

While the material culture of operative fetoscopy (transabdominal, minimally invasive) is similar to diagnostic embryofetoscopy and amniocentesis, the fact that it is a therapeutic technique makes it necessary to consider it in light of other tools, such as open fetal surgery. (It is also important to recognize that, like open fetal surgery, operative fetoscopy is a lengthy procedure in which the woman may be placed under general anesthesia.)[17] Like diagnostic comparisons, it would be an overstatement that all theorists accept these comparisons or pursue them. Yet physicians who present operative fetoscopy procedures commonly reference open fetal surgery referring to its high rates of maternal morbidity and fetal mortality (for social analysis of open fetal surgery, see Casper 1998). As opposed to open fetal surgery, operative fetoscopy utilizes small incisions to access the fetus. For example, Ruben A. Quintero, who introduced the term *operative fetoscopy,* uses 2–3 mm incisions through which he conducts surgery (Quintero, personal communication). Many proponents of operative fetoscopy laud the substantially smaller incisions. Comparing operative fetoscopy's access to that of open fetal surgery, one group clearly explains that "the extreme invasiveness of this therapeutic option [open fetal surgery] has severely limited its application to only one or two centers world-wide [citations offered]. . . . Recently, however, endoscopy and video-endoscopic surgery have undergone revolutionary changes. These changes, and a mounting frustration with the problems of open fetal surgery, have paved the way for the concept of endoscopic fetal surgery" (Luks and Deprest 1993, 1).[18] In this regard, a potential goal of operative fetoscopy is to reduce surgical trauma to both the woman and fetus.

Yet not all physicians view the smaller incisions as a clear advantage, and some caution that the tool is not yet proven: "If fetoscopic surgery is to become an alternative to open fetal surgery, this approach must allow safe, monitored, and reproducible access to the fetus" (Luks et al. 1994, 1008). Another paper reminds readers that the terms *access* and *invasive* are not synonymous: "But before minimal *access* surgery is accepted as an alternative to open fetal surgery, it will have to prove minimally *invasive* to the fetus, the uterus and, ultimately, the mother" (italics in original, Luks and Deprest 1993, 1). These physicians suggest that potential trauma may include more than the point of entry and caution that excitement and anticipation should be tempered with rigorous testing to demonstrate safety and usefulness (Luks and Deprest 1993). Future problems may stem from the fact that the tool is associated with rupture of the membranes, and one group warns, "This problem may become operative fetoscopy's Achilles' heel, just as preterm labour was for open fetal surgery" (Deprest, Lerut, and Vandenberghe 1997, 1256). To this end, they remind other physicians that maternal safety must be the central issue that drives whether or not operative fetoscopy is deemed acceptable.

Along with concerns for safety, operative fetoscopy has a distinct set of limits and implications. As a therapeutic technology, operative fetoscopy requires a diagnosis amenable to surgical intervention. Such diagnosis might come from other reproductive technologies such as amniocentesis and ultrasound. Also fetoscopic surgery requires the creation of a variety of surgical tools to be used along with endoscopic access (e.g., Dreyfus et al. 1996; Quintero and Evans 1995). Beyond the material limitations of operative fetoscopy, as a second or third trimester surgical tool, it may have legal or other policy limitations regarding when and how it can be performed (e.g., abortion law and hospital guidelines). Generally, medical risks are presented in relation to a specific medical procedure; however, as a therapeutic tool physicians must also weigh the contextual risk of not intervening (which may lead to pregnancy loss), or possibly waiting until the fetus is born, and having the baby undergo surgery at that time.

Whether physicians are using embryofetoscopy, operative fetoscopy, or both, reports in medical journals frequently address the risks of the procedures. For example, risks may stem from trauma to the amniotic sac, amniotic fluid leakage, or harm to the fetus. Over time, and with animal experiments, physician are not only attempting to identify risks but also investigating ways to overcome the risks (i.e., some groups are exploring methods for controlling amniotic fluid leakage). Other investigations have explored whether or not the endoscopic light harms developing fetal eyes. Two groups indicate that eye damage is unlikely: on chick embryos, see Quintero, Crossland and Cotton (1994); on fetal lambs, see Deprest et al. (1999). Physicians are working to understand and minimize the risks associated with the new developments in fetoscopy. While these tools may offer advantages to physicians and patients seeking diagnoses and therapies, like other reproductive technologies, material and interpretative limitations encumber them.

IMPLICATIONS SUGGESTED BY CURRENT REPRODUCTIVE TECHNOLOGY ANALYSES

If social scientists wish to understand current fetoscopy developments and anticipate future implications, it is useful to consider whether analyses of other reproductive technologies might suggest avenues for critical analysis of fetoscopy. When turning to social analyses of amniocentesis, ultrasound, and open fetal surgery, many issues are relevant to fetoscopy. For the purpose of this work, I highlight three issue areas: timing dilemmas, fetus as separate from a woman-mother, and pregnancy loss. By analyzing these issues in light of fetoscopy, social scientists may arrive at new understandings to assist physicians, patients, and their companions when interacting with, thinking about, or constructing fetoscopy.

Timing Dilemmas

Social analyses of pregnancy experiences have been critical of timing issues associated with reproductive technology use. Many reproductive technologies imply that women must wait to take a test, and in some cases she must wait again to receive results. During these periods, anxious women struggle to define who they are and what they wish as "would-be" mothers (Layne 1992, 32; Rothman 1986; Rapp 1988a, 1999). When pursuing fetoscopy, timing issues occur before, during, and following procedures.

Whether patients pursue diagnostic or operative procedures, their pregnancies do not follow the presumed linear narrative of unproblematic conception, gestation, and birth.[19] These pregnancies are high risk. Following this assessment, patients must identify a method for continuing or not continuing the pregnancy. Diagnosis and timing merge within diagnostic embryofetoscopy to open a host of new clinical possibilities in the early stages of pregnancy. As a second or third trimester therapeutic tool, operative fetoscopy also implies difficult issues for patients and their families.

Given clearer visual access, researchers are no longer limited to procedures that may take more than a week to culture and analyze; instead, like ultrasound, diagnostic embryofetoscopy researchers are able to generate "real-time" diagnoses by analyzing the physical structures of an embryo-fetus (e.g., Rapp 1998). Certainly, concerned parents may appreciate the immediacy of results; however, real-time tests do not ensure unambiguous results. While physicians may look for fetal structures, as with ultrasound, their appearance may not be clear, and physicians may find themselves debating the image on the monitor. This may be particularly problematic if such discourse occurs while the woman is awake. Physicians using visual diagnoses are limited to how they perceive the monitor and interpret its meaning. While physicians work to interpret the images, women strive to make sense of their pregnancies.

A patient choosing to undergo fetoscopic intervention may find the period before her procedure particularly difficult as she struggles to determine whether her pregnancy is "in danger" and when it might be "out of danger." Many patients referred to their pregnancy experiences as being on a "roller-coaster" with "ups and downs" depending upon whom they last saw or what they last read. When I asked one patient, Monica Rivera, how she dealt with going from physician to physician and prognosis to prognosis, she laughed a bit and explained:

> Well, it wasn't a fun thing. It's very stressful. . . . Well, we really didn't know
> what to think. We thought, well, okay, all bad news. Then we thought, well,
> the DNA tests are good, that's good news. And then we thought, surgery,
> that's good news. But then they said, well, no, we shouldn't do surgery, so
> that's bad news. And then [the doctor] said, well, maybe we can. We'll try
> this new method. . . . Then we thought, well, is that good news? I guess. . . .
> It's been a long road, it seems. A very long pregnancy, and it's not over yet.

In this case, and many like it, patients worked to make sense of their precarious pregnancies. How they react to the fetus, understand its current and potential health problems, and potentially position it within a family context is in flux. So, too, are their decisions of whether or not to pursue fetoscopy and what to do following a procedure.

Situating the pregnancy within a family context is particularly difficult when parents later realize that they did not fully understand an earlier ill-ness or its prognosis. This may be particularly relevant when parents diagnosed with little-known diseases turn to lesser-known tools for intervention. Angela March, whose twin fetuses were diagnosed with twin to twin transfusion syn-drome (uneven sharing of blood in the placenta by identical twin fetuses, lead-ing to harm or death of one or both fetuses), found it hard to "follow" which of her fetuses was sick:

> [My husband] and I were a little confused. First of all, I thought . . . pretty much one baby would be fine. And the other baby—that was smaller—would, could die. So there was a possibility of that, which would be devastat-ing. But I thought well . . . we'll still have one healthy baby, God willing. No. I mean, you get home and after talking to [the physician], they're not going to both live. They're either both gonna die or one's gonna die—but you can-not just let it go, or they're both gonna die.

Angela had trouble understanding what exactly the disease meant in relation to the possible death of one or both of her babies.

Like Angela, patients diagnosed with troubled twin pregnancies not only had to endure the ups and downs of a high-risk pregnancy but also often struggled to (re)define their pregnancies. For parents of a single fetus, illness was a shock. For parents of twin fetuses, twins were a shock; illness, more so. One patient, Abby Nates, explained the difficulty of these transitions:

> **Abby Nates:** We found out we were pregnant. We were excited about it. It went pretty normal through the first few weeks. . . . [Then we] got to the triple screen test, and the results came back abnormal. And at that point we knew something was wrong. And we found out we were having twins. . . . It was the first sonogram we had ever seen as well, when we went and found we were having twins. They said, "There's two." And we said, "Two what?" (She laughs a bit.)
> **Deborah Blizzard:** Did you really? (I laugh a bit, too.)
> **Abby Nates:** Yeah. *Two what?* . . . Suddenly you realize that you know noth-ing about what you're doing, and about your body and babies. . . . I could tell immediately [something was wrong] because the person doing the sono-gram was not very talkative. . . . People are usually real excited about your pregnancy, and I thought that if someone found out that you were having twins, and everything was normal, that they would be excited, you know? But she immediately saw that one was smaller. . . . They really just didn't know. They couldn't see, based on the equipment they had. So we were excited, I think, to find out we were having twins, but scared to death

because, you know, you go from one, to thinking that you have a problem with one, to twins, that you may have problems with both, you know?

Over time, what constituted this pregnancy shifted. Not only did Abby have to come to terms with a troubled pregnancy, but she had to keep track of what constituted the pregnancy and whether or not it (as a pregnancy, fetus, or fetuses) was healthy.

Unlike purely diagnostic technologies, given appropriate timing, operative fetoscopy offers patients the chance to alter their pregnancies. With operative fetoscopy, the pregnancy is "far enough along" that parents can intervene, but it's not "far enough along" that the fetus is viable. Operative fetoscopy implies a liminal state for parents: They are somewhere between having, and not having, a baby. This may be particularly difficult for parents of twins (or other multiples) who face the decision of whether or not to ligate (tie off an umbilical cord to a dying fetus) in an effort to save the other twin from harm. Emily and Peter, who chose to ligate a dying twin, explained their situation:

> **Peter:** We just happen to fit right into that 16- to 26-week block where you don't have the vanishing twin and you don't have an intervention where they go in and do a C-section. We fit right into that.
> **Emily:** They're not viable, you know.
> **Peter:** Yeah, it's not viable. . . . We did what we thought was best for all.

In these predicaments, some patients may see themselves as similar to parents who "naturally" lose part of a pregnancy while continuing to carry a healthy embryo or fetus. Emily and Peter's procedure made it possible to try to save one fetus from harm by ligating the other. Without the ligation, it is possible that the healthier fetus would have suffered neurological damage or death from the effects of the co-twin's death. Because of the timing, Emily and Peter were able to intervene. The full impact of this decision may not be clear until much later.

Following a surgery in which one twin fetus dies, parents must simultaneously mourn a loss and anticipate a "new baby." During a "tentative pregnancy" in which a woman awaits amniocentesis results, she lives as both a potential mother to a baby and potential carrier of a genetic mistake (Rothman 1986). "Simultaneously distanced and substantiated, the pregnancy is suspended in time and status, awaiting a medical judgment of quality control" (Rapp 1998, 45). Depending upon the outcome of her test, and her reaction to it, she may or may not continue the pregnancy. A similar liminality was apparent in fetoscopy procedures involving the death of a fetus. Following fetal demise, a woman exists as both a carrier of a deceased fetus and caregiver to a potential baby. The difficulty of reconciling these relationships and emotions exist for all involved in the procedure (*myself included*). While we offered condolences for one fetus and best wishes for the other, it remained that the parents had to make sense of their new situation. Abby and Brett Nates explained these tensions:

> **Abby:** It's hard to decide what to do at this point. . . . [It] weighs heavily on my mind that [I] continue to carry a baby that's dead. We saw it moving. You know, we saw it alive and well except for the fact that, you know, it's small and getting too much, or not getting enough, blood. You know, that's hard. We had named it. I mean, we had named both . . .
> **Brett:** We saw it today and they didn't mention it.
> **Abby:** Yeah . . .
> **Brett:** You know, through the sonogram we could tell . . . we think.
> **Abby:** Yeah, [the operator] said, "Let's look at the fundus," and he went over and you could see it . . .
> **Brett:** And you know he wasn't going to say, "Well, there's your deceased baby," I mean, but you could tell . . .
> [recording inaudible]
> **Abby:** . . . It's not a big deal. It's just that you know something is missing, that something's gone. . . . [If we] are fortunate enough to have a healthy little girl, every time we look at that little girl we'll know there was another one, too, you know? And that's sad.

Like other patients who underwent ligations, Abby and Brett were both happy and saddened to have the opportunity to intervene:

> **Abby:** I'm just thankful that we had the procedure. . . . I can't believe that there are people who miss out on this opportunity. . . . That's exactly what it was, an opportunity for us to try to save one baby, or to try to save two—but that just didn't happen. But without this procedure, then there's nothing. There's no hope, and that's what people have is no hope, that don't know about this. So, I would do it again.

Later in the interview they returned to their feelings about intervening and the possibility of saving one baby:

> **Abby:** I just think if we can have one, then that's just a blessing . . .
> [I ask her husband]
> **Brett:** Ditto. Yeah, I mean, exactly. I don't feel any differently than that. I mean, we're happy to have the baby girl . . .

Abby: We were excited about twins—
Brett: A week ago, a week ago yesterday—
Abby: We were having nothing.
Brett: We were having nothing.

While they may have lost a fetus, they saved (part of) a pregnancy. They believe they had made the right choice, and they accepted that its future impact was not yet realized.

The timing issues in fetoscopy are complex, and current social analyses of reproductive technologies may shed light upon fetoscopy issues. Social analyses should investigate how fetoscopy affects the ways in which patients construct themselves as women and mothers over time (e.g., Layne 1999, and forthcoming). When analyzing amniocentesis, Rayna Rapp asks if the technology "offer[s] women a 'window of control,' or an anxiety-provoking responsibility, or both?" (Rapp 1988a, 109). Fetoscopy patients seemed relieved to have a procedure that both increased their knowledge of, and control over, their pregnancies. However, in gaining information and intervening, it is possible that some parents lessened some anxieties only to have new ones appear. In the medical literature, women undergo diagnostic embryofetoscopy for reasons that include wanting the earliest possible diagnosis or having a condition that is only diagnosed through refined visualization. Although reasons vary, a woman choosing to undergo the procedure may face difficult decisions regarding the continuation or termination of her pregnancy. On the other hand, with the information gained, she may feel more knowledgeable in making such decisions. Anxiety also accompanies operative fetoscopy intervention. To illustrate, during my ethnographic work I was repeatedly instructed that when a twin dies it is important to recognize that the woman *remains* a mother of twins, and the surviving baby *is* a twin. If a tentative pregnancy takes into account the tensions of being a mother and a carrier, how might similar analyses further explain or highlight the experience of a patient who chooses to lose one twin while continuing to gestate the other? How might legal requirements for disposing (e.g., burial or cremation) of a dead fetus affect the ways in which parents form relationships with it and surviving babies? Might these interactions inform policy recommendations on when and how to pursue fetoscopy?

Fetus as Separate from the Woman-Mother

Social scientists are critical of increasing public awareness of fetal images and the subsequent construction of the public fetus and fetal patient (e.g., Taylor 1992; Casper 1998). Familiarity with utero images has led to a level of comfort with, and social assumptions about, the meaning and value of the fetus as a cultural object. The public fetus belongs to everyone and anyone; it exists separately from a particular mother and is readily identified in a number of potentially political contexts (e.g., Taylor 1992; Petchesky 1987). As an "autonomous" entity (sometimes featured on billboards or pro-life placards), this fetus is constructed as not reliant on, or connected to, a particular woman or mother (e.g., Stabile 1992; Franklin 1991; Rothman 1989). Thus, when a Volvo advertisement featured a sonogram with the caption, "Is something inside telling you to buy a Volvo?" the question was directed not at a specific pregnant woman but at a society and culture that mobilizes around the rights and protection of the individual, including the public fetus (Taylor 1992, 68; on individualism, see, e.g., Franklin 1991; Rothman 1989; Rapp 1988a). Like the public fetus, the fetal patient may also divert attention from a woman and redirect it toward a "new subject" that may be at odds with its "container" (e.g., Hartouni 1991; Casper 1998). Today, women undergoing fetoscopy do so in a medical and legal context that has precedence to place a woman's decisions after the assumed needs of a fetal patient (e.g., Pringle 1986; Evans, Johnson, and Holzgreve 1990).[20] The "unborn" has become a patient whose presence may challenge women's claims to their own bodies (Casper 1998).

With the advent of ultrasound and other reproductive technologies, many women are becoming familiar with their pregnancies earlier in gestation (e.g., Duden 1993; Rapp 1998; Petchesky 1987; Taylor 1998). This may be problematic when these tools actually offer a medicalized "window" to the otherwise invisible fetal patient. Yet this window is not transparent, and some tools (e.g., ultrasound) must be medically translated to a woman because the image is not obvious—it is a technological rendering that must be explained, pointed out, and introduced. Although seeing the fetus and bonding with it may be an enjoyable experience, the entrance of the fetal patient into early pregnancy may challenge a woman's ability to define her own pregnancy experience and decide whether or not to continue the pregnancy (this may be particularly problematic if "bonding" is stressed as a natural process or an essentialized relationship between a mother and her baby). Similarly, theorists caution that tests such as amniocentesis are also problematic because they allow the choice to terminate fetus(es) at a relatively late stage in pregnancy (this concern is also reflected in some physician articles). Monitoring and surveillance techniques, whether visual or chromosomal, that occur both early and late in the pregnancy, potentially alienate a woman from her body and gestation by introducing a "new" patient with particular needs into the pregnancy experience.

When using both diagnostic embryofetoscopy and operative fetoscopy, a woman may bond with a potentially ill fetal patient. In addition, many women who undergo fetoscopy have undergone other procedures (e.g., ultrasound and amniocentesis) that may have already laid the social foundation for maternal-fetal bonding and fetal patienthood. While previous interactions do not remove the potential for fetoscopy to encourage *further* bonding or social separation of a woman and her fetus, women seeking fetoscopy may do so because they have *already* established a bond with their fetuses. Previous bonding and separation notwithstanding, fetoscopic images in the face of potential loss are powerful devices. For example, some fetoscopy patients received copies of their in utero pictures (taken during the procedure). These "baby pictures," as one nurse referred to them, were often of toes, fingers, or facial features. At first, I was concerned that the pictures might encourage bonding with critically ill fetuses in high-risk pregnancies. Yet over time it became clear that the photos symbolized many things to the patients and were highly valued (e.g., some patients planned to take the photos home and put them with other baby things).

Meeting and bonding with a fetus may be further exacerbated when the image through which parents "interact" with their fetus is a well-refined fetoscopic picture requiring little translation. While not all fetoscopic images are clear, in many cases, fetal appendages and features can be identified by parents, social scientists, and others not trained to interpret the images. (To be clear, operative fetoscopy images show only parts of a fetus. Although the entire fetus is too large to fit in one photo, it is possible to see complete fetal hands, profiles, toes, etc.) Certainly the pictures may have added to the creation and separation of the fetal patient while increasing bonding between a woman and her fetus; however, parents were frequently surprised and happy to receive the pictures, even when warned that the pregnancy might not "make it."

Although many parents enjoyed the photos, fetal images and their subsequent imaginings may create particular tensions for patients who choose to ligate one fetus while continuing to gestate the co-twin.[21] Peter and Emily found seeing a sonogram the day after surgery to ligate the umbilical cord to one of their twin fetuses particularly difficult. Peter explained, "I'm going to have a real hard time with this next couple of months because of the fact [that] I have this image in my head of two floating around, so I don't know where it's going to go from there, but it's just . . . I just gotta keep my mind off . . . the, you know, the negatives of it, and just [think of the] positives of it." Later in the interview Peter and Emily returned to the difficulties of reconciling past fetal images within a new context:

> **Emily:** That was one of the [difficult] things today, the sonogram . . . after four or five of those things . . . watching them for hours, you know you're not seeing the same things as the techs and the doctors, but you know what you're looking at, and you can see and identify, and—
> **Peter:** You weren't even looking—
> **Emily:** Huh?

Peter: She placed the wand down in that area and you started getting glassy-eyed. You knew where she was.

Emily: Oh, I know. I know where she was looking.

Peter: . . . Well, you may not have been looking with your eyes—but your mind is [there].

Emily: Well, but I also know what we've done and I know what [her] state is and her situation. But you have a visual in your head, and right now I want to keep that visual. . . . I'm not quite prepared to see her without a heart-[beat]. It's just part of the whole process.

Emily was not prepared to face the ultrasound "window" to see her dead fetus. At the same time this decision kept her from seeing or "visiting" her healthier fetus. The images produced by fetoscopy and the ensuing ultrasounds are problematic. In some instances they were reaffirming and comforting. In other cases they were painful reminders of what was lost in both body and hope.

Bonding is not static; woman-fetal and mother-baby relationships are complex. While concerns about the potential for visualizing technologies to promote bonding and fetal patienthood are useful, as suggested earlier, such relationships may also rely on the time at which the test is administered. In the past, women relied on various cultural and biological markers to indicate pregnancy (e.g., swollen breasts and quickening). These experiences remain powerful components in the construction of pregnancy. "Low-tech" experiences affect patient decisions to use "high-tech" tools. On the realization that both of her fetuses might die if she did not intervene, Angela March explained: "I've already become attached to these. Even though they're just—I'm just five months pregnant—I've felt movement, and it's just, it's just very—they're very real to me." Angela's experience of her fetuses as "real" informed her decision to undergo fetoscopy. It is likely that operative fetoscopy patients have not only undergone other reproductive procedures (e.g., amniocentesis and ultrasound) that add to the construction of a fetus as a separate individual or patient but that a woman may already think of herself as pregnant and possibly a mother.

Fetoscopic intervention and the early social introduction of fetuses within the pregnancy experience may lead to earlier bonding between a woman and her fetus, increase familiarity with the public fetus, and reinforce fetal patienthood. At the same time, the pictures may prove useful artifacts through which patients interpret their own pregnancy experiences. Might needing less translation to understand or interpret her fetus or test prove empowering for a woman? Alternatively, women who have already lost a pregnancy may feel ambivalent toward fetal images, and in some cases may protect themselves from getting attached to future fetuses (Layne 1992). Would these patients find the fetoscopic image more troubling than those unfamiliar with pregnancy loss?

Could an unanticipated loss following a procedure prove more traumatic after seeing and bonding with a fetus or baby? Could seeing and bonding with her fetus or baby affect a woman's ability to either accept or refuse future testing or termination?

Pregnancy Loss

Pregnancy loss is being altered by reproductive technologies and has been studied in the social science literature.[22] Increasingly, tools such as amniocentesis and ultrasound are becoming regular parts of normal pregnancy experiences. With these and other procedures, women are becoming aware of their pregnancies earlier in gestation and those wishing to remain pregnant acquire tokens (such as amnio reports and sonogram "photos") throughout their pregnancies in their attempts to establish and substantiate fetal well-being (e.g., Layne 1992). Through these and other activities, a pregnant woman (and her partner) may slowly come to think of the fetus as a baby, while they construct themselves as parents (Layne 1999, and forthcoming). Following this cultural transformation, pregnancy loss occurs between parents and their babies. These contexts and terms are difficult to reconcile; as indicated earlier, referring to an in utero fetus as "baby" may threaten women's claims to their bodies. Pregnancy loss is problematic as a source of grief because it may further entrench the fetus as an object of public value. This aside, women who lose their pregnancies may find themselves in a bind—they have not only lost a pregnancy (or baby) but there is little social assistance when expressing their grief or gaining bereavement support (e.g., Layne 1997). To make a painful situation worse, these women are often "comforted" with explanations that it was an "act of nature," "for the best," or that they can always "try again" (e.g., Layne 1990). It is not enough to compare fetoscopy to social analyses of reproductive tools; it is also necessary to place it within a theoretical context that places pregnancy loss within a culturally situated pregnancy experience that is, in part, mediated and constructed by reproductive technologies (e.g., Layne 1990, 1992, 1997; Rapp 1999; Taylor 1998).

Although each patient and case was unique, one thing they shared was they did not want to lose their pregnancies. Unfortunately, in some cases loss did occur, and each was traumatic. Pregnancy loss is linked to fetoscopy procedures in three ways: women undergo a diagnostic procedure to assist in their decisions to continue or terminate a pregnancy, women use operative fetoscopy to ligate a nonviable or dying fetus in an effort to save the other twin from harm, and women undergo fetoscopy hoping for no fetal demise, only to have it occur in the future. During my research, I met women who experienced each of these losses. In these cases, the loss was distinct, and the woman, her family, and hospital staff grieved. While the potential for loss always existed, all of the patients wished for successful outcomes (it is important to note that "successful" differed from patient to patient).

Ligation cases were particularly problematic as women, their companions, and the medical staff continually worked through the tensions and inconsistencies of grieving for a lost fetus while anticipating a new baby. Rick Taylor, father of a ligated fetus, explained this quandary: "And the proponents of the procedure are going to say we saved the life of the one baby not through the death of the other one but by stopping what was happening, which the end result was the death of Baby A. The opponents to it are going to say, 'Who has made you God . . . to change the course of Nature . . . as to who's going to live and who's not going to live?'" This couple not only identified the range of others' judgments but they also realized the ambiguity in their own interpretations. When explaining how their situation was similar or dissimilar to abortion issues, Marcie and Rick hit an ontological impasse:

> **Marcie:** I still believe in the right for the woman to choose [abortion]. . . . But I know that, down underneath, my personal thing is I can't do that. So that it was so hard for me . . . to say yes to Baby A going so that Baby B can survive.
> **Rick:** The moral issue is, and the reality of it is, we have killed a baby. . . . We just assisted with what was actually already happening . . .
> **Marcie:** I don't look at it the way that you look at it. I do not look at it . . . that I've killed something. I do not look at it at all that way. In my mind it's just that I know that this baby has died, but I don't look at it that I've killed something.
> **Rick:** . . . I think what we're both having a hard time struggling with is there was a heartbeat . . .
> **Marcie:** There was movement . . .

While the couple agreed that the situation was grave, and that ligation was their best option, they could not fully agree on what it was they had done.

Given the potential trauma of having to "let go" of one baby to "save" the other, some parents found support through family and spiritual networks. In some cases, family members continued to have relationships with ligated fetuses. Abby and Brett, who chose to ligate a dying fetus to protect its twin, believed that Abby's recently deceased mother might look after their newly deceased baby:

> **Abby:** You know, I've told you that my mom died, and I guess I feel like, that you know, she'll take care of this baby, that this baby's with her . . .
> **Brett:** Spoiling her.

Abby: Spoiling her. And that comforts me. She loved kids. She was so excited about [me being pregnant]. She did not know I was pregnant before she died, but that's what she would tell all her nurses, is that she was waiting on me to have a grandchild before she died. And so she didn't make that, but now she'll have one of her own . . .

Although the loss of her mother is still painful, the belief that her baby is with her mother is a comfort to her. Another patient, Emily, also invoked family relationships following the ligation of one of her twins. When asked about the ligation she solemnly told me that through the death of one, the other could live. Through her surviving sister, the dead twin would continue to be with them. Abby and Emily grieved for their lost babies, but both found some comfort in knowing the baby was with someone close, a loved one.

Fetoscopic procedures and photos that result from attempts to intervene may prove useful artifacts to substantiate the very real loss experienced by parents. In this light, the "baby pictures" may be empowering tools for women who have lost their pregnancies in a social and cultural setting where often their loss is not recognized, discussed, or deemed important.[23] If fetal images and other tokens acquired during gestation show the loss was real, they may help women demonstrate the significance of their loss. Considering early loss, Layne warns that "the 'reality problem' . . . is greatly heightened. . . . Sonogram images may be one of the only things available to testify to the fact that a 'real baby' ever existed" (Layne forthcoming) This problem may also exist for those who lose a fetus later in pregnancy.[24] In the fetoscopic image, skin tones, finger nails, eyebrows, and other "baby parts" are relatively clear and may prove more convincing than a fuzzy black-and-white sonogram or fetal monitor tape. When I asked one patient, Mary Evans, why she wanted the photos, she stressed that they would be evidence for family members critical of her desire to continue a troubled pregnancy: "You have to give people something where they can kind of get a, you know, visual image . . . something to show people, [and say,] 'This is what we went through all that for.'. . . Seeing is believing." The photos substantiated her procedure and her pregnancy. Fetoscopic images may prove powerful devices when mobilized by an otherwise marginalized woman or mother.

While pregnancy loss (of any sort) is painful, ligation is also problematic; parents choose to undergo the procedure. Whether parents lose a twin early or later in gestation, they live with the paradox of a pregnancy ending in life and death (Perfect Sychowski 1998). According to one nursing journal, "When one twin dies perinatally, mothers and fathers have a very confusing, ambivalent introduction into new parenthood. Congratulations and condolences, birth and death announcements, baptismal gowns and caskets are all a part of the first few postpartum weeks" (Swanson-Kauffman 1988, 81). Parents who choose to ligate a twin face two complex situations: they end a wanted gestation, fetus, or baby, at the same time that they lose the outward appearance of being parents of twins. In other words, parents who have prepared for twins must now return to having only one bassinet, only one highchair, half the diapers, etc. Whether parents are trying to avoid loss (laser or shunting) or minimize it (ligation of one), pregnancy loss is a part of every fetoscopy procedure. In some cases, it was a background issue: it *could* happen. In other cases, it was part of the procedure: it *did* happen. To understand fetoscopy, it is necessary to investigate the many ways in which pregnancies are lost and constructed through fetoscopic procedures. Might fetoscopic "baby pictures" substantiate parental grief following their loss? Do the parents' (and others') experience of pregnancy loss differ if the loss was "natural" or "by consent"? Also, in the case of ligation it is important to investigate how parents of ligated fetuses construct relationships with the dead fetus-baby as well as with the surviving fetus-baby, and even more, how they position or construct a relationship between the twins. In what ways are choosing to terminate a fetus with a disability (following a positive amniocentesis) similar or dissimilar to choosing to ligate a dying fetus in an effort to save its co-twin from harm? In both cases, parents decide to stop a particular gestation. While the reasons for intervention may differ, the tensions parents face while making the decision and living with the outcome may be similar. Reflecting upon parent decisions following a positive diagnosis from amniocentesis, Rapp observes: "While most women . . . go on to abort, the solutions people choose are in part dependent on the specific diagnosis and their cultural background" (Rapp 1988a, 110). Even when termination is desired, "chosen loss" is still *a loss* (Rapp 1999, 225). Women who wish to abort may still find the experience difficult (e.g., Hubbard 1988). At my site, fetoscopic ligation occurred not because a baby would be disabled but because a fetus was dying or nonviable and its situation threatened the health of its co-twin. It is reasonable to consider if other sites follow this pattern. What are the culturally situated understandings of *termination, loss,* and *ligation*? What does it mean to save a pregnancy and how might that differ from saving a fetus or baby?

CREATING FETOSCOPY: OPENINGS FOR SOCIAL SCIENCE

Social analyses have demonstrated that reproductive technologies are outcomes of social and cultural interactions and are critical of technologies developed and implemented in ways that privilege or marginalize certain groups. A survey of diagnostic embryofetoscopy articles indicates that future development may lead to procedures that occur earlier in gestation, are minimally invasive, identify more anomalies, and offer treatment for some of the problems encountered. Likewise, physicians indicate that operative fetoscopy use will continue to expand in the hope of lowering fetal mortality and maternal morbidity. Certainly fetoscopy embodies both hope and concern for physicians and patients alike (although their hopes and concerns may differ). In her early work on amniocentesis, Rayna Rapp wrote, "This new technology has potentials that are at once both emancipatory and socially controlling, depending on the context in which its use is shaped and practiced" (Rapp 1988b, 155). Today, fetoscopy is newly developing. How might fetoscopy reflect, entrench, or challenge sociocultural interactions and understandings? What should the role of social scientists be in this process? What conditions warrant examination? What constitutes an acceptable level of health? Who has access to the tool? How will it be used? How will developments occur? What perspectives will be considered along the way? At this point in fetoscopy development, these questions have yet to be fully answered. Unlike well known and used reproductive tools, what fetoscopy is, and what it can be, remains uncertain. Instead of waiting for the tool to "fully" develop and then analyze it, this is a unique opportunity for social scientists to draw upon criticisms already suggested for other tools and ask if these criticisms are relevant to fetoscopy. Might social scientists, patients, and physicians use existing analyses to make fetoscopy (the tool and policies that surround it) more responsive to the varying concerns and hopes of a variety of people?

It is worthwhile to revisit reproductive technology analysis and ask how fetoscopy development might affect the ways in which women interact with other technologies. How might seeing the embryo-fetus alter or affect the ways that women make sense of other reproductive technologies? How might seeing her embryo-fetus through diagnostic embryofetoscopy limit or enhance a woman's decision to use other reproductive tools such as amniocentesis? How might a woman react to ultrasounds following an operative fetoscopic procedure to tie off an umbilical cord in a troubled twin pregnancy? Does fetoscopy development effectively reconstruct existing technologies? This analysis suggests new areas for theoretical exploration of other reproductive tools.

Within the medical journals, fetoscopy researchers appear excited over the diagnostic and therapeutic potentials of their developing tools. As such, many position fetoscopy as a logical extension of already accepted prenatal technology and find that its continued use and development will lead to better pregnancy outcomes (e.g., Reece 1999). Some of these views are accompanied by physician concern for the social effects of the tool and calls for caution (e.g., Hobbins 1996; Reece and Homko 1994; Quintero, personal communication). According to Reece and Homko,

The most recent and perhaps most exciting advance in maternal-fetal medicine . . . is embryoscopy, which now opens the frontier to intervention and fetal therapy. The possibility of actually being able to treat previously terminal or debilitating fetal disorders before birth gives an entirely new meaning to prenatal diagnosis [citation offered]. The ability to correct fetal defects will lead to a renewed interest in fetal diagnosis, fetal pathophysiology, and techniques of fetal intervention. However, the possibility of fetal therapy raises complex ethical questions about risks and benefits, and about the rights of the mother and fetus as patients. . . .

Undoubtedly, many ethical, legal, and regulatory questions must be addressed before the full potential of embryoscopy is realized. The responsibility for the judicious use of this powerful technology for prenatal intervention therefore will have to be shared by the scientific community as well as a well-informed public. (1994, 720–21, 724)

Referring to operative fetoscopy, Deprest, Lerut, and K. Vandenberghe concluded:

Fetoscopy is giving fetal surgical therapy a new stimulus. . . . Fetoscopy may become an instrument for new therapies, such as organ targetted gene therapy. It has also become a reality for some conditions. Despite that optimism, operative fetoscopy should not be considered as a clinical achievement. . . . The procedures are delicate and should not be attempted without proper training and experience, without a formal protocol, and appropriate consent procedure. (1997, 1257)

While many fetoscopy physicians are excited about current advances and potential developments, this excitement is frequently tempered with concerns for the contexts in which the tools are (or could be) used. I found that medical workers at the hospital where I conducted my ethnography (and others that I contacted) were interested in social analyses and believed these analyses useful in furthering their own understanding of the tool. My ethnographic work indicated that while physicians may publish articles with determinist phrasing, these assumptions are rarely reflected in the fetoscopy procedures and actual fetoscopy workers were critical and cautious of forwarding the tool too quickly and certainly without judgment. Based upon the medical literature and ethnographic work, there are at least two "openings" for social analysis: current medical articles offer a useful, if limited, analogy between fetoscopy and other reproductive technologies, and people at the sites appear willing to incorporate social analyses in their work.

The future of fetoscopy is not clear. Physicians are debating the ways in which the tool could and should be used in prenatal care.[25] They agree that advances in fetoscopy can be likened to a "vast and promising horizon" (Quintero, Puder, and Cotton 1993, 563) or "new era" (Reece and Homko 1994, 709) for prenatal diagnosis and therapy. Following these claims some call for ethical, legal, and social analyses of fetoscopy. These analyses might ask what price will these technologies bring; how might our worldviews be altered by fetoscopy; and further, how might our worldviews alter the technology? Physicians have urged interest and invited comment from parties outside of their research groups, it is worthwhile to reply. The early development of the tool, and the apparent willingness of physicians to engage in social analysis of it, position fetoscopy as an excellent project for the social construction of a reproductive technology.

NOTES

This material is based upon work supported by the National Science Foundation under Grant N. 9710783. Any opinions, findings, and conclusions or recommendations expressed in this material are those of the author and do not necessarily reflect the views of the National Science Foundation (NSF).

I would like to thank the many patients, nurses, physicians, and others who have shared their stories with me. Their honesty, sympathy, and curiosity make this research possible. I would especially like to thank the members of the fetoscopy team where I conducted my research. Their assistance (both during the ethnography and subsequent analysis) in translating medical reports and explaining medical devices has increased my understanding of these complex tools and the social networks that create them. I would also like to thank Linda Layne and Ann Saetnan for their constructive comments throughout the creation of this chapter. This research derives from an ongoing project to analyze the sociocultural construction of fetoscopy. An earlier version of this work was presented at the 1995 annual meeting of the Society for Social Studies of Science, Bielefeld, Germany.

1. Ruth Schwartz Cowan (1994) has shown that it is useful to analytically separate reproductive technology creation into development and diffusion. During development, the technology is flexible and alters rapidly, whereas in diffusion the tool is spreading, changing only slightly, and becoming routine. The distinction is important because it highlights the fact that those who have the ability to alter the tool early in development are different from those who may come in contact with it later. When applied to fetoscopy construction, the smaller and more limited development stage might include physicians and engineers, emphasizing the physical construction of the tool. The diffusion stage might include social scientists and policymakers, unaware of the issues that may have been voiced or overcome in the earlier developmental phases.

2. Many theorists in science and technology studies analyze the social (e.g., Bijker, Hughes, and Pinch 1987) or cultural (e.g., Hess 1995) construction of technology. These analyses often highlight the contextual, social relationships that cooperate and conflict when building technologies. Theorists may use terms such as *socially construct* to emphasize the sociocultural embeddedness of technology development. For example, Ruth Schwartz

Cowan analyzes how users or consumers of technology help to shape the technology through their decisions and consumption practices (e.g., Cowan 1987, 1994).

3. There are a number of approaches for anticipating the effects of fetoscopy and constructing the tools. The following suggestions might be useful starting points for increasing public and social scientific understandings of fetoscopy:

> **a.** Compare recent developments with existing reproductive technologies.
> **b.** Question how the insurance and cost of the procedure may be implemented.
> **c.** Identify the location of professional research networks.
> **d.** Identify who will be an acceptable patient.
> **e.** Conduct ethnographic study of development sites.
> **f.** Attend professional meetings to form dialogues with medical workers.
> **g.** Apply political pressure to hasten or limit development or diffusion.
> **h.** Create conferences or public forums that draw together professionals, activists, patients, and others to discuss the potential and current uses of the technology.

This short list offers various approaches for persons when analyzing fetoscopy development and diffusion; clearly, it is not an exhaustive list, and persons may wish to create their own approaches or merge some of those offered here. The above approaches bring inquirers directly into contact with the researchers and clinics that are developing the tools. Through interaction with these research groups, social scientists can increase their understandings of the technologies and, in so doing, may affect development.

4. While most reports on fetoscopy are published in medical journals, fetoscopy has appeared in the popular press. Examples of coverage include Kolata 1993, Kase 1994, and Schneider 1994. The recent use of operative fetoscopy to treat amniotic band syndrome was covered in a variety of publications in late January 1998. Fetoscopy was also highlighted in the *Dateline NBC* segment "Blood Relatives" (October 12, 1998) in which fetoscopy was presented as a treatment option for twin to twin transfusion syndrome.

5. During my fieldwork and subsequent analysis, I have found the limits of terms problematic. While interacting with patients, physicians, and others, I often struggled to find ways to talk about what was occurring and to whom it occurred. As many have noted, in cases where women undergo reproductive procedures and testing, there are at least two patients (more in multiple gestations): the woman and the fetus. During my research, it was clear that this was the case. However, it is interesting to note that when hospital workers referred to "the patient," they generally meant the woman. When speaking of the fetus, patients and medical workers generally used the term *baby*. Linda Layne has argued that a pregnant woman and her partner may come to think of their fetus as a baby at the same time that they construct themselves as parents (Layne 1999, and forthcoming). I find this approach of making babyhood and parenthood during gestation useful for understanding the relationships and rhetoric that I encountered. Each fetoscopy case brought new patients, parents, fetuses, and babies. The degrees to which anyone or anything was more or less a parent or baby varied. Within this chapter I use the term *patient* to refer to a woman seeking fetoscopy. I use the terms *parent* and *baby* if the interaction described relies upon an already constructed relationship between the woman-patient and fetus as evident in that context.

6. Ligation is different than "natural" or "noncontrolled" in utero demise. When two or more fetuses share blood (through the placenta), there is a chance that the spontaneous death of one will harm the other(s). The harm derives from the possibility of a living fetus bleeding into the dead one. Tying off the umbilical cord stops the blood from reaching the other fetus, therefore minimizing potential harm to the surviving fetus(es) (Quintero, personal communication). For examples of surgical fetoscopy procedures, see Deprest et al. 1997; Ville et al. 1995; Quintero, Romero, et al. 1996.

7. The patient names I use are pseudonyms. Recent analysis of reproductive technologies argue that culture and class (e.g., ethnicity and profession) affect how people construct their reproductive experiences. I agree with this perspective and believe that fetoscopy experiences should be examined in light of particular contexts. However, at this time, due to the limited number of fetoscopy sites and patients worldwide, I am only using pseudonyms in an effort to extend as much anonymity as possible. (Similar concerns for anonymity and privacy have been expressed in a recent social analysis of open fetal surgery; see Casper 1998, 28–29.) As the research continues and more informants are gained, I will expand this analysis to include explicit culture and class components.

Some of the examples included in this work, however, require details regarding the procedure (i.e., diagnosis and treatment option). Where appropriate, I give that information. To better understand the context from which I cite examples, the following lists indicate the types of procedures I observed and the informants I interviewed while conducting the ethnography. (I use the phrase "three or fewer" in an effort to extend anonymity.)

I observed the following procedures: three or fewer diagnostic cases, three or fewer shunting cases (inserting a small catheter to drain fluids), three or fewer biopsy cases (removing a small sample of embryo-fetal tissue), three or fewer ligations for acardiac twins (the presence of a nonviable fetus having a number of abnormalities including an absent, or nearly absent, heart threatens the viability of the otherwise "normal" twin), four laser surgeries for twin to twin transfusion syndrome (identical twins share blood disproportionately through the placenta, leading to fetal distress and possible harm or demise to one or both fetuses), and five ligations for twin to twin transfusion syndrome.

I interviewed one or more persons associated with the following procedures: three or fewer diagnostic cases, three or fewer shunting cases, three or fewer biopsy cases, three or fewer ligations of acardiac twins, four laser surgeries for twin to twin transfusion syndrome, and five ligations for twin to twin transfusion syndrome.

8. During my ethnographic research I also formally interviewed and informally spoke with hospital workers (e.g., physicians, nurses, chaplains, social workers, ultrasound technicians), reporters, and technology manufacturers. Although these interactions inform my understanding of fetoscopy, I do not explicitly draw from these interviews and discussions in this work. Also, this analysis is part of an ongoing study that will include "past patients," who underwent fetoscopy before I began the ethnography. For the purposes of this work, I draw from interviews and observations of "current patients" who underwent their procedures while I conducted the ethnography.

9. Not all forms of "in utero visualization" infer that sampling the embryo-fetus is possible. For a discussion of physiological development and potential tool placement, see Ville et al. 1997.

10. Within the fetoscopy literature, physicians commonly cite others to substantiate their claims. These citations can be lengthy (more than one source), but they are important because they help to make visible the professional networks creating fetoscopy. For the purposes of this work I use [citation(s) offered] to indicate that physicians are citing others within a passage.

11. While reading reports of diagnostic cases, I found one article in which it appears that physicians did not use anesthesia: "Embryoscopy was performed in the following manner. Under continuous ultrasound guidance a 20-gauge spinal needle was inserted into the amniotic cavity without local anesthesia or sedation after the abdomen was cleansed with a Betadine solution" (Ginsberg, Zbaraz, and Storm 1994, 373). Most reports mention some sort of anesthesia.

12. The usefulness of endoscopic access for reproductive diagnoses are demonstrated in a handful of cases when physicians have ultrasound assessments and then use the tool to affirm or reject a previous diagnosis (e.g., Reece et al. 1995b; Hobbins et al. 1994; Ginsberg, Zbaraz, and Storm 1994; Quintero, Abuhamad et al. 1993; Dumez et al. 1994). For example, one group recently demonstrated the usefulness of "needle embryofetoscopy" in the in utero diagnosis of Robert's syndrome. Robert's syndrome is a genetic abnormality characterized by severe facial deformity and growth deficiency. "Most infants with Robert's syndrome are still-born or die very early in infancy. The survivors have marked growth deficiency and many have severe mental deficiencies as well [citation offered]" (Reece et al. 1997, 138). In this case, a patient who had already given birth to a child with Robert's syndrome chose to undergo the procedure in the hope that physicians could identify if her developing twelve-week fetus had the abnormalities associated with the disease. The physicians viewed the fetus and found no apparent abnormalities. The parents continued the pregnancy and gave birth to "a normal full-term male" (Reece et al. 1997a, 138). In this case, physicians relied solely upon the visual capacities of the tool to make a diagnosis that was impossible with other reproductive technologies, including amniocentesis.

13. At the 1994 annual meeting of the Society of Perinatal Obstetricians, Quintero and colleagues announced in an oral plenary presentation that they had accomplished embryofetoscopy on continuing pregnancies.

14. There are always risks with an invasive procedure. With real-time ultrasound, the risks of unintended fetal loss with amniocentesis are thought to lie around 1:200 and are considered "reasonable" (e.g., Sokol, Jones, and Pernoll 1994; David and Steiner-Grossman 1995). Physicians generally accept that with proper techniques (and practice) a physician should be able to minimize fetal loss *and* control a crisis (Sokol, Jones, and Pernoll 1994). While risks vary depending on the skill of the physician and time at which the test is administered, amniocentesis is generally presented in the medical literature as a reasonably safe prenatal diagnostic technology.

15. I purposefully choose the austere term *statistical risk* instead of *safety* because the latter may imply a larger umbrella including psychological welfare and overall good for the woman, both of which are debated by physicians and social theorists (e.g., Sokol, Jones, and Pernoll 1994; Stenchever and Jones 1994; Cullen et al. 1990; Rothman 1986).

16. The continued use and development of amniocentesis has been extensive, leading physicians to separate it into two tools: early amniocentesis and midtrimester amniocentesis. According to one physician, "Midtrimester amniocentesis is most commonly performed between 15 and 17 weeks' gestation; however, early amniocentesis is done between 10 and 14 weeks" (Reece 1997b, 72).

17. While an analogy between operative fetoscopy and amniocentesis is not pursued in the medical literature, this comparison may prove useful for social scientists and patients more familiar with amniocentesis and less familiar with operative fetoscopy. In particular, analogies may be especially helpful for patients who have already undergone amniocentesis before operative fetoscopy. For example, like amniocentesis, operative fetoscopy may be used in the second trimester with a transabdominal point of entry. Although this point is larger than for amniocentesis, it is still "minimally invasive" when compared with many forms of surgery, including open fetal surgery.

18. Fetal surgery and other forms of fetal diagnosis and treatment are rapidly developing practices. As such, Luks and Deprest's 1993 assessment of one or two centers offering open fetal surgery may be dated. In her 1998 work on open fetal surgery, Monica Casper reports that "there are only about fifteen centers in five or six countries pursuing invasive fetal treatments such as fetal surgery" (8). She notes, "Fetal surgery has been attempted in the United States, the Netherlands, France, Germany, Italy, Japan, the United Kingdom, and a handful of other countries, all with mixed success" (227).

19. Linear narratives of progress and success are common to pregnancy experiences. Linda Layne (1996) analyzed the tensions and paradoxes between these narratives and the lived experience of parents when her son was treated in a neonatal intensive care unit. Linear narratives of progress for both gestation and neonatal periods may prove particularly problematic for fetoscopy patients who have "high-risk" pregnancies that may end in the birth of a sick or premature baby.

20. Some physicians affiliated with fetoscopy programs are extremely aware of the legal tensions and cultural assumptions that exist between the woman patient and fetal patient (e.g., Reece and Homko 1994; Evans et al. 1994). For example, Evans, Johnson, and W. Holzgreve (1990, 31) state: "The 1980s saw instances of obstetricians seeking judicial sanction to force women to undergo cesarean sections against their will for the supposed benefit of their viable fetus. Numerous such cases have now been catalogued, and analysis reveals that in many instances patients subjected to such court orders either did not speak English well or were of minority groups and of lower socioeconomic status. In at least one instance the husband of a woman who was forced to undergo a cesarean section against their wishes actually committed suicide soon thereafter." They warn: "As physicians in centers heavily involved in developing novel interventive fetal therapeutic modalities, we might easily become victims of our own zeal and consequently be tempted to impose our will on such patients. . . . Without regard for the basic rights of the mother in decisions of potentially invasive interventions inflicted on her body, impassioned physicians who unilaterally focus on the fetus as the individual, solitary patient could even unintentionally do great harm to the hard-fought gains of women in the last two decades" (32–33).

21. In a recent analysis, Janelle Taylor argues that ultrasound creates a "prenatal paradox" when it encourages bonding and reassurance while it is used to help parents make decisions regarding the outcomes of their pregnancies. Taylor's analysis also considers the tensions and inconsistencies between "bonding" and "reassurance." According to Taylor, the fetus "is constructed more and more as a consumer commodity, and pregnancy as a 'tentative' condition [citation offered (Rothman 1986)] *at the same time and through the same means* that pregnancy is also constructed more and more as an absolute and unconditional relationship, and the fetus as a person from the earliest stages of development" (italics in original, Taylor 1998, 16). Taylor's insights can be applied to fetoscopy analyses and expanded to investigate the ongoing tensions (continual paradox) that parents face following a ligation or in utero death of one fetus while the co-twin continues to develop.

22. For examples of how reproductive technologies alter women's experiences of pregnancy loss, see, e.g., Layne 1990, 1992, 1997; on "chosen loss" following an amniocentesis, see, e.g., Rapp 1999; on ultrasound leading to parental bonding and reassurance while constructing the pregnancy as a conditional or tentative matter, see, e.g., Taylor 1998.

23. At the hospital where I conducted my ethnography, the social services department ran a bereavement program designed to assist patients through pregnancy loss. This program was for all pregnancy loss, including those not associated with fetoscopy. Among other services offered, patients who lost pregnancies were given photos, baby blankets, footprints, and other keepsakes.

24. Although most pregnancy loss occurs during the first trimester, Layne found that the majority of contributions to pregnancy loss support group newsletters refer to a later loss (Layne 1997). Fetal loss following operative fetoscopy, whether or not attributed to the procedure, takes place in middle and later stages of pregnancy. Although each contributor to a newsletter will have her or his own reasons for so doing, it may be significant that a large percentage of contributions come from a comparatively small percentage of overall loss. The reactions of parents who lose pregnancies in the second and third trimesters may assist fetoscopy workers and inform policy for helping parents through their losses.

25. A European working group has created the Eurofetus Programme 1997 to identify the usefulness of developments in fetoscopy. Goals include designing a registry of fetoscopy sites and evaluating procedures (e.g., controlled trials). Although based in Europe, the site is accessible via the Internet, and clinics and researchers from around the world are able to join the registry (Deprest, Lerut, and Vandenberghe 1997)

REFERENCES

Benzie, R. J.:
  1980 Amniocentesis, Amnioscopy, and Fetoscopy. *Clinics in Obstetrics and Gynaecology* 7(3): 439–60.
Bijker, W. E., T. P. Hughes, and T. Pinch:
  1987 *The Social Construction of Technological Systems: New Directions in the Sociology and History of Technology.* Cambridge: MIT Press.
Casper, M. J.:
  1998 *The Making of the Unborn Patient: A Social Anatomy of Fetal Surgery.* New Brunswick, N.J.: Rutgers University Press.
Cowan, R. S.:
  1987 The Consumption Junction: A Proposal for Research Strategies in the Sociology of Technology. In Wiebe E. Bijker, Thomas P. Hughes, and Trevor Pinch (eds.), *The Social Construction of Technological Systems: New Directions in the Sociology and History of Technology,* 261–80. Cambridge: MIT Press.
  1994 Women's Roles in the History of Amniocentesis and Chorionic Villi Sampling. In K. H. Rothenberg and E. J. Thomson (eds.), *Women and Prenatal Testing: Facing the Challenges of Genetic Technology,* 35–48. Columbus: Ohio State University Press.
Cullen, M. T., E. A. Reece, J. Whetham, and J. C. Hobbins:
  1990 Embryoscopy: Description and Utility of a New Technique. *American Journal of Obstetrics and Gynecology* 162(1): 82–86.
David, K. L., and P. Steiner-Grossman:
  1995 Genetic Counseling. In R. P. Epps and S. C. Stewart (eds.), *Women's Complete Healthbook: The American Medical Women's Association Up-to-the-Minute Medical Information on the Issues That Concern Women Most,* 189–208. New York: Delacorte Press.
DeLia, J. E.:
  1996 Surgery of the Placenta and Umbilical Cord. *Clinical Obstetrics and Gynecology* 39(3): 607–25.

Deprest, J., T. E. Lerut, and K. Vandenberghe:
  1997 Operative Fetoscopy: New Perspective in Fetal Therapy? *Prenatal Diagnosis* 17(13):
        1247–60.
Deprest, J., F. I. Luks, K. H. E. Peers, and R. van Ginderdeuren:
  1999 Natural Protective Mechanisms against Endoscopic White-Light Injury in the Fetal
        Lamb Eye. *Obstetrics and Gynecology* 94(1): 124–27.
Dreyfus, M., F. Becmeur, C. Schwaab, J. J. Baldauf, L. Philippe, and J. Ritter:
  1996 The Pregnant Ewe: An Animal Model for Fetoscopic Surgery. *European Journal of
        Obstetrics and Gynecology and Reproductive Biology* 71: 91–94.
Duden, B.:
  1993 *Disembodying Women: Perspectives on Pregnancy and the Unborn.* Cambridge: Har-
        vard University Press.
Dumez, Y., M. Dommergues, M. Gubler, V. Bunduki, F. Narcy, M. Lemerrer, L. Mandel-
brot, and R. Berkowitz:
  1994 Meckel-Gruber Syndrome: Prenatal Diagnosis at Ten Menstrual Weeks Using Em-
        bryoscopy. *Prenatal Diagnosis* 14: 141–44.
Evans, M. I., N. S. Adzick, M. P. Johnson, A. W. Flake, R. Quintero, and M. R. Harrison:
  1994 Fetal Therapy—1994. *Current Opinion in Obstetrics and Gynecology* 6: 58–64.
Evans, M. I., M. P. Johnson, and W. Holzgreve:
  1990 Fetal Therapy: The Next Generation. *Jacobs Institute of Women's Health* 1(1): 31–
        33.
Franklin, S.:
  1991 Fetal Fascinations: New Dimensions to the Medical-Scientific Construction of Per-
        sonhood. In S. Franklin, C. Lury, and J. Stacey (eds.), *Off Centre: Feminism and
        Cultural Studies,* 190–205. London: HarperCollins Academic.
Ginsberg, N. A., D. Zbaraz, and C. Storm:
  1994 Transabdominal Embryoscopy for the Detection of Carpenter Syndrome during the
        First Trimester. *Journal of Assisted Reproduction and Genetics* 11(7): 373–75.
Grannum, P. A., and J. A. Copel:
  1990 Invasive Fetal Procedures. *Radiologic Clinics of North America* 28(1): 217–25.
Hartouni, V.:
  1991 Containing Women: Reproductive Discourse in the 1980s. In C. Penley and A. Ross
        (eds.), *Technoculture,* 27–56. Minneapolis: University of Minnesota Press.
Hess, D. J.:
  1995 *Science and Technology in a Multicultural World: The Cultural Politics of Facts and
        Artifacts.* New York: Columbia University Press.
Hobbins, J. C.:
  1996 The Future of First-Trimester Embryoscopy. *Ultrasound in Obstetrics and Gynecology*
        8: 3–4.
Hobbins, J. C., O. W. Jones, S. Gottesfeld, and W. Persutte:
  1994 Transvaginal Ultrasonography and Transabdominal Embryoscopy in the First-
        Trimester Diagnosis of Smith-Lemi-Opitz Syndrome II. *American Journal of Obstet-
        rics and Gynecology* 171(2): 546–49.
Hubbard, R.:
  1988 Eugenics: New Tools, Old Ideas. *Medical Anthropology Quarterly* 13(1–2): 225–35.
Kase, L.:
  1994 Do Pregnant Women Need All Those Tests? *Redbook* (August).

Kolata, G.:
  1993 Miniature Scope Gives the Earliest Pictures of a Developing Embryo. *New York Times,* July 6, C1-C3.

Layne, L. L.:
  1990 Motherhood Lost: Cultural Dimensions of Miscarriage and Stillbirth in America. *Women and Health* 16(3–4): 69–98.
  1992 Of Fetuses and Angels: Fragmentation and Integration in Narratives of Pregnancy Loss. In L. Layne and D. Hess (eds.), *Knowledge and Society: The Anthropology of Science and Technology,* vol. 9, 29–58. Greenwich, Conn.: JAI Press.
  1996 How's the Baby Doing? Struggling with Narratives of Progress in a Neonatal Intensive Care Unit. *Medical Anthropology Quarterly* 10(4): 624–56.
  1997 Breaking the Silence: An Agenda for Feminist Discourse of Pregnancy Loss. *Feminist Studies* 23(2): 289–315.
  1999 "I Remember the Day I Shopped for Your Layette": Consumer Goods, Fetuses, and Feminism in the Context of Pregnancy Loss. In L. M. Morgan and M. W. Michaels (eds.), *Fetal Subjects, Feminist Positions.* Philadelphia: University of Pennsylvania Press.
  Forth- Baby Things as Fetishes? Memorial Goods, Simulacra, and the "Realness" Problem
  coming of Pregnancy Loss. In H. Ragone and W. Twine (eds.), *Ideologies and Technologies of Motherhood.* New York: Routledge.

Luks, F. I., and J. A. Deprest:
  1993 Endoscopic Fetal Surgery: A New Alternative? *European Journal of Obstetrics and Gynecology* 52: 1–3.

Luks, F. I., J. A. Deprest, K. Vandenberghe, I. A. Brosens, and T. Lerut:
  1994 A Model for Fetal Surgery through Intrauterine Endoscopy. *Journal of Pediatric Surgery* 29(8): 1007–9.

Luks, F. I., K. H. Peers, J. A. Deprest, T. E. Lerut, and K. Vandenberghe:
  1996 The Effect of Open and Endoscopic Fetal Surgery on Uteroplacental Oxygen Delivery in the Sheep. *Journal of Pediatric Surgery* 31(2): 310–14.

Oakley, A.:
  1984 *The Captured Womb: A History of the Medical Care of Pregnant Women.* Oxford: Basil Blackwell.

Pennehouat, G. H., Y. Thebault, Y. Ville, P. Madelenat, and K. H. Nicolaides:
  1992 First-Trimester Transabdominal Fetoscopy. *Lancet* 340: 429.

Perfect Sychowski, S. H.:
  1998 Life and Death: In the All at Once. *Mother Baby Journal* 3(1): 33–39.

Petchesky, R.:
  1987 Fetal Images: The Power of Visual Culture in the Politics of Reproduction. *Feminist Studies* 13(2): 263–92.

Pringle, K. C.:
  1986 Fetal Surgery: It Has a Past, Has It a Future? *Fetal Therapy* 1: 23–31.

Quintero, R. A., A. Abuhamad, J. C. Hobbins, and M. J. Mahoney:
  1993b Transabdominal Thin-Gauge Embryofetoscopy: A Technique for Early Prenatal Diagnosis and Its Use in the Diagnosis of a Case of Meckel-Gruber Syndrome. *American Journal of Obstetrics and Gynecology* 168(5): 1552–57.

Quintero, R. A., W. J. Crossland, and D. B. Cotton:
  1994 Effect of Endoscopic White Light on the Developing Visual Pathway: A Histologic,

Histochemical, and Behavioral Study. *American Journal of Obstetrics and Gynecology* 171(4): 1142–48.

Quintero, R. A., and M. I. Evans:

1995   Bringing Surgery to the Fetus. *Lancet* 346 (suppl): 18.

Quintero, R. A., W. J. Morales, J. Phillips, C. S. Kalter, and J. L. Angel:

1997   In Utero Lysis of Amniotic Bands. *Ultrasound in Obstetrics and Gynecology* 10(5): 316–20.

Quintero, R. A., K. S. Puder, and D. B. Cotton:

1993   Embryoscopy and Fetoscopy. *Obstetrics and Gynecology Clinics of North America* 20(3): 563–81.

Quintero, R. A., H. Reich, K. S. Puder, M. Bardicef, M. I. Evans, D. B. Cotton, and R. Romero:

1994   Brief Report: Umbilical-Cord Ligation of an Acardiac Twin by Fetoscopy at Nineteen Weeks Gestation. *New England Journal of Medicine* 330(7): 469–71.

Quintero, R. A., R. Romero, H. Reich, L. Goncalves, M. P. Johnson, C. Carreno, and M. I. Evans:

1996   In Utero Percutaneous Umbilical Cord Ligation in the Management of Complicated Monochorionc Multiple Gestations. *Ultrasound in Obstetrics and Gynecology* 8(1): 16–22.

Rapp, R.:

1988a   Moral Pioneers: Women, Men, and Fetuses on a Frontier of Reproductive Technology. *Medical Anthropology Quarterly* 13(1–2): 101–16.

1988b   Chromosomes and Communication: The Discourse of Genetic Counseling. *Medical Anthropology Quarterly* 2: 143–57.

1998   Real-Time Fetus: The Role of the Sonogram in the Age of Monitored Reproduction. In G. L. Downey and J. Dumit (eds.), *Cyborgs and Citadels: Anthropological Interventions in Emerging Sciences and Technologies,* 31–48. Santa Fe, N.M.: School of American Research Press.

1999   *Testing Women, Testing the Fetus.* New York: Routledge.

Reece, E. A.:

1997a   Embryoscopy and Early Prenatal Diagnosis. *Fetal Diagnosis and Therapy* 24(1): 111–21.

1997b   Early and Midtrimester Genetic Amniocenteses: Safety and Outcomes. *Fetal Diagnosis and Therapy* 24(1): 71–81

1999   First Trimester Prenatal Diagnosis: Embryoscopy and Fetoscopy. *Seminars in Perinatology* 23(4): 424–33.

Reece, E. A., I. Goldstein, A. Chatwani, R. Brown, C. Homko, and A. Wiznitzer:

1994   Transabdominal Needle Embryofetoscopy: A New Technique Paving the Way for Fetal Therapy. *Obstetrics and Gynecology* 84, no. 4, pt. 1: 634–36.

Reece, E. A., and C. J. Homko:

1994   Embryoscopy, Fetal Therapy, and Ethical Implications. *Albany Law Review* 57: 709–30.

Reece, E. A., C. J. Homko, I. Goldstein, I. and A. Wiznitzer:

1995a   Toward Fetal Therapy Using Needle Embryofetoscopy. *Ultrasound in Obstetrics and Gynecology* 5: 281–85.

Reece, E. A., C. J. Homko, S. Koch, and L. Chan:

1997   First-Trimester Needle Embryofetoscopy and Prenatal Diagnosis. *Fetal Diagnosis and Therapy* 12(3): 136–39.

Reece, E. A., C. J. Homko, A. Wiznitzer, and I. Goldstein:
  1995b Needle Embryofetoscopy and Early Prenatal Diagnosis. *Fetal Diagnosis and Therapy* 10: 81–82.
Reece, E. A., S. Rotmensch, J. Whetham, M. Cullen, and J. C. Hobbins:
  1992 Embryoscopy: A Closer Look at First-Trimester Diagnosis and Treatment. *American Journal of Obstetrics and Gynecology* 166(3): 775–80.
Reece, E. A., J. Whetham, S. Rotmensch, and A. Wiznitzer:
  1993 Gaining Access to the Embryonic-Fetal Circulation via First- Trimester Endoscopy: A Step into the Future. *Obstetrics and Gynecology* 82(5): 876–79.
Rothman, B. K.:
  1986 *The Tentative Pregnancy: Prenatal Diagnosis and the Future of Motherhood.* New York: Penguin Books.
  1989 *Recreating Motherhood: Ideology and Technology in a Patriarchal Society.* New York: W. W. Norton.
Schneider, P.:
  1994 Beyond Ultrasound. *Parents* (March): 34.
Simpson, J. L., and S. Elias:
  1996 Fetoscopy, Fetal-Tissue Sampling and the ESHRE Guidelines on Prenatal Diagnosis. *Human Reproduction* 682.
Sokol, R. J., T. B. Jones, and M. L. Pernoll:
  1994 Methods of Pregnancy Assessment for Pregnancy at Risk. In A. H. DeCherney and M. L. Pernoll (eds.), *Current Obstetric and Gynecologic Diagnosis and Treatment*, 275–303. East Norwalk: Appleton and Lange.
Stabile, C. A.:
  1992 Shooting the Mother: Fetal Photography and the Politics of Disappearance. *Camera Obscura* 28: 179–205.
Stenchever, M. A., and H. W. Jones:
  1994 Genetic Disorders and Sex Chromosome Abnormalities. In A. H. DeCherney and M. L. Pernoll (eds.), *Current Obstetric and Gynecologic Diagnosis and Treatment*, 93–123. East Norwalk: Appleton and Lange.
Swanson-Kauffman, K.:
  1988 There Should Have Been Two: Nursing Care of Parents Experiencing the Perinatal Death of a Twin. *Perinatal and Neonatal Nursing* 2(2): 78–86.
Taylor, J. S.:
  1992 The Public Fetus and the Family Car: From Abortion Politics to a Volvo Advertisement. *Public Culture* 4(2): 67–80.
  1998 Image of Contradiction: Obstetrical Ultrasound in American Culture. In S. Franklin and H. Ragone (eds.), *Reproducing Reproduction: Kinship, Power, and Technological Innovation*, 15–45. Philadelphia: University of Pennsylvania Press.
Ville, Y., J. P. Bernard, S. Doumerc, O. Multon, H. Fernandez, R. Frydman, and G. Barki:
  1996 Transabdominal Fetoscopy in Fetal Anomalies Diagnosed by Ultrasound in the First Trimester. *Ultrasound in Obstetrics and Gynecology* 8: 11–15.
Ville, Y., J. Hyett, K. Hecher, and K. Nicolaides:
  1995 Preliminary Experience with Endoscopic Laser Surgery for Severe Twin-Twin Transfusion Syndrome. *New England Journal of Medicine* 332(4): 224–27.
Ville, Y., A. Khalil, T. Homphray, and G. Moscoso:
  1997 Diagnostic Embryoscopy and Fetoscopy in the First Trimester of Pregnancy. *Prenatal Diagnosis* 17(13): 1237–46.

Contributors

Franca Bimbi is an associate professor of sociology at the University of Padua. She has chaired the Equal Opportunities Commission for the Government of the Veneto Region (1992–95) and served as a consultant to the minister of social solidarity and family.

Deborah Blizzard is a Ph.D. candidate in science and technology studies at Rensselaer Polytechnic Institute, Troy, New York. Her doctoral project analyzes the sociocultural construction of fetoscopy.

C. H. Browner is a professor of psychiatry and biobehavioral science and a professor of anthropology at UCLA. Her recent work focuses on women's autonomy and knowledge regarding reproductive medicine.

Adele E. Clarke is a professor of sociology and history of health sciences at the University of California, San Francisco. She is the author of *Disciplining Reproduction: Modernity, American Life Sciences, and "the Problems of Sex"* (1998). She also edited *Revisioning Women, Health, and Healing: Feminist, Cultural, and Technoscience Perspectives* with Virginia L. Olesen (1999) and *Women's Health: Complexities and Differences* (1997) with Sheryl Burt Ruzek and Virginia L. Olesen.

Eugenia Georges is an associate professor of anthropology at Rice University. Since 1990 she has been conducting research on Greek women's and physicians' development, particularly the involvement of users in technology development and gender issues.

Jyotsna Agnihotri Gupta is a freelance consultant in the areas of gender, health, and development and has carried out assignments for, among others, the International Commission of Jurists and the World Health Organization in Geneva. Her Ph.D dissertation (Leiden University, 1996) is forthcoming under the title *New Freedoms, New Dependencies: New Reproductive Technologies, Women's Health, and Autonomy.*

Marta Kirejczyk is an assistant professor in the Faculty of Philosophy and Social Sciences at the University of Twente, Enschede, Netherlands. Her research focuses on the shaping of gender in public debates and political regulation of preimplantation diagnosis, intracytoplasmatic sperm injection, human embryo research, and cloning.

Lise Kvande is a Ph.D. candidate at the Center for Technology and Society at Norwegian University of Science and Technology. Her doctoral project is a study of the history of ultrasound in obstetrics and cardiology in Norway.

Françoise Laborie has been a sociologist at the CNRS since 1976. She is a member of the research group GEDISST. She has been called as an expert in several audits for French and international public organizations, including the World Health Organization.

Lara Marks has published widely on the history of maternal and child health, including *Model Mothers: Jewish Mothers and Maternity Provision in East London, 1870–1939* (1994) and *Metropolitan Maternity: Maternal and Infant Welfare Services in Early Twentieth-Century London* (1996). She has also coedited books, including *Migrants, Minorities, and Health* (1997) with Michael Worboys. She is based at the Centre for the History of Science Technology and Medicine, Imperial College, London.

Lisa M. Mitchell teaches anthropology at the University of Victoria, British Columbia. Her research focuses on biomedical and parental narratives and experiences of fetal anomaly and perinatal loss.

Lynn M. Morgan is a professor of anthropology at Mount Holyoke College. She is author of *Community Participation in Health: The Politics of Primary Care in Costa Rica* (1993) and coeditor of *Fetal Subjects, Feminist Positions* (1999) with Meredith W. Michaels. She has also written numerous articles on the political economy of health and the social construction of personhood. She is currently investigating the social history of embryology and the material fetal body.

Federico Neresini is a researcher at the University of Padua. His main research areas are sociology of science and bioethics.

Nelly Oudshoorn is a professor of gender and technology in the Faculty of Philosophy and Social Sciences at the University of Twente and an assistant professor in the Department of Behavioral and Social Sciences at the University of Amsterdam. She is the author of *Beyond the Natural Body: An Archaeology of Sex Hormones* (1994).

Naomi Pfeffer is a senior lecturer in health studies at the University of North London and editorial adviser to the *Journal of Medical Ethics*. She is the author of *The Stork and the Syringe: A Political History of Reproductive Medicine* (1993).

H. Mabel Preloran is an assistant research anthropologist in the Department of Psychiatry and Biobehavioral Science at UCLA. She has written numerous articles on gender, health, and economy.

Ann Rudinow Saetnan is an associate professor in the Department of Sociology and Political Science at the Norwegian University of Science and Technology. Her research focuses on medical technologies and gender.

Jessika van Kammen is a Ph.D. candidate in the Department of Science and Technology Dynamics, University of Amsterdam. Her research interests include medical technology development, in particular the involvement of users and gender issues. She worked for four years in Nicaragua for the Dutch government, in the field of women and health.

Author Index

Subject Index

abortion, 56–57, 117n. 23
  health issues, 268
  induced, 358, 373, 400; access to, 261, 267, 268–69, 371; opposition to, 106, 116–17n. 20, 117n. 23, 229, 230, 269, 330n. 22, 399, 400–401, 429; regulation of, 180, 209, 227, 250, 261, 264–65, 267–69, 274n. 4; support for, 128, 129, 230, 258, 259, 429
  selective: embryonic reduction in multiple pregnancies, 293, 300n. 12, 412, 422–24, 426–30, 435–36n. 6; following fetal diagnoses, 316–17, 322, 323, 326, 329n. 21, 364, 371, 374, 375, 377, 380, 425, 428, 430, 431; for sex selection, 241, 248
  spontaneous, 150, 307, 358, 360, 418–19, 422, 428
  as unintended consequence of other interventions, 293, 371, 376, 381n. 1, 414, 417, 418, 428, 437n. 15
adoption: IVF preferred to, 249; laws regulating, 188, 192, 193, 249, 258; in response to infertility, 212, 240, 244
alfa-fetoprotein (AFP) testing, 308
  access to, 370
  acceptance/rejection of follow-up amniocentesis, 372–81, 381n. 3; abortion attitudes, 374, 375, 377, 380; anxiety levels, 375, 377–78; interpretation of AFP, 376; interpretation of sonogram, 376, 378–79; medical authority, 377, 378, 380; reproductive self-confidence, 375, 376–77, 378, 380; risk of complications, 375–76, 379, 380
  follow-up testing, 370–71
  See also fetal diagnostics

amniocentesis, 321, 324, 371, 437n. 15; gender relations of, 372; complications/spontaneous abortion following, 371, 381n. 1, 417, 437n. 16; selective abortion following, 316, 371. See also fetal diagnostics
andrology, 104, 131, 280
animal testing, 111, 112, 118n. 33–34, 150, 162, 168n. 16, 283, 419; calls for, 278, 281–82, 283, 286, 287, 294–96; detailed description, 153–54; disputed value of, 281, 282; relation to clinical (human) testing, 118n. 33, 284–85, 294–96
assisted fertilization: access to, 227, 229–30, 231, 246; artificial insemination, 241; ethical issues, 316, 321; gender relations of, 214, 215, 222, 224, 227, 230, 240, 241; health risks, 240; homologous/heterologous, 211, 222, 223, 230, 235n. 4; sex selection, 180, 239, 241, 244, 246, 248, 250; social and economic costs, 246–47, 248, 251; social construction of, 208–10, 211, 213, 248. See also ICSI; IVF

Baker, John R., 46, 63
Bartelmez, George, 44
Baulieu, Etienne-Emile, 56–57
birth control
  movement for, 37, 39, 41, 42, 44, 48, 57–58, 66, 94, 128, 147–48
  as subject of controversy, 151, 158, 171n. 73; economic development arguments, 103, 115n. 7; emancipation arguments, 147–48; health arguments, 49, 116–17n. 20, 151; moral arguments, 38, 42, 44–45, 93, 146, 156

WOMEN AND HEALTH SERIES: CULTURAL AND SOCIAL PERSPECTIVES
Rima D. Apple and Janet Golden, Editors

The series examines the social and cultural construction of health practices and policies, focusing on women as subjects and objects of medical theory, health services, and policy formulation.

Mothers and Motherhood: Readings in American History
Edited by Rima D. Apple and Janet Golden

Modern Mothers in the Heartland: Gender, Health, and Progress in Illinois, 1900–1930
Lynne Curry

Making Midwives Legal: Childbirth, Medicine, and the Law, second edition
Raymond G. DeVries

A Social History of Wet Nursing: From Breast to Bottle
Janet Golden

Travels with the Wolf: A Story of Chronic Illness
Melissa Anne Goldstein

The Selling of Contraception: The Dalkon Shield Case, Sexuality, and Women's Autonomy
Nicole J. Grant

Women in Labor: Mothers, Medicine, and Occupational Health in the United States, 1890–1980
Allison Hepler

Crack Mothers: Pregnancy, Drugs, and the Media
Drew Humphries

And Sin No More: Social Policy and Unwed Mothers in Cleveland, 1855–1990
Marian J. Morton

Women and Prenatal Testing: Facing the Challenges of Genetic Technology
Edited by Karen H. Rothenberg and Elizabeth J. Thomson

Women's Health: Complexities and Differences
Edited by Sheryl Burt Ruzek, Virginia L. Olesen, and Adele E. Clarke

Motherhood in Bondage
Margaret Sanger

Listen to Me Good: The Life Story of an Alabama Midwife
Margaret Charles Smith and Linda Janet Holmes